FORENSIC GENETICS

Kruger Brentt
Publishers

FORENSIC GENETICS

Volume 1

Marly Cardoso
Eduardo Penna

Kruger Brentt
Publishers

2025

Kruger Brentt Publishers UK. LTD.
Company Number 9728962

Regd. Office: 68 St Margarets Road, Edgware, Middlesex HA8 9UU

ISBN: 978-1-78715-331-8 (Vol. 1)

For information on all our publications visit our website at http://krugerbrentt.com/

PREFACE

"Forensic Genetics" delves into the fascinating intersection of genetics and forensic science, offering readers a comprehensive exploration of the principles, techniques, and applications that define the field of forensic genetics. This book serves as an essential resource for students, researchers, forensic scientists, law enforcement professionals, and legal practitioners seeking to understand the role of genetics in criminal investigations, identification of individuals, and the administration of justice.

Forensic genetics utilizes genetic information, such as DNA analysis, to solve crimes, identify victims, exonerate the innocent, and establish biological relationships in legal proceedings. With advances in technology and the increasing availability of genetic data, forensic genetics has become an indispensable tool in criminal justice systems worldwide, revolutionizing the way investigations are conducted and evidence is analyzed.

The primary objective of this book is to provide readers with a comprehensive overview of forensic genetics, covering key topics such as DNA extraction and profiling, forensic DNA databases, kinship analysis, forensic genealogy, molecular autopsy, and ethical considerations in genetic testing. Each chapter offers insights, case studies, and practical examples to help readers understand the fundamental principles and applications of forensic genetics in real-world scenarios.

Contributions from leading experts in the field explore various aspects of forensic genetics, including the use of DNA evidence in criminal investigations, mass disaster victim identification, missing persons cases, paternity testing, and the challenges of interpreting complex genetic data in court. Special emphasis is placed on emerging technologies and methodologies, such as next-generation sequencing, single nucleotide polymorphism (SNP) analysis, and probabilistic genotyping algorithms.

As forensic genetics continues to evolve and expand its capabilities, it is essential for practitioners and stakeholders to stay abreast of the latest developments, ethical considerations, and legal implications in the field. By fostering collaboration, transparency, and interdisciplinary approaches, we can ensure that forensic genetics remains a reliable and powerful tool for achieving justice and truth in the criminal justice system.

We extend our sincere gratitude to the contributors whose expertise and dedication have enriched this book. It is our hope that "Forensic Genetics" will serve as a valuable resource and catalyst for dialogue, innovation, and collaboration in advancing the science and practice of forensic genetics worldwide.

Marly Cardoso

Eduardo Penna

CONTENTS

VOLUME-2

01 EVALUATING THE FORENSIC SIGNIFICANCE OF DNA EVIDENCE DERIVED FROM Y CHROMOSOMES AND MITOGENOMES

1. QUANTIFICATION OF THE WEIGHT OF EVIDENCE FOR LINEAGE MARKER PROFILES

Conventional DNA profiles utilize autosomal DNA, which is passed down from both parents. In this context, our attention is directed towards DNA profiles derived from the Y chromosome and the mitochondrial genome (mitogenome/mtDNA), which are exclusively inherited from the father and mother, respectively. Due to the transmission of DNA exclusively from one parent to the next throughout multiple generations, these genetic profiles are referred to as lineage markers. We elucidate the forensic significance of lineage markers in a comprehensive manner, providing a concise historical overview and critical analysis of evaluation techniques, while also offering suggestions for enhanced implementation. An important point to note is that the increased mutation rates of the most recent generation of Y chromosomal short tandem repeat (STR) profiles amplify the shortcomings of previous analytic approaches. However, comprehending these consequences can help identify potential solutions. The mutation rate of the entire mitogenome is comparatively lower. However, knowledge gained from studying high-mutation-rate scenarios is similarly valuable for assessing and conveying the strength of evidence.

We focus on the simplest scenario in which there is a good-quality, single-contributor DNA profile (either Y or mitogenome) obtained from an evidence sample, and a matching reference profile from a known individual Q who is alleged to be the source of the evidence sample (sometimes Q is called the person of interest, PoI). Hypotheses of interest are:

$$H_Q : \text{the evidence profile came from } Q,$$
$$H_X : \text{the evidence profile came from } X,$$

where X is an alternative to Q as the source of the DNA whose profile is not available. The likelihood ratio (LR) comparing the strength of the DNA profile evidence for HQ relative to HX is then

$$\text{LR}(X,Q) = \frac{\text{P(profile evidence} \mid H_Q)}{\text{P(profile evidence} \mid H_X)} = \frac{1}{\text{P}(X \text{ has profile } q)}, \tag{1}$$

where q is the profile of Q. We omit background information and other evidence from the notation; see [1] for a discussion. The denominator of (1) is a probability for the unknown profile of X, given the observed q and possibly a database of profiles.

1.1. The Effect of Relatedness and Mutation Rate on the LR

For lineage markers, the relatedness of two individuals is fully captured by a single number, G, of generations (or germline transfers, or meioses) that separate X and Q, following either female-only or male-only ancestors. Degree-1 (*G*=11) relative pairs are parent/offspring, *G*=22 for siblings and grandparent/grandchild, while *G*=3 for avuncular relationships such as aunt/niece as well as great-grandparent/great-grandchild. As G increases, the relatedness becomes less likely to be known, but there is a female-lineage G and a male-lineage G for all pairs of individuals, "unrelated" only means that G is large and/or unknown.

Given *G*=*g* for X and Q, we can approximate (1) by

$$\text{LR}(X,Q) = \frac{1}{(1-\mu)^g} \approx e^{g\mu} \tag{2}$$

where μ is the profile mutation rate, which is the probability that parent and child have non-matching profiles. For Y-STR loci with mutation rates μl,=1,...,L, and assuming independence of mutation events across loci, we have

$$\mu = 1 - \prod_{l=1}^{L}(1-\mu_l) < \sum_{l=1}^{L} \mu_l \,. \tag{3}$$

For the mitogenome, the lower mutation rate, larger number of sites, and possible germline selection events as part of the mitochondrial bottleneck [2] make it impractical to use (3) at individual sites, but it can be employed over genome regions [3,4].

The LR Formula (2) is not exact for at least two reasons. Firstly, it assumes that μ is constant over generations and independent of the current profile state. In fact, accurate estimates are hard to obtain but the STR mutation rate is likely to depend on the allele sequence (including its length and presence of a partial repeat) [5]. However, these effects are relatively unimportant for the total mutation rate over many loci. Secondly, it is based on assuming no mutations in the lineage path connecting X and Q, whereas a match can also arise following an even number of mutations between X with Q such that the effect of each mutation is reversed by another mutation. However, profiles consisting of many loci and with multiple possible mutation events at each locus are very unlikely to match if there is any mutation between X and Q [6,7].

For G unknown, in place of (**2**), we have (see also [**8**]):

$$\mathrm{LR}(X,Q) = \frac{1}{\sum_{g=1}^{\infty}(1-\mu)^g \mathrm{P}(G=g)} \qquad \text{where} \quad \sum_{g=1}^{\infty} \mathrm{P}(G=g) = 1. \tag{4}$$

Equation (**4**) requires a probability distribution for G, which can be informed by population genetic models and by the available information about alternative possible sources of the DNA profile. We introduced X as a specific alternative individual but, in practice, there are usually many alternative sources of the DNA. In either case, P(G=g) can be interpreted as the probability that the unknown alternative source of the DNA is a degree-g relative of Q. If, for example, it is known that all of the degree-g relatives of Q are excluded as possible sources, then P(G=g)=0P in (**4**), and the other values must be assigned to maintain $\sum_{g=1}^{\infty} \mathrm{P}(G=g) = 1$.

Although we can rarely compute it accurately, (**4**) tells us how to evaluate a lineage marker profile match: we need to assess, given the known circumstances, the probability that an alternative source of the DNA has relatedness g with the alleged source Q, and weight this probability by (1-μ)g, which means that individuals with $g \gg 1/\mu$ contribute little to the LR.

Most presentations of lineage marker DNA profile evidence mention something like "maternally-related individuals will share the same mitochondrial DNA profile" and then proceed to assess weight of evidence assuming that X and Q are unrelated. This practice is potentially misleading, because we are all maternally related and we are also all paternally related, what is important is the degree g of the relatedness (or that $g \gg 1/\mu$).

1.2. *The Significance of Databases in Assessing Evidence*

The approaches discussed below utilize a profile database to get data on population profile frequencies. When there are many databases to choose from, it is generally advisable to select the one that has the closest ancestral relationship to Q [9,10], unless the database is relatively small and there is a bigger alternative database available that is taken from a population with similar ancestry.

Databases typically do not consist of random samples [7,11] and are not derived from the population that is pertinent to a particular instance. The significance of relatedness in lineage markers suggests that the sampling method used for the database might greatly influence the inferences made. Database sampling may exhibit bias by favoring the inclusion of groupings of related persons, such as when relatives of a suspected contributor are also considered as suspects. Conversely, certain databases enforce a policy of barring immediate family members.

For Y and the mitogenome, the most important international databases, both highly respected for their data quality [**12**], are available online at **www.YHRD.org**

(accessed on 1 August 2021) [**13**] and **www.EMPOP.online** (accessed on 1 August 2021) [**14,15**]. In July 2021, EMPOP had 48,572 mtDNA sequences (of which 4289 cover the entire mitogenome, the rest span some or all of the control region, which is the most variable part of the mitogenome [**15**]). YHRD had 337,449 minimal (8 STR loci) profiles, of which 97,087 were 27-locus Yfiler Plus profiles. Both databases consist of samples from various global populations, which may include numerous subpopulations in certain instances.

1.3. Profile Matching Probability

Equation (4) has significant ramifications for the involvement of databases in computing the LR. The set of potential profiles for any of the lineage markers listed in Table 1 is so immense that it is highly improbable for two separate lineages to produce the exact same (full) profile by neutral mutations. While it has been observed that males with different single-nucleotide polymorphism (SNP) subhaplotypes can have matching Y-STR profiles, this has only been observed in cases where the males were from the same geographic region and were likely to be related. It is important to note that the Y chromosome undergoes several single-nucleotide mutations in each generation. Unless the value of μ is extremely small, the likelihood of a match occurring between individuals who are distantly related is insignificant compared to the much more probable occurrence of a match between pairs of persons who are closely linked enough to produce the match, but not recognized as being related. Autosomal profiles are similarly influenced by relatedness, but the effects are diminished by recombination, particularly in the situation of monozygotic twins [19].

Table 1. Estimations of μ for lineage marker profiles. The annual mitogenome mutation rates in [3,4] have been multiplied by a generation time of 25 years.

Type	Markers	Profile Mutation Rate μ [% Per Generation]	Reference
Ychr	PowerPlex Y (12 loci)	2.5%	[**7,20**]
Ychr	Yfiler (17 loci)	4.4%	[**7,20**]
Ychr	PowerPlex Y23 (23 loci)	8.3%	[**7,20**]
Ychr	Yfiler Plus (27 loci)	13.5%	[**7,20**]
Mitogenome	16,070 sites	0.3–1.9%	[**3,21**]
Mitogenome	16,494 sites	0.4–2.3%	[**4,21**]

For the mitogenome, μ is estimated to be approximately 1 per 70 generations (**Table 1**). Thus, alternative sources X will almost certainly be female-line relatives of Q with G up to a few hundred [**21**]. This is greatly beyond the known relatives of Q, but is still closer than a random pair of individuals in a large population, who are typically separated by thousands of generations [**21**]. For older Y profile kits, μ is a small multiple of the mitogenome value; but for more recent Y profile kits, μ can be an order of magnitude higher, approximately 1 per 7.5 generations for Yfiler Plus profiles (**Table 1**). In that case, profile matches occur between pairs of individuals separated by at most a few tens of generations [7].

Therefore, the majority of profiles in broadly-defined databases such as YHRD or EMPOP are drawn from individuals that are too distantly related to Q to be relevant to a particular case. The frequency of q can depend sensitively on the choice of population, according to its average relatedness with Q. Alternative sources of the DNA may be concentrated in the same subpopulation as Q, defined by geographical origin and/or social factors such as ethnicity and religion. A relevant consideration is that if Q is in fact not the source of the DNA, the false allegation may in part be due to Q resembling the true source in some characteristics such as appearance, place of residence, or social background, which tends to increase $P(G=g)$ for small values of g.

2. EVALUATION METHODS REVIEW

The majority of approaches have failed to include the essential impacts of relatedness, mutation rate, and database sampling frame that were previously mentioned. We shall examine the techniques under the assumption, as the majority of authors have done, that the database at hand is suitable. We will revisit these matters in the subsequent discussion.

2.1. Adjusted Database Counts

The denominator of the LR (**1**), is often assumed to equal the match probability, πq, the relative frequency of q in a population of alternative sources of the DNA. Many approaches aim to estimate πq based on the count kq of q in a database of size n. The database relative frequency kq/n has long been recognised as an unsatisfactory estimator of πq, because we often have kq=0 and yet Q has the profile and so πq>0.

Further, the requirement to avoid overstatement of evidence converts here to preferring a "conservative" over-estimate of πq rather than an under-estimate. Overly cautious behavior results in the squandering of knowledge, and our objective should be to assess the facts with utmost precision, while being cautious not to adopt an anti-conservative stance. Nevertheless, meeting the latter condition is challenging, and there is no consensus over the degree to which we should strive to eradicate any potential for being anti-conservative.

Various adjustments to kq and n have been proposed to avoid zero estimates and introduce an upward bias. We will discuss them in order of increasing conservativeness as measured by $\hat{\pi}\, q$ when kq=0.

2.1.1. Database Frequency Spectrum-Based Adjustment

Brenner's κ (kappa) estimate [22] (based on [23]) is $\hat{\pi}\, q$=(1-κ)/n when kq=0, where κ is the fraction of singleton profiles (observed only once in the database). Intuitively, a large κ corresponds to high profile diversity, which justifies a low estimate for πq. The estimator can be very small if the database consists mainly of singletons, which is the case for high-mutation-rate Y profiles. In particular, if the database consists only of singletons, then κ=1 and $\hat{\pi}\, q$=0. Cereda's estimators [24,25] are based on the numbers of both singletons and doubletons (profiles observed exactly twice). All of these approaches take no account of individuals that share profile q due to relatedness with Q, and the estimates can be strongly influenced by the way the database is sampled, as discussed above.

2.1.2. Augmenting the Database

If we compute the database relative frequency after adding q, then both kq and n are augmented by one to obtain $\hat{\pi}\, q$=(kq+1)/(n+1). If we add two copies of q to the database, corresponding to the profiles of both Q and X under HX, we obtain [26]

$$\hat{\pi}_q = \frac{k_q + 2}{n + 2}. \tag{5}$$

Other methods can be modified similarly by augmenting the database with one or two copies of q. Use of (5) is conservative in the sense that we do not know whether we have observed one or two individuals with q (that is, we do not know whether HX is true). Both the above estimators can alternatively be derived as Bayesian posterior probabilities given a uniform prior for πq, the first using the original database, while (5) uses the database augmented with one copy of q. A uniform prior is conservative in that it assigns weight to unrealistically high values of πq.

2.1.3. Upper Confidence Limit (UCL)

An alternative to (5) is an upper confidence limit (usually 95%) for πq [27,28]. This is the smallest binomial "success" probability π such that the probability of observing up to kq successes in n trials is ≤0.05. That is, the UCL is the largest π such that

$$\sum_{x=0}^{k_q} \binom{n}{x} \pi^x (1-\pi)^{n-x} \leq 0.05 \tag{6}$$

which is sometimes called the Clopper–Pearson formula [29]. The UCL represents a standard scientific approach to controlling the risk of overstating the evidence: it provides an answer to the question of how big the unknown πq could reasonably be, given observations kq and n. The 95% UCL is larger (more conservative) than (5). For example, when kq=0, from (6) and ln(0.05)≈-3(0.05)≈-3, the UCL is just under 3/n3/, whereas (5) is just under 2/n2/.

2.2. The Discrete Laplace Method

The Discrete Laplace method [**30,31**] models πq for all possible q, making it also useful for model-based clustering and mixture analyses [**32,33)**Based on the information in the database profiles, clusters are found that correspond to the descendants of a recent common ancestor. Probabilities are then calculated to determine the likelihood of the observed profiles belonging to each cluster. The forebears are regarded as unconnected, hence their profiles are considered independent. Profile probabilities are calculated by assuming that profiles descend separately from each ancestor, following a Discrete Laplace (double geometric) distribution.

2.3. *Population substructure is accounted for by the use of coancestry adjustment.*

The population genetic parameter *FST,* often referred to as θ in forensic DNA profiling, has been widely used to correct match probabilities for autosomal DNA profiles [**34**]. An analogous adjustment for lineage marker profiles [**1,35**] is

$$\mathrm{LR} = \frac{1}{\theta + (1-\theta)\pi_q} \tag{7}$$

There are several interpretations of θ—one is that it represents the average level of relatedness of individuals within a subpopulation, relative to a larger population. In forensic settings, the larger population can be interpreted as the population from which the available profile database was drawn, while the subpopulation is not usually well defined but it is assumed to include Q and some or all of the alternative possible sources of the evidence sample. The denominator of (7) can be loosely interpreted as follows. Under *HX*, there is probability θ that X is a relative of Q, sufficiently close that a match is very likely, while with probability 1-θ1-, X comes from the broader population which includes more distant relatives of Q such that the match probability is well estimated by the database relative frequency.

Equation (**7**) can be used in conjunction with the Discrete Laplace or adjusted database count methods to estimate πq. However, θ cannot be directly estimated because the value will depend on the available case-specific background information as well as the population that the reference database was drawn from. For example, if the database is drawn from a broad population that extends greatly beyond the population relevant to the case, then a larger θ would be needed than if the database came from a smaller more homogeneous region that includes most alternative donors of the DNA in a particular case.

Population-genetic estimates of θ have been reported for many human subpopulation-population pairs [**36,37**] and from simulation scenarios [**9**]. Most available estimates of θ are for autosomal loci. For lineage markers, the smaller effective population size (there are 4 copies of each autosome for every Y chromosome) tends to increase the value of θ, but the higher mutation rate of the Y tends to act in the opposite direction. Many population genetic studies do not estimate θ relative to a forensic database, but instead use a hypothetical ancestral reference population which leads to smaller estimates. Further, few studies are available at the fine geographical scale relevant for many cases.

In general, every alternative X can have a different value of θ reflecting their level of ancestry shared with Q relative to the database population. However, rather than try to choose a distribution of θ values appropriate for the alternative contributors in a case, usual practice is to take a single value from the upper tail of that distribution. Ref. [**36**] argued for θ=0.03=0.03 as a conservative, default value for autosomal profiles, finding through simulations based on real data that it remains appropriate even if X in fact comes from a different continent than the database population.

2.4. Estimating the Number of Matches in the Population

If we knew that Kq individuals have a profile matching Q, and these are well-mixed in a population of alternative sources of the DNA of size N, then the LR would equal the inverse of the match probability, which is

$$\mathrm{LR} = \frac{N}{K_q}. \tag{8}$$

We have noted above that this is not directly useful in practice, in contrast with the central role of the LR in the interpretation of autosomal profiles, because the choice of population and hence the value of N is problematic for lineage marker profiles. As we consider larger suspect populations, Kq tends to increase at a slower rate than N, because the matching individuals are relatives of Q and they are expected to form a smaller proportion of the population when it is more broadly defined.

An alternative to reporting the LR is to report estimates of Kq. A precise estimate is not usually possible, but probability distributions for Kq can be obtained using simulation under different population genetic models [**7,21,38**], which can include various mutation rates and mechanisms, and demographic factors such as population growth and structure, as well as variance in offspring number. The simulations can also take into account database frequencies, provided the database sampling scheme is known, which is only feasible in practice if the database can be assumed to be a random sample from the population. Often conditioning on kq and n from a database does not greatly alter the distribution of Kq, since it merely confirms that the profile is rare, as expected from the mutation rate [**7**].

A further advantage of the simulation approach is that it can easily incorporate available information about the numbers of close relatives of Q, and about their profiles if available [**38**].

Using the malan (MAle Lineage ANalysis) software [**20**], the distribution of Kq was found in high-mutation-rate settings to be insensitive to the modelling assumptions [**7**,**38**]. In the case of Yfiler Plus, the number of matching males is typically <10 and rarely more than a few tens. This approach has been extended to mitogenomes [**21**], but due to their lower mutation rate, the distribution of Kq was spread over a wider range, and was more sensitive to the population genetic model. While there remains merit in reporting to jurors an estimate of Kq, the arguments for this are less compelling than in high-mutation-rate settings, and conversely problems with the match probability and LR are lessened.

Given the estimates of Kq, a juror can assess how likely it is that one of these matching individuals was the source of the evidence profile, rather than Q. The population size N may play some role in these considerations, but is relatively unimportant. Since Kq is a count, it is likely to be more interpretable to a juror than an LR or a match probability [**39**]: it can be presented using phrases such as "the number of individuals with profile q is unlikely to be more than...".

2.5. Methods Not Widely Used

2.5.1. Population Genetic Modelling Using the Coalescent

The first method for computing match probabilities using an explicit genetic model was based on a genealogical tree with n+2 leaves, representing the database augmented with one copy of q plus a leaf node representing an unobserved profile [**40**]. A Markov chain Monte Carlo algorithm is used to update the tree structure, branch lengths, and profiles at the internal nodes and unobserved leaf node of a given mutation model and demography model that describes population size, growth rates, and structure. The estimation of profile distribution in the population is derived from the equilibrium frequencies at the unobserved leaf. The method shown strong performance relative to contemporaneous methods [41], however, it is computationally intensive, especially for extensive databases. This occurs because the entire range of profiles is examined, yet just the probability of q is necessary for forensic identification.

2.5.2. Frequency Surveying method

The frequency surveying approach [42,43,44] relies on calculating pairwise distances, expressed in mutational steps, between the Y profiles of individual i and j. Subsequently, an exponential regression is employed using these distances to form a Beta prior distribution within a Bayesian model that has a binomial likelihood. An inherent drawback of this strategy is its disregard for the variations in mutation rates among Y-STR loci, and its tendency to overlook valuable information by solely focusing on the count of mutational steps. This method is still available at **www.YHRD.org** (accessed on 1 August 2021) [**13**], but is no longer recommended [**11**].

2.5.3. Graphical Statistical Models

The Y profile models [45,46] are characterized by their computational efficiency and ability to incorporate intermediate alleles, a feature that is not possible in the population-genetic models mentioned earlier. However, they do not effectively utilize a significant amount of genetic information, and alleles are simply presumed to belong to distinct groups.

3. GUIDANCE FROM FORENSIC EXPERTS

For Y profiles, the Discrete Laplace method (**Section 2.2**) is currently recommended in the Philippines [**47**] and in Germany [**48**], where it was first used in court in a case from 2015 [**49**]. In that case, profiles were available for some male-line relatives of the suspected contributor, which can be taken into account in assessing the strength of the evidence by the malan simulation approach [**38**] (**Section 2.4**). The Polish Speaking Working Group of the International Society for Forensic Genetics (ISFG) [**50**] currently recommends using the κ method (**Section 2.1.1**). The UK Forensic Regulator has recently commended use of (**5**), the adjusted database frequency [**10**].

Here, we provide a concise overview and analysis of suggestions from two additional forensic experts.

3.1. Scientific Working Group on DNA Analysis Methods (USA, Canada)

3.1.1. Y Profiles

The SWGDAM 2014 guidelines [**51**] note that "the profile probability is not the same as the match probability", but they do not distinguish between low- and high-mutation-rate profiles. They recommend that the profile probability is estimated by the unadjusted database relative frequency kq/n, or with a UCL (**Section 2.1.3**), and that this value be used within (**7**) to adjust for population structure (**Section 2.3**).

The guidelines also discuss the importance of identifying the relevant population(s) and the difficulty in choosing an appropriate θ value, and they suggest default values for three kits. For PowerPlex Y23, the most discriminatory (highest profile mutation rate) of the three, they suggest θ=2×10−5 for African Americans, Asians, Caucasians and Hispanics; and θ=3×10−4 when Native Americans are considered.

3.1.2. mtDNA

The SWGDAM 2019 guidelines for mtDNA [**52**] are similar to those for Y profiles [**51**], except for the θ adjustment. They write: "It is recognized that population substructure exists for mtDNA haplotypes. However, determination of an appropriate theta (θ) value is complicated by the variety of primer sets, covering different portions of HV1 and/or HV2, which may be applied to forensic casework. SWGDAM has not yet reached consensus on the appropriate statistical approach to estimating θ for mtDNA comparisons".

3.2. International Society for Forensic Genetics (ISFG)

3.2.1. Y Profiles

The ISFG 2020 guidelines [**11**] state that "Information on the degree of paternal relatedness in the suspect population as well as on the familial network is, however, needed to interpret Y chromosome results in the best possible way" but did not delineate how to achieve this. The guidelines focus on estimating a profile relative frequency from a database, for which they recommend the Discrete Laplace method (**Section 2.2**), which we support in low-mutation-rate settings, but the guidelines do not distinguish low- and high-mutation-rate settings. They note arguments for avoiding estimates of the match probability πq, referencing [7], but they write "the appropriate wording for statements not relying on population databases need to be validated in the context of the national guidelines".

3.2.2. mtDNA

The ISFG 2014 guidelines on mtDNA [**15**] focus on estimates of πq. They do not recommend a particular estimator, but they mention (**5**) (**Section 2.1.2**) and the UCL (**Section 2.1.3**).

4. SOME FURTHER ISSUES

4.1. Combination with Autosomal Evidence

Lineage marker profiles bear resemblance to a single locus of an autosomal profile in several aspects. However, they exhibit a higher mutation rate, resulting in increased allelic variety compared to ordinary autosomal loci. Notably, lineage marker profiles only possess one allele, as opposed to the usual two alleles. The problem of the strong role for relatedness that we have highlighted in this review also arises at a single autosomal locus, although, due to diploidy, there are four lineages connecting Q and X at an autosomal locus, one for each pairing of an allele from Q with one from X.

It is possible to compute a combined LR for autosomal and lineage marker profiles that both match Q. Practically speaking, this is seldom carried out, possibly due to the fact that an autosomal profile match usually provides such significant information that the relatively minor increase in evidential strength from the lineage marker match is overshadowed by the added complexities in interpretation. One possible approach would be to multiply a conservative estimate of Kq by the autosomal match probability, to obtain an estimate of the expected number of individuals matching Q at both lineage marker and autosomal profiles. Alternatively, if the lineage marker profile mutation rate is low, it may be acceptable to multiply autosomal and lineage marker LRs, each obtained using a suitable value of θ.

4.2. Locus Order for Duplicated Y Loci

The STR loci that form a Y profile have known locations on the Y chromosome, except for the ordering of some pairs of duplicated loci including DYS385a and DYS385b. Two males with the same pair of alleles DYS385a/b may or may not match because of the unknown order. When the two alleles from Q are the same as those from the evidence profile, the evaluation problem can be overcome by omitting the duplicated loci, which tends to underestimate evidential strength, or by assuming a match at both loci, which tends to overstate evidential strength, by at most a factor of two and arguably much less.

4.3. Consistency

A consistency principle has been proposed requiring that the strength of evidence for a Y profile cannot be less than that for any of the subprofiles obtained by omitting one or more loci [**53**]. This reasonable requirement is not enforced by most of the methods discussed here, because a Y profile is treated as a single allele and subprofiles are not considered. The problem can be important when there is a good sample size for a particular DNA profiling kit, but a reduced sample size for a more detailed profile that includes additional loci [**10,51**]. The method of **Section 2.4** based on the distribution of the number Kq of matching individuals does respect the principle, because adding additional loci to a profile increases the mutation rate, and hence stochastically reduces Kq.

4.4. Partial Profiles

Often the DNA from a contributor of interest is at a very low level and/or degraded, so that a partial profile can arise if no allele is observed at some Y-STR loci, due to allele drop-out and/or masking by the alleles of a known contributor. The principles of interpretation are unchanged, using only the loci at which an allele is observed. The fewer the loci observed, the lower the profile mutation rate, which increases the number of matching individuals and decreases their average relatedness with Q. These quantities can be assessed using simulation including only the observed loci [**20,54**].

4.5. Mixtures

Several evidence profiles often originate from multiple unidentified contributors. When there is a significant difference in the quantities of DNA, it is feasible to separate the mixture (attribute alleles to separate, unidentified donors) by analyzing the heights of the peaks. Examples of mixtures, along with information about the height of their peaks, can be found in reference [55].

Remarkably, when dealing with Y profiles that have a high rate of mutation, a profile created by a blend of two males, where q is completely represented, is nearly as effective as observing q as a single-source evidence profile [38]. While there are numerous potential Y profiles that could explain the observed combination, the vast majority of these profiles are not present in the global human population, which is far less compared to the immense number of possible profiles. Given the presence of q in the population, the probability of the pair of profiles containing q is significantly higher compared to all other profile pairs, unless one or more of the other profiles have been detected in a database [38].

For low-mutation-rate Y profiles, the Discrete Laplace method (**Section 2.2**) can be used to deconvolve mixtures using estimated population frequencies [**33**].

A "profile-centred" (HC) method [**55**] is based on (**4**) and focusses on the number of generations G in the lineage linking Q with alternative contributor X. Beyond some threshold on G, the method assumes that the match probability is low and uses a population frequency estimator similar to the Discrete Laplace method. The HC method assumes a constant-size, random mating population of size N to assign weights for the mixture donors (using formulas for the probability that two random persons are g generations apart). The HC method uses the κ method (**Section 2.1.1**) for calibration, so that these methods are the same in the special case of good-quality single-source profiles.

5. DISCUSSION

Our analysis of techniques for evaluating the forensic significance of DNA evidence derived from lineage markers, specifically Y profiles and mitogenomes, has highlighted the crucial importance of the mutation rate of the profiles and the degree of relatedness G, whether through the male or female line. These factors are often not sufficiently considered in many existing methodologies. In particular, it is unsatisfactory to inform courts that, for example, a Y profile match is likely for male-line relatives and then to proceed as if the alleged contributor Q is unrelated to the alternative contributors, because (**4**) highlights that the evidential weight depends on the relatedness of Q with each alternative source of the evidence sample DNA profile.

Values of G are typically unknown in actual populations except when G is very small, but the distribution of G can be investigated via simulation in population genetic models (**Section 2.4**). There are also some well documented actual human populations that can be studied in more detail. To date these are relatively isolated and not typical of many cosmopolitan urban populations. A national-scale project is underway in Denmark aimed at tracing lineages over a century for almost the whole population [**56**]. At this time-depth, lineage paths up to about G=8 for two contemporary young adults can be traced, provided that there are no migrants in the lineage.

When the profile mutation rate is low (say below 0.05 per generation, which holds for the mitogenome and older Y-STR profiling kits), most of the individuals with profiles matching Q are separated by at least several tens of generations. There are typically hundreds of matching individuals—in some cases, thousands of them [**21**]. That is enough individuals and at sufficient genetic distance that many of them will differ from Q in many characteristics, thus lessening the problems discussed above. In these cases, methods based on estimating the population match probability πq, such as the Discrete Laplace method recommended by the ISFG (**Section 2.2**) may be acceptable, provided that the role of relatedness is also adequately explained possibly through a θ adjustment. As discussed in **Section 2.3**, appropriate values for θ can depend on case-specific details and the reference database.

For high-mutation-rate profiles (say above 0.10.1 per generation), most males matching Q are related to him within a few generations, and there seems no satisfactory alternative to summarising to a court the distribution of the number of close relatives of Q expected to match, as well as their degree of relatedness (**Section 2.4**). The UCL, for example, will be conservative if the alternative sources of the DNA include few close relatives of Q, but without addressing that question directly we cannot be sure. Methods that rely on a database may be affected by a non-conservative bias, because a broad database population may have lower average relatedness with Q than the alternative sources of the DNA in a particular case, and they may be adversely affected by the role of relatives in the database sampling frame.

Enhanced models and more accurate estimations for mutation will enhance the simulation-based method for calculating the quantity of individuals that match. While some data exists, there is limited research on the relationship between mutation rate and the current profile state, especially in the context of mitogenomes. Previous studies have explored mutation models that consider allele-specific mutation rates [5]. However, the existing data were inadequate for reliably estimating the parameters of the model.

We are confident that the difficulties of relatedness, mutation, and database that we have emphasized may be effectively resolved, and that a fair and easily understandable assessment of lineage marker profile evidence is now achievable.

6. SUMMARY

Y chromosome and mitochondrial DNA profiles have long been presented in court as evidence. However, the matter of assessing the precise significance of this evidence has not been adequately resolved. Unlike standard autosomal DNA profiles, which are inherited from both parents, both markers in this case are lineage markers, meaning they are inherited from just one parent. This presents unique challenges in interpretation. We analyze techniques for evaluating lineage marker profiles in forensic identification, with a focus on the essential roles of kinship (beyond known relatives) and the pace of profile mutation. Higher mutation rates imply a reduced number of individuals that meet the criteria of an alleged contributor, however they will still exhibit stronger associations. This complicates the evaluation of whether one of these matched persons could be the authentic origin, as relatives may be unlikely alternative contributors and may not be uniformly spread throughout the society. Decreased genetic similarity with the alleged donor may result in bigger populations having a lower occurrence rate, therefore diminishing the usefulness of profile databases obtained from a wide group. The impact of distant relatedness has become more apparent with the latest generation of Y profiles that have significant mutation rates. However, many evaluation methodologies fail to adequately consider this factor.

REFERENCES

1. Balding, D.J.; Steele, C.D. Weight-of-Evidence for Forensic DNA Profiles, 2nd ed.; Wiley: Chichester, UK, 2015. **[Google Scholar]**

2. Johnston, I.; Burgstaller, J.; Havlicek, V.; Kolbe, T.; Rülicke, T.; Brem, G.; Poulton, J.; Jones, N. Stochastic modelling, Bayesian inference, and new in vivo measurements elucidate the debated mtDNA bottleneck mechanism. Elife **2015**, 4, e07464. **[Google Scholar] [CrossRef] [PubMed] [Green Version]**

3. Rieux, A.; Eriksson, A.; Li, M.; Sobkowiak, B.; Weinert, L.A.; Warmuth, V.; Ruiz-Linares, A.; Manica, A.; Balloux, F. Improved Calibration of the Human Mitochondrial Clock Using Ancient Genomes. Mol. Biol. Evol. **2014**, 31, 2780–2792. **[Google Scholar] [CrossRef] [PubMed] [Green Version]**

4. Översti, S.; Onkamo, P.; Stoljarova, M.; Budowle, B.; Sajantila, A.; Palo, J.U. Identification and analysis of mtDNA genomes attributed to Finns reveal long-stagnant demographic trends obscured in the total diversity. Sci. Rep. **2017**, 7, 6193. **[Google Scholar] [CrossRef] [Green Version]**

5. Jochens, A.; Caliebe, A.; Rösler, U.; Krawczak, M. Empirical Evaluation Reveals Best Fit of a Logistic Mutation Model for Human Y-chromosomal Microsatellites. Genetics **2011**, 189, 1403–1411. **[Google Scholar]** **[CrossRef]** **[PubMed]** **[Green Version]**

6. Brenner, C.H. Understanding Y haplotype matching probability. Forensic Sci. Int. Genet. **2014**, 8, 233–243. **[Google Scholar]** **[CrossRef]**

7. Andersen, M.M.; Balding, D.J. How convincing is a matching Y-chromosome profile? PLoS Genet. **2017**, 13, e1007028. **[Google Scholar]** **[CrossRef]** **[Green Version]**

8. Caliebe, A.; Krawczak, M. Match probabilities for Y-chromosomal profiles: A paradigm shift. Forensic Sci. Int. Genet. **2018**, 37, 200–203. **[Google Scholar]** **[CrossRef]**

9. Steele, C.D.; Balding, D.J. Choice of population database for forensic DNA profile analysis. Sci. Justice **2014**, 54, 487–493. **[Google Scholar]** **[CrossRef]** **[Green Version]**

10. Forensic Science Regulator. Guidance for Y-STR Analysis Delivered into the Criminal Justice System in England and Wales: Forensic Science Regulator Guidance Y-STR Profiling (FSR-G-227). 2021. Available online: **https://www.gov.uk/government/publications/y-str-profiling** (accessed on 1 August 2021).

11. Roewer, L.; Andersen, M.M.; Ballantyne, J.; Butler, J.M.; Caliebe, A.; Corach, D.; D'Amato, M.E.; Gusmão, L.; Hou, Y.; de Knijff, P.; et al. DNA commission of the International Society of Forensic Genetics (ISFG): Recommendations on the interpretation of Y-STR results in forensic analysis. Forensic Sci. Int. Genet. **2020**, 48, 102308. **[Google Scholar]** **[CrossRef]** **[PubMed]**

12. Zimmermann, B.; Röck, A.; Huber, G.; Krämer, T.; Schneider, P.M.; Parson, W. Application of a west Eurasian-specific filter for quasi-median network analysis: Sharpening the blade for mtDNA error detection. Forensic Sci. Int. Genet. **2011**, 5, 133–137. **[Google Scholar]** **[CrossRef]** **[PubMed]** **[Green Version]**

13. Willuweit, S.; Roewer, L. The New Y Chromosome Haplotype Reference Database. Forensic Sci. Int. Genet. **2015**, 15, 43–48. **[Google Scholar]** **[CrossRef]**

14. Parson, W.; Dür, A. EMPOP—A forensic mtDNA database. Forensic Sci. Int. Genet. **2007**, 1, 88–92. **[Google Scholar]** **[CrossRef]**

15. Parson, W.; Gusmão, L.; Hares, D.; Irwin, J.; Mayr, W.; Morling, N.; Pokorak, E.; Prinz, M.; Salas, A.; Schneider, P.; et al. DNA Commission of the International Society for Forensic Genetics: Revised and extended guidelines for mitochondrial DNA typing. Forensic Sci. Int. Genet. **2014**, 13, 134–142. **[Google Scholar]** **[CrossRef]**

16. Larmuseau, M.; Vanderheyden, N.; Van Geystelen, A.; van Oven, M.; de Knijff, P.; Decorte, R. Recent Radiation within Y-chromosomal Haplogroup R-M269 Resulted in High Y-STR Haplotype Resemblance. Ann. Hum. Genet. **2014**, 78, 92–103. **[Google Scholar] [CrossRef] [PubMed]**

17. Solé-Morata, N.; Bertranpetit, J.; Comas, D.; Calafell, F. Recent Radiation of R-M269 and High Y-STR Haplotype Resemblance Confirmed. Ann. Hum. Genet. **2014**, 78, 253–254. **[Google Scholar] [CrossRef] [PubMed] [Green Version]**

18. Balanovsky, O. Toward a consensus on SNP and STR mutation rates on the human Y-chromosome. Hum. Genet. **2017**, 136, 575–590. **[Google Scholar] [CrossRef] [PubMed]**

19. Tvedebrink, T.; Morling, N. Identical twins in forensic genetics—Epidemiology and risk based estimation of weight of evidence. Sci. Justice **2015**, 55, 408–414. **[Google Scholar] [CrossRef] [PubMed]**

20. Andersen, M.M. malan: MAle Lineage ANalysis. J. Open Source Softw. **2018**, 3. **[Google Scholar] [CrossRef] [Green Version]**

21. Andersen, M.M.; Balding, D.J. How many individuals share a mitochondrial genome? PLoS Genet. **2018**, 14, e1007774. **[Google Scholar] [CrossRef] [Green Version]**

22. Brenner, C.H. Fundamental problem of forensic mathematics—The evidential value of a rare haplotype. Forensic Sci. Int. Genet. **2010**, 4, 281–291. **[Google Scholar] [CrossRef]**

23. Robbins, H.E. Estimating the Total Probability of the Unobserved Outcomes of an Experiment. Ann. Math. Stat. **1968**, 39, 256–257. **[Google Scholar] [CrossRef]**

24. Cereda, G. Impact of model choice on LR assessment in case of rare haplotype match (frequentist approach). Scand. J. Stat. **2017**, 44, 230–248. **[Google Scholar] [CrossRef] [Green Version]**

25. Cereda, G. Bayesian approach to LR assessment in case of rare type match. Stat. Neerl. **2017**, 71, 141–164. **[Google Scholar] [CrossRef]**

26. Balding, D.J. Weight-of-Evidence for Forensic DNA Profiles, 1st ed.; Wiley: Chichester, UK, 2005. **[Google Scholar]**

27. Holland, M.; Parsons, T. Mitochondrial DNA Sequence Analysis—Validation and Use for Forensic Casework. Forensic Sci. Rev. **1999**, 11, 21–50. **[Google Scholar] [PubMed]**

28. Budowle, B.; Ge, J.; Chakraborty, R. Basic Principles for Estimating the Rarity of Y-STR Haplotypes Derived from Forensic Evidence. In 18th International Symposium on Human Identification; Promega: Madison, WI, USA, 2007; Available online: **https://www.promega.com/products/pm/genetic-identity/ishi-conference-proceedings/18th-ishi-oral-presentations-mvc/** (accessed on 1 August 2021).

29. Clopper, C.; Pearson, E. The use of confidence or fiducial intervals illustrated in the case of the binomial. Biometrika **1934**, 26, 404–413. **[Google Scholar] [CrossRef]**

30. Andersen, M.M.; Eriksen, P.S.; Morling, N. The discrete Laplace exponential family and estimation of Y-STR haplotype frequencies. J. Theor. Biol. **2013**, 329, 39–51. **[Google Scholar] [CrossRef] [Green Version]**

31. Andersen, M.M. Discrete Laplace mixture model with applications in forensic genetics. J. Open Source Softw. **2018**, 3. **[Google Scholar] [CrossRef]**

32. Andersen, M.M.; Eriksen, P.S.; Morling, N. Cluster analysis of European Y-chromosomal STR haplotypes using the discrete Laplace method. Forensic Sci. Int. Genet. **2014**, 11, 182–194. **[Google Scholar] [CrossRef] [PubMed] [Green Version]**

33. Andersen, M.M.; Eriksen, P.S.; Mogensen, H.S.; Morling, N. Identifying the most likely contributors to a Y-STR mixture using the discrete Laplace method. Forensic Sci. Int. Genet. **2015**, 15, 76–83. **[Google Scholar] [CrossRef]**

34. Balding, D.J.; Nichols, R.A. DNA profile match probability calculation: How to allow for population stratification, relatedness, database selection and single bands. Forensic Sci. Int. **1994**, 64, 125–140. **[Google Scholar] [CrossRef]**

35. Buckleton, J.; Krawczak, M.; Weir, B. The interpretation of lineage markers in forensic DNA testing. Forensic Sci. Int. Genet. **2011**, 5, 78–83. **[Google Scholar] [CrossRef] [Green Version]**

36. Steele, C.D.; Syndercombe Court, D.; Balding, D.J. Worldwide Estimates Relative to Five Continental-Scale Populations. Ann. Hum. Genet. **2014**, 78, 468–477. **[Google Scholar] [CrossRef] [Green Version]**

37. Buckleton, J.; Curran, J.; Goudet, J.; Taylor, D.; Thiery, A.; Weir, B. Population-specific FST values for forensic STR markers: A worldwide survey. Forensic Sci. Int. Genet. **2016**, 23, 91–100. **[Google Scholar] [CrossRef] [Green Version]**

38. Andersen, M.M.; Balding, D.J. Y-profile evidence: Close paternal relatives and mixtures. Forensic Sci. Int. Genet. **2019**, 38, 48–53. **[Google Scholar] [CrossRef] [PubMed] [Green Version]**

39. Hoffrage, U.; Lindsey, S.; Hertwig, R.; Gigerenzer, G. Communicating Statistical Information. Science **2000**, 290, 2261–2262. **[Google Scholar] [CrossRef] [PubMed] [Green Version]**

40. Wilson, I.J.; Weale, M.E.; Balding, D.J. Inferences from DNA Data: Population Histories, Evolutionary Processes and Forensic Match Probabilities. J. R. Stat. Soc. Ser. A **2003**, 166, 155–201. **[Google Scholar] [CrossRef]**

41. Andersen, M.M.; Caliebe, A.; Jochens, A.; Willuweit, S.; Krawczak, M. Estimating trace-suspect match probabilities for singleton Y-STR haplotypes using coalescent theory. Forensic Sci. Int. Genet. **2013**, 7, 264–271. **[Google Scholar] [CrossRef]**

42. Roewer, L.; Kayser, M.; de Knijff, P.; Anslinger, K.; Betz, A.; Caglia, A.; Corach, D.; Füredi, S.; Henke, L.; Hidding, M.; et al. A new method for the evaluation of matches in non-recombining genomes: Application to Y-chromosomal short tandem repeat (STR) haplotypes in European males. Forensic Sci. Int. **2000**, 114, 31–43. **[Google Scholar] [CrossRef]**

43. Krawczak, M. Forensic evaluation of Y-STR haplotype matches: A comment. Forensic Sci. Int. **2001**, 118, 114–115. **[Google Scholar] [CrossRef]**

44. Willuweit, S.; Caliebe, A.; Andersen, M.; Roewer, L. Y-STR frequency surveying method: A critical reappraisal. Forensic Sci. Int. Genet. **2011**, 5, 84–90. **[Google Scholar] [CrossRef]**

45. Andersen, M.M.; Curran, J.; de Zoete, J.; Taylor, D.; Buckleton, J. Modelling the dependence structure of Y-STR haplotypes using graphical models. Forensic Sci. Int. Genet. **2018**, 37, 29–36. **[Google Scholar] [CrossRef]**

46. Andersen, M.M.; Caliebe, A.; Kirkeby, K.; Knudsen, M.; Vihrs, N.; Curran, J.M. Estimation of Y haplotype frequencies with lower order dependencies. Forensic Sci. Int. Genet. **2020**, 46, 102214. **[Google Scholar] [CrossRef]**

47. Rodriguez, J.; Laude, R.; De Ungriaa, M. An integrated system for forensic DNA testing of sexual assault cases in the Philippines. Forensic Sci. Int. Synerg. **2021**, 3, 100133. **[Google Scholar] [CrossRef] [PubMed]**

48. Willuweit, S.; Anslinger, K.; Bäßler, G.; Eckert, M.; Fimmers, R.; Hohoff, C.; Kraft, M.; Leuker, C.; Molsberger, G.; Pich, U.; et al. Joint recommendations of the project group "Statistical analysis of DNA" and the German Stain Commission on the statistical analysis of Y-chromosomal DNA typing results. Rechtsmedizin **2018**, 28, 138–142. **[Google Scholar] [CrossRef]**

49. Roewer, L. Y-chromosome short tandem repeats in forensics—Sexing, profiling, and matching male DNA. WIREs Forensic Sci. **2019**, 1, e1336. **[Google Scholar] [CrossRef] [Green Version]**

50. Rębała, K.; Branicki, W.; Pawłowski, R.; Spólnicka, M.; Kupiec, T.; Parys-Proszek, A.; Woźniak, M.; Grzybowski, T.; Boroń, M.; Wróbel, M.; et al. Recommendations of the Polish Speaking Working Group of the International Society for Forensic Genetics on forensic Y chromosome typing. Arch. Forensic Med. Criminol. **2020**, 70, 1–18. **[Google Scholar] [CrossRef]**

51. SWGDAM. SWGDAM Interpretation Guidelines for Y-Chromosome STR Testing. 2014. Available online: **https://www.swgdam.org/publications** (accessed on 1 August 2021).

52. SWGDAM. SWGDAM MtDNA Interpretation Guidelines. 2019. Available online: **https://www.swgdam.org/publications** (accessed on 1 August 2021).

53. Cowell, R.G. Consistent estimation of Y STR haplotype probabilities. Forensic Sci. Int. Genet. **2020**, 49, 102365. **[Google Scholar] [CrossRef]**

54. Andersen, M.M. mitolina: MITOchondrialLINeage Analysis. J. Open Source Softw. **2019**, 4, 1266. **[Google Scholar] [CrossRef]**

55. Taylor, D.; Curran, J.M.; Buckleton, J. Likelihood ratio development for mixed Y-STR profiles. Forensic Sci. Int. Genet. **2018**, 35, 82–96. **[Google Scholar] [CrossRef]**

56. Using Artificial Intelligence for Mapping the Danish Genealogy and Strengthening Research. Available online: **https://novonordiskfonden.dk/en/news/kunstig-intelligens-skal-kortlaegge-danskernes-stam-trae-og-styrke-forskning/** (accessed on 17 June 2021).

02 ADVANCING THE APPLICATION OF FORENSIC DNA PHENOTYPING TO PREDICT VISIBLE TRAITS IN CANINES

1. INTRODUCTION

The application of DNA phenotyping in forensic science was created as a valuable improvement to conventional human DNA profiling, which primarily relies on the use of STRs for individual identification [1,2]. Forensic DNA phenotyping (FDP) is used when DNA profiles do not align with a suspect's profile or a criminal DNA database record. Its purpose is to anticipate the outwardly observable traits of an individual by examining appropriate DNA markers. It generates fresh investigative leads regardless of the existence of any additional information, such as eyewitness accounts [1]. DNA-based prediction of physical appearance in forensic science began in the early 2000s [3]. Since then, tests on human iris, hair, and skin pigmentation have been effectively verified for regular casework investigations [1,4,5,6,7,8]. Their incorporation into the legislative systems of several countries is currently being extensively debated [9].

The objective of this study is to propose a method for Canine DNA phenotyping in forensic contexts, with the purpose of investigating the feasibility of applying the concept of FDP (Forensic DNA Phenotyping) to non-human DNA. Initially, we produced preliminary data to investigate methods and potential for creating a molecular genetic tool that may forecast observable characteristics of canines based on DNA tailored specifically for forensic purposes. The domestic dog was selected due to its exceptional range of physical characteristics and its importance in forensic investigations.

The varied physical characteristics of dogs are the outcome of a prolonged and thorough domestication process. Although still being discussed with controversial arguments, it is broadly accepted that all contemporary dogs were domesticated from the Eurasian grey wolf (Canis lupus) and that they accompanied humans over millennia [**10,11,12,13,14,15,16,17,18,19,20,21**]. Dogs have performed a variety of roles starting from ancestral dogs that were primarily valued for their hunting or protective skills [22,23]. The desire to develop dogs with particular physical traits was the driving force behind selective breeding practices. During the last 200 years, the focus of breeding changed from working ability to outward appearance and resulted in the formation of modern dog breeds [24,25,26]. At present, more than 400 breeds exist, and this diversity is even leveraged by inter-breeds and mongrels. Dogs exhibit a vast array of phenotypic traits, with varying body sizes, skull shapes, hair structure, coat colours, etc. [27,28,29,30,31,32,33,34,35,36,37,38,39,40,41,42, 43,44,45,46,47,48,49,50,51,52,53,54,55,56]. As a result, even an untrained eye can easily identify and describe some significant characteristics of a dog. This leads one to expect that the output of a canine DNA phenotyping test could provide practical information about the appearance of a dog of interest, which is comparable to an eye-witness testimony.

Currently, the global population of dogs is estimated to be between 700 million and 1 billion [57,58]. The distribution of dogs varies significantly between countries, with notably higher populations observed in the United States and Europe [57]. Dogs in these cultures are primarily confined to the home, emphasizing their significant function as companions. This elucidates the significance of utilizing material derived from canines in various forensic investigations. Dogs have the potential to cause accidents or engage in aggressive behavior towards humans, wildlife, and domestic animals. To obtain a current summary of dog-related deaths, refer to reference [59]. Cases involving the transfer of canine DNA evidence are particularly relevant in forensic analysis and pose greater challenges. These occurrences can establish connections between victims, suspects, and/or crime scenes, hence aiding in the production of evidence in human forensic cases. Canine transfer samples can be abundant as a result of frequent interaction with humans. Examples of this may encompass spit stains on trousers or strands of hair left on the rear seat of a vehicle. Due to the increased rate of hair shedding in dogs compared to people, the likelihood of discovering dog hairs is greater than finding hairs from the dog's owner.

DNA fingerprinting techniques offer compelling evidence for the specific identification of the implicated dog(s). Several methods have been documented that utilize specific genetic markers in dogs to identify individual dogs from evidence found at crime scenes [60,61,62,63,64,65,66,67,68]. Additionally, guidelines have been created to determine the necessary validation for these forensic techniques [69,70]. STR profiling enables the determination of whether a particular dog was responsible for an attack or if the hair detected on the victim came from the suspect's dog. Nevertheless, instances of crime scene DNA not aligning with a suspected dog or where reference material is unavailable are common. Therefore, examples of useful leads would include remarks such as "the attack was carried out by a sizable canine with a black coat color" or "the hair originates from a dog with a black and white spotted pattern and long fur." Typically, these assertions originate from accounts given by those who have directly witnessed the event. Nevertheless, the availability of eyewitness testimony is not constant and it can be subjective or incorrect [71,72,73,74]. Utilizing DNA analysis, specifically focused on canine DNA phenotyping, can overcome these restrictions by providing answers to issues similar to the aforementioned examples using an unbiased and measurable approach.

2. MATERIALS AND METHODS

2.1. Sampling, Documentation and DNA Extraction

The establishment of our sample collection was conducted through direct solicitations to individual dog owners, as well as by attending dog exhibitions, dog schools, and dog breeders. The dog owner collected buccal swabs to minimize any disruptive impact on the animals. Distinct alphanumeric sample IDs were utilized to ensure clear and unequivocal assignment of samples. Furthermore, the Institute for Veterinary Pathology at Justus-Liebig-University Gießen, Germany, gathered tissues from deceased dogs, as outlined in reference [61]. A total of 84 canine samples were included in the investigation.

DNA was extracted from buccal swabs according to routine procedures on a Qiagen EZ1 Advanced XL Nucleic Acid Automated Purification System (Qiagen, Hilden, Germany) using the DNeasy Blood & Tissue Kit (Qiagen) or using GentraPuregene reagents and protocols (Qiagen), according to the manufacturers' recommendations. The DNA of the tissue samples was extracted in a class 2 biological safety cabinet using the GentraPuregene Tissue Kit (Qiagen, Hilden, Germany) [**61,75**]. Nuclear DNA quantities were determined with a spectral photometer (Nanodrop 2000; Peqlab GmbH, Erlangen, Germany) or by applying a quantitative real-time PCR assay according to [**76**]. The assay was performed in a total volume of 10 μL on an AB 7500 Fast Real-Time PCR System (Thermo Fisher Scientific [TFS], Waltham, MA, USA).

2.2. *Selection of markers and design of the study*

A total of 21 markers were selected, comprising 15 SNPs and six INDELS. The latter two were microINDELS (each with a length of 3 bp), one was of intermediate-size (167 bp) and three belong to SINE insertions. The complete marker set is listed in **Table 1**, which contains relevant molecular genetic information as well as metadata regarding the related phenotypes.

The execution of the proof of concept study was partitioned into three sequential phases or experimental trials that progressively expanded upon each other: the preliminary trial, the indicator trial, and the concealed trial. For each test, Sanger sequencing was performed on a group of canine DNA samples to generate genetic data for interpreting phenotypes in subsequent analyses.

2.3. PCR Amplification and Sanger Sequencing

Whenever feasible, primer sequences were either directly obtained from published data or modified to minimize the length of amplicons. The creation of primers was conducted using the OligoAnalyzer Tool from Integrated DNA Technologies, located in Coralville, IA, USA. The reference sequences used were from CanFam3.1, obtained from EMBL-EBI in Hinxton, Cambridgeshire, UK. Additionally, the primers were examined for the production of secondary structures using Mfold, developed by the University at Albany in NY, USA.

PCR amplifications were carried out in 20 μL assays, containing 0.4 μL 50X Advantage 2 Polymerase Mix, 2 μL 10X Advantage 2 PCR Buffer (both Takara, Kyoto, Japan), 0.25 mg/mL BSA (Serva, Heidelberg, Germany), 200 μM each dNTP (TFS), 0.6 μL of each 10 μM primer. Two to 30 ng of DNA extract were used for amplification. Thermal cycling was performed on a DNA Engine Dyad thermal cycler (Bio-Rad, Hercules, CA, USA) or a Gene Amp PCR System 9700 (TFS), comprising initial denaturation at 95 °C for 2 min, followed by 37 cycles of 95 °C for 15 s, 58 to 67 °C for 30 s and 72 °C for 45 s. PCR products were purified using ExoSAP-IT (Amersham, Bucks, UK) according to the manufacturer's recommendations.

Sanger sequencing was accomplished by combining 2 μL of BigDye Terminator v1.1 Ready Reaction Mix, 2 μL 5X Sequencing Buffer (both TFS), 1 μL 5 μM amplification primer and 5 μL amplification product to a total volume of 10 μL. Cycling conditions were 95 °C for 2 min, and 30 cycles of 96 °C for 1 min, 50 °C for 5 s and 60 °C for 4 min. Products were purified using the Performa DTR Ultra 96-Well Plate Kit (EdgeBio, San Jose, CA, USA) according to the manufacturer's recommendations. Capillary electrophoresis was performed on an AB 3500xl Genetic Analyzer using POP6, 50 cm capillary arrays and default instrument settings (all TFS). Sequencing data were analysed using Sequencing Analysis Version 5.4 (TFS) and Sequencher Version 5.1 (GeneCodes, Ann Arbor, MI, USA). SNP data were formatted in Excel 2016 (Microsoft Corporation, Redmond, WA, USA).

The genotypes used to predict observable features consisted of single nucleotide polymorphisms (SNPs) and insertion/deletion markers (INDELS), which included short interspersed nuclear elements (SINEs). The polymorphic locations were examined using sequence analysis of the amplified DNA fragments. The determination of the allelic states at homozygous and heterozygous SNP locations was unequivocal. This also applied to brief insertions or deletions (INDELS) of up to three nucleotide base pairs. Nevertheless, the presence of lengthy INDEL markers, ASIP SINE, MITF SINE, PMEL SINE, and the RSPO2 insertion resulted in raw data that was challenging to understand when in a heterozygous state. In these instances, the short and long amplicon sequences, originating from both the allele lacking an insertion and the allele containing an insertion, intersected and resulted in incongruent sequence data. To interpret the heterozygous status, we analyzed the overlapping nucleotides in the chromatogram, which represent both sequence variants.

3. RESULTS

In order to provide a detailed description of individual dogs, genetic markers were chosen for six specific traits: (1) coat color, (2) coat pattern, (3) coat structure, (4) body size, (5) ear shape, and (6) tail length. A total of 21 markers were utilized, as indicated in Table 1. Figure 1 presents a diagram illustrating the potential observable characteristics that might be inferred from this set of markers. The information provided is derived from the reported explanatory capacity of the markers, as indicated in Table 1. Overall, our findings validated the documented impact of genetic variants at the examined genetic regions on the observable characteristics of canines.

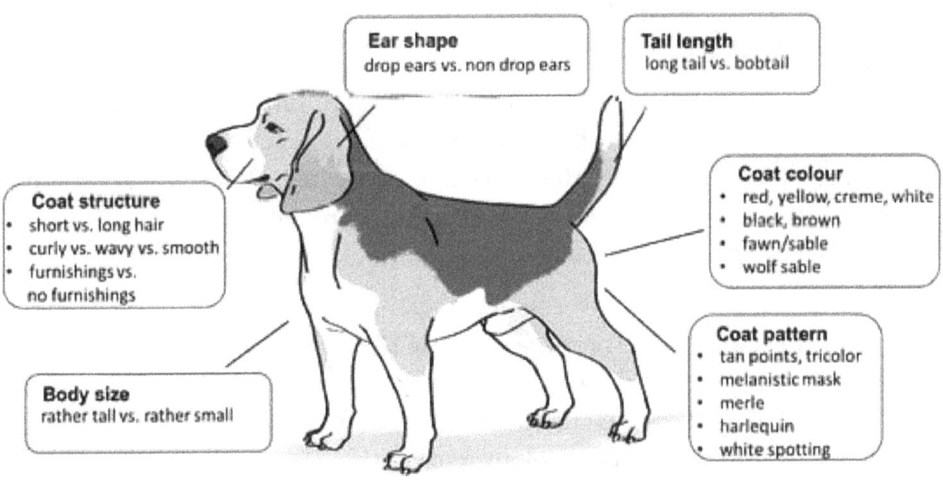

Figure 1. Schematic illustration of the trait categories selected to deduce a dog's appearance by applying canine DNA phenotyping. The six trait categories include the most obvious characteristics of a dog that can easily be recognized and described even by an untrained eyewitness. Each box refers to onc trait category and contains clearly distinguishable externally visible characteristics predictable from a particular genotype. The listings should provide an overview of the standardized terminology used here to characterize the appearance. vs.—versus (picture copyright: Larissa Hasenheit).

3.1. Pilot Test

The pilot study involved DNA samples from twelve dogs chosen from a sample pool consisting of around 1200 dogs [75]. A total of 12 samples were examined for genetic analysis using 21 markers, resulting in a total of 252 genotypes. The purpose of this test was to confirm the accuracy of the SNP and INDEL sites mentioned in the literature. Additionally, it aimed to improve the laboratory process by optimizing the conditions for PCR and sequencing, and redesigning primers if required. All 21 markers were successfully sequenced and all SNPs/INDELS could be unambiguously assigned. In all but three markers (PMEL, PSMB7, and T-box), all previously described allelic states were found within the pilot test sample set.

3.2. Marker Test

The marker test assessed the accuracy of predicting the phenotype for each of the 21 markers that represented the six trait categories. Therefore, the test samples were selected from the full sample collection (n = 1200) with respect to the phenotypical appearance of the dogs to include the different phenotypic manifestations of a particular trait.

The marker test outcomes are presented alongside an outline of the genetic underpinnings and generally used terminology for each feature.

3.2.1. Coat Colour and Coat Pattern

The nomenclature for the genetics of coat colours and coat patterns in dogs is based on the system established by [77] and with later adaptations (e.g., [**38**,**55**,**78**,**79**]). The term "Locus" is preceded by an alphabetical character which refers to the main characteristic realized by the particular locus (e.g., A-Locus: "A" stands for "Agouti"). Since the introduction of this naming convention by Little (1957) [**77**], all loci were assigned to genes, as described below.s

As in most mammals, the synthesis of eumelanin (black, brown) or phaeomelanin (yellow, red) is regulated by the two genes MC1R (E-Locus) and ASIP (A-Locus). In addition to these two genes, CBD103 (K-Locus) is of particular importance for black fur [**28**,**80**,**81**]. The genes MITF (S-Locus), MLPH (D-Locus), PMEL (M-Locus), and PSMB7 (H-Locus) modify the coat colour and pattern that is provided by the three main loci described above and are therefore called "modifiers" [**82**].

For testing the coat colour markers, one set of sixteen dog samples was used. It consisted of five solid brown, two solid black, two fawn/sable with white spotting, and two brown dogs with white spotting, as well as one wild type agouti, one brown sable, one black with white spotting, one black merle, and one blue (grey) dog.

E-Locus ("Extension"); The MC1R (Melanocortin 1 receptor) gene is epistatic to the K- and A-loci and responsible for a red, yellow, creme, and sometimes white coat colour in dogs (genotype: e/e) [**31,32,33,34,83**]. Alleles of the E-Locus are the dominant E (establishing a brown or black coat colour), and the recessive e. The allele for the coat pattern "melanistic mask" E^m is dominant over the E allele. Therefore, a melanistic mask is present in all E^m dogs, even if phenotypically not so well recognizable as in solid black dogs [**79**].

K-Locus ("dominant black"); The CBD103 (β-defensin) gene is responsible for black coat colour [**28**]. The effect of the K-Locus is dependent on the E-Locus and is only expressed when at least one E allele is present in a genotype. The dominant K^B allele inhibits the expression of the A-Locus. That results in solid coloured phenotype when no modifier gene (e.g., MLPH) is expressed [**40,79**]. The coat pattern "brindle" (K^{br}), in which stripes of red-yellow hair alternate with black-brown hair, was not included in this study.

A-Locus ("Agouti"); The Agouti signaling protein gene has four alleles identified so far, hierarchically ordered according to their dominance: A^y (fawn/sable) > a^w (agouti/wild type- wild type, black banded hairs) > a^t (tan points) >a (recessive black) [**27,29**]. The A-Locus is expressed when the K-Locus is homozygous for the recessive k^y allele. The coat pattern "sable" arises from hairs with tips darker in colour than the light-coloured base. Three main sable patterns are common in dog breeds: (1) clear sable—completely fawn dogs with just a few eumelanin (black/brown) hairs; (2) tipped sable—fawn dogs with eumelanin (black/brown) hairs usually on the back, head, ears and tail; (3) shaded sable—fawn dogs with eumelanin (black/brown) hairs covering the top of the head, ears and back; shading can be very light or very dark and distinct [**http://www.doggenetics.co.uk/tan.html#sable**] (accessed on 10 June 2021).

Agouti (a^w—"w" stands for "wild type") is characterized by hairs showing alternating colours along the hair shaft ("banding"; Fawn/black or brown).

B-Locus ("Brown"); The gene TYRP1 (Tyrosinase-related protein 1) affects only eumelanin, causing all black areas to turn to a brownish colour [**33,55**]. Brown is expressed by recessive alleles. It can be expressed when two of the three brown alleles are present in a genotype (b^s/b^s, b^s/b^d, b^s/b^c, b^d/b^d, b^d/b^c, b^c/b^c) [**55**]. The gene also affects the colour of the nose and eyes, making them brownish (liver).

D-Locus ("Dilution"); The MLPH (Melanophilin) gene affects both eumelanin and phaeomelanin [**30,56,84**]. As the allele causing dilution is recessive, a dilution is only expressed when a dog is homozygous for this allele. In this case, a black dog will become dark grey (also called "blue"), and a brown dog will become pale cream-brown ("Isabella").

S-Locus ("Spotting"); The MITF gene (microphthalmia associated transcription factor) is associated with one or more spotting patterns in dogs [**47,55,85**]. The range of spotting patterns is large, starting from no spotting and minimal white spotting, known as wild type (S/S), pseudo irish spotting (S/S^p), to piebald spotting and extremely white spotting (S^p/S^p). This is mainly caused by a SINE insertion on the MITF gene [**85**].

M-Locus ("Merle"); The premelanosome protein (PMEL) gene is responsible for merle coats described by the following features: (1) a light, diluted base colour and (2) random patches of fully pigmented fur of various size and location [**39,40,41**]. As the variant is semi-dominant, heterozygous individuals have at least a mild dilution of eumelanin areas, whereas m/m animals are normally pigmented and M/M individuals are mainly white (the latter occasionally exhibit deafness and ocular problems) [**79**]. A variety of merle phenotypes is known among dog breeds, such the classic, double, hidden, harlequin, cryptic and dilute forms. The hidden form possesses the M allele but the phenotypic merle pattern is invisible due to the epistatic impact of the e allele at the MC1R gene, when homozygous [**39,41,86**].

H-Locus ("Harlequin"); The PSMB7 (Proteasome 20S Subunit β7) gene is a dominant modifier gene of the merle SILV gene (M-Locus) that removes the dilute pigment and increases the size of the fully pigmented regions (dark spots on a white background) [**37**]. Harlequin is only expressed on a Merle background and is a well-known and easily recognizable coat pattern almost exclusively found in Great Danes.

Applying the just-described genetic foundations of coat colour traits to the results of the marker test, in 12 out of 16 analysed dogs, the genotypes predicted the expected phenotypes correctly.

For six of the 16 dogs, the phenotypic interpretation of the genotypic data obtained was straightforward, and for the other six dogs, heterozygous alleles in Q331 (b^s) were detected. Three of the latter group had a brown coat colour, one had a black coat colour and one showed a grey coat that is in accordance with the recessive inheritance of the coat colour modifier gene MLPH. One dog had an "e/e" MC1R genotype and a "B/b^s" TYPR1 genotype and showed brown eye rims and brown nose leather, which is in accordance with the description given in [**55**].

For three dog samples, the sequence analyses failed in the ASIP SINE markers. However, due to the hierarchical gene expression of the coat colour genes, it was deducible that the ASIP gene was of no account in these cases. Dog DE02_20 showed an e/e genotype at the E-locus and both dogs DE01_006 and DE01_052 had a K^B/K^B genotype at the K-locus.

The only discrepancy within the group of 16 dogs refers to the genotype interpretation of markers TYRP1_Q331ter and TYRP1_345delP, which refer to a black coat colour instead of actually brown (dog individuals AT0282, DE01_006, DE01_052, and DE02_017).

For the coat pattern trait, consistent results for all tested samples between the genotypic data and the physical visible traits of the dogs were achieved. Only individual AT0134 showed no results in both MITF markers.

It should be noted that three dogs (AT0062, AT0183, AT0257) were heterozygous at the K-Locus (K^B/k^y), indicating that their coat pattern could be brindled [**80**], but this pattern was not observed in these individuals. AT0062 showed a black with white spotting phenotype and AT0183 and AT0257 had a solid black phenotypic appearance.

The markers of the remaining trait categories were tested with 10 dog samples each. For each category, the dogs were selected by their appearance, in order to include both manifestations of the particular phenotypic characteristics in question, e.g., smooth vs. curly dogs, small vs. tall dogs.

3.2.2. Coat Structure

Three genes, RSPO2, FGF5, and KRT71 (encoding for R-spondin–2, fibroblast growth factor–5, and keratin-71, respectively), together account for most coat structure phenotypes. The RSPO2 gene is strongly associated with wired hair as well as the "furnishings", phenotypically characterized by a moustache and pronounced eyebrows as well as increased hair growth on the face and legs [**36,87**]. Variations in the FGF5 gene control the hair length in many dog breeds, the short hair mutation being of dominant inheritance [**40**]. The KRT71 gene is found to be associated with a curly hair phenotype. As the mutation is semi-dominant, animals heterozygous for this gene have an at least so-called "wavy" coat [**40**].

The analyses for the three above-mentioned **coat structure trait** markers were straight forward and the genotype data were in accordance with the phenotypical appearance of all 10 dogs.

Table 1. Detailed information on the selected 21 phenotype-specific markers allocated to the respective trait category. For the coat colour and coat pattern markers, the commonly used locus (Locus) and allele names (Allele) are listed (see, for example, reviews [38,40]). Upper case letters of an allele refer to dominant inheritance, lower case letters to recessive inheritance. For a detailed description of external visible traits (phenotype), see Section 3.2.1, Section 3.2.2 and Section 3.2.3. Additionally, the phenotypic manifestation is given as well as the corresponding references.

Trait Category	Marker ID	Locus	Allele	Marker Type	Nucleotide	Dominance (x)	Phenotype	Reference
Coat colour, coat pattern	MC1R_306ter	E (extension)	e	SNP	T		red, yellow, cream, white	[33,34,35,36,37,38,39,40,41,42,43,44,45,46,47,48,49,50,51,52,53,54,55]
			E		C	x	black, brown	
	MC1R_M264V	E (extension)	E	SNP	A		**no melanistic mask (black, brown)**	[32,34]
			E^{m}		G	x	melanistic mask (black, brown)	
	CBD103_S54	K (from 'dominant black')	k^{y}	INDEL	GGG		yellow—expression of agouti alleles	[28,80]
			K^{B}		DelGGG	x	black, brown, blue	
	CBD103_S53	K (from 'dominant black')	k^{y}	SNP	G		**yellow—expression of agouti alleles**	[28,80]
			K^{B}		C	x	black, brown, blue	
	ASIP S82	A (agouti)	A^{y}	SNP	T	x	fawn/sable	[27]
			a^{w}		G		wild type/agouti (black, brown)	

Trait Category	Marker ID	Locus	Allele	Marker Type	Nucleotide	Dominance (x)	Phenotype	Reference
Coat colour, coat pattern	**ASIP H83**	**A (agouti)**	A^y	**SNP**	**A**	**x**	**fawn/sable**	[27]
			a^w		G		wild type/agouti (black, brown)	
	ASIP_SINE	A (agouti)	a^t	SINE	SINE		tan points (black, brown), tricolour	[29]
			a^w		no SINE		wild type/agouti (black, brown)	
	ASIP_R96	A (agouti)	a^t	SNP	C		**tan points (black, brown), tricolour**	[27]
			a		T		recessive black	
	TYRP1_Q331ter	B (brown)	B	SNP	C	x	black	[33,55]
			b^s		T		brown	
	TYRP1_345delP	**B (brown)**	**B**	**INDEL**	**CCT**	**x**	**black**	[33,55]
			b^d		DelCCT		brown	
	MLPH_157471_c. -22G>A	D (dilutes eumelanin)	D	SNP	G	x	not diluted pigmentation	[30,56,84]
			d		A		diluted pigmentation	
	MITF_SNP	S (spotting)	S	SNP	A	**not clarified**	**solid colorred, minimal white spotting**	[47]
			S		G		white spotting	

Trait Category	Marker ID	Locus	Allele	Marker Type	Nucleotide	Dominance (x)	Phenotype	Reference
Coat colour, coat pattern	MITF_INS	S (spotting)	S	SINE	no SINE		solid coloured, minimal white spotting	[85]
			S^p		SINE		white spotting (S^p—piebald)	
			S/S^p				pseudo irish spotting	
	PMEL	**M (merle)**	**M**	**SINE**	**SINE**	**semi dominant**	**merle**	[39,40,41,46]
			m		no SINE		no merle	
			M/m		SINE/no SINE		mild merle	
	PSMB7	H (harlequin)	H	SNP	G	x	harlequin	[35,37]
			h		T		no harlequin	
	FGF5	**n.a.**	**n.a.**	**SNP**	**G**	**x**	**short hair**	[36]
					T		long hair	
	RSPO2	n.a.	n.a.	INDEL	no Ins		no furnishings	[36]
					Ins	x	furnishings	
	KRT71	**n.a.**	**n.a.**	**SNP**	**A**	**semi minant**	**smooth coat**	[36,40]
					G		curly coat	
					A/G		wavy coat	
Tail length	T-Box_C295G	n.a.	n.a.	SNP	G	x	bobtail	[48,54]
					C		long tail	
Ear shape	**BICFPJ1062878**	**n.a.**	**n.a.**	**SNP**	**G**	**not clarified**	**non drop ears**	[89]
					A		drop ears	
Body size	IGF1R	n.a.	n.a.	SNP	G		rather tall	[49]
					A	x	rather small	

3.2.4. Ear Shape

Wild canines have upright ears, whereas hanging ears are a characteristic of dog domestication. The marker IGF2BP2_BICFPJ1062878 used for ear shape determination was described in [**89**] .

The interpretation of this single ear shape marker included in the marker set proved to be unreliable. Only two dogs reflected the genotype in their phenotypical appearance. One dog did not show drop ears as genotypically indicated. No clear interpretation was possible for the six heterozygote dogs, as three of them had drop ears, and the other three exhibited non-drop ears. For one sample, no sequence data were obtained (AT0274).

3.2.5. Body Size

The insulin-like growth factor 1 receptor (IGF1R) has a strong effect on the size of a dog. The allele "A" of the nonsynonymous SNP at 41,849,479 (CanFam 3.1) is a causal mutation for small body size in dogs and is present in many tiny breeds [**49**].

IGF1R could be successfully genotyped for all dogs in the marker study. Even though only this single body size marker was included in the marker set, an accurate prediction of the body size in seven out of 10 dogs was possible.

3.3. Blind Test

In the course of the blind test, nine samples from dogs of blinded phenotypes were analysed with the 21-marker set, resulting in 189 genotypes. For this test, nine canine DNA extracts (D4925–D4931, D4933–D4934) were collected and prepared in a second lab—which also recorded the associated metadata including a photographic documentation—and were sent to the laboratory performing the tests. All samples were successfully genotyped in all markers. Subsequently, sketches of the nine dogs were drawn based on the genetic information obtained and compared to the dogs' phenotypes as displayed on photos, which were disclosed after the completion of the genetic analyses and the drawing of the sketches. **Figure 2** shows a comparison between the photographical documentation and the images drawn based solely on the genetic data. Additionally, the outcome of the test is summarized as a heatmap.

Three dogs had an identical genotype for all markers (D4926, D4928 and D4931) except for the ear shape marker, which showed a heterozygous state in D4931. Indeed, their phenotypical appearance was very similar, as all three individuals had black and tan points and minimal white spotting (S/S and a^t/a^t) fur, long smooth hair, a long tail, and a rather tall body size. In all three cases, the ear shape could not be traced by the provided photo documentation.

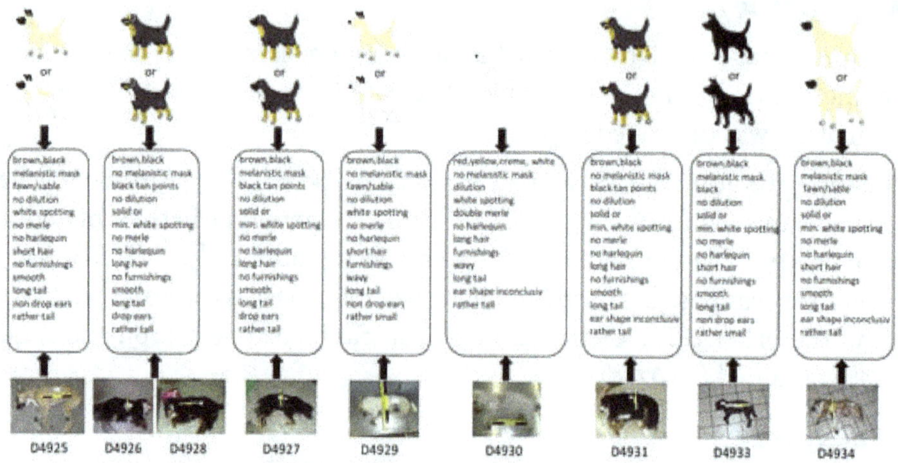

Figure 2. Results of the blind test: Identikit pictures (sketches) were drawn based on the genotypes and subsequently compared with photos of the nine tested dogs. Uncertainties in the manifestation of some visible characteristics required up to two versions of the identikit pictures. For all but one dog (D4930), two versions were necessary in order to reflect the possible phenotypes obtained from the genotype data. Dogs D4926 and D4928 showed the same genotype and therefore identical sketches. In general, identikit pictures and photos showed high levels of similarity. min. = minimal.

Dog D4927 showed a very similar genotype as the three dogs described above except the two E-locus markers, both being heterozygous, resulting in a correctly predicted "black tan points" fur including a melanistic mask (**Figure 2**).

For dog D4925, a high genotype–phenotype concordance was observed, except for the tail length. The genotype indicates a long tail, which is in contrast to the tail on the reference photo. However, the tail seemed to be artificially cropped.

For the light-coloured dog, D4929, with obvious upright ears, a high correspondence between genotypic prediction and phenotypic appearance could be achieved.

D4930 showed, in all but two markers, a high concordance between the genotypic predication and phenotypic appearance. The state of the body size marker suggested a tall body size that obviously did not match the dog's appearance. The heterozygous state at the ear shape marker led to inconclusive phenotypic interpretation.

Five of the six physical visible traits of D4933 were successfully predicted by the genetic data. Only the ear shape—non-drop ears—could not be unambiguously identified based on the reference photo. The K-Locus showed a heterozygous allelic state (K^B/k^y), which in some cases would indicate a brindle coat pattern, but the coat pattern of this individual was black with white spotting.

D4934 had a high correspondence between genotypic predication and phenotypic appearance for coat colour, coat pattern and coat structure, but for the body size, tail length, and ear shape, the assignments were discrepant or inconclusive, respectively.

4. DISCUSSION

The canine DNA phenotyping method described here is based on existing knowledge mostly obtained from genome-wide association studies [49,50,90,91,92,93,94] and recent advancements in canine genetics, including the sequencing of the dog genome [24,95,96,97]. Therefore, there was no need to seek out novel candidate markers that could potentially be linked to morphological features. Instead, a set of markers that had already been published was chosen, as outlined in Table 1. The genotyping of several observable characteristics in dogs has already been established for medical research purposes [98] or to assist in breeding efforts within specific breeds [82,99]. Current applications of genomic prediction, including those that are commercially accessible, primarily aim to authenticate pedigrees or breeds, choose specific phenotypes based on market demands or studbook policies, and prevent the occurrence of hereditary disorders. The objectives of these methodologies clearly vary from the requirements of forensic analysis. An essential concern pertains to the quality of the sample. Evaluating DNA evidence at crime scenes can be particularly challenging due to the limited amount and/ or quality of DNA, as well as the potential for contamination with other DNA sources or chemicals, such as PCR inhibitors. Hence, the objectives of the pilot test encompassed the enhancement of the laboratory workflow and the validation of the documented SNP or INDEL positions. This optimization stage involved modifying multiple previously published PCR primers, leading to the production of shorter amplicons. Shortened amplicons are known to yield better results when analyzing degraded DNA [100,101,102]. The pilot test's successful completion served as the methodological foundation for the succeeding trials.

The work utilized a proof of concept approach, focusing on a limited set of 21 genetic markers that have been identified in the literature as either causative or strongly associated with externally observable features. The marker test was used to ascertain the accuracy of predicting the phenotype. Considering the limited number of markers discussed in this context, the potential to distinguish observable characteristics proved to be encouraging. Nevertheless, the accuracy of the individual markers in accurately predicting specific trait categories exhibited significant variability. The selection of 15 markers for the categories of coat colour and coat structure was found to be sufficient, as evidenced by the high level of accuracy in predicting these traits for the majority of dogs in this study. The coat color and shape of almost all canines were accurately predicted, as indicated in Table

S5. Nevertheless, the test findings indicate that enhancing the predictions could be achieved with a focused augmentation of the markers. An illustration of this claim can be provided using the TYRP1 gene. Schmutz et al. [55] provided a description of three TYRP1 alleles, namely Q331ter, 345delP, and S41C, which result in the expression of a brown coat color when any two of these recessive TYRP1 alleles are combined. The marker set we used consisted solely of the two markers TYRP1_Q331ter and TYRP1_345delP. This limited selection of markers may account for the suboptimal accuracy in predicting color under certain combinations of alleles. Hence, using a minimum of three TYRP1 markers, specifically the allele "bc" which involves a nucleotide alteration in exon 2 resulting in a serine to cysteine exchange (S41C; c.121T>A), is likely to enhance the precision of coat color estimation. In addition, there is a possibility that there are other uncommon variations of the TYRP1 gene that result in brown coat color, which were not identified in our first examination of dogs. However, it is expected that these variations would be infrequent. Conversely, the coat category structure appears to be comprehensively represented by the three markers in our marker collection. All samples in this category were accurately allocated in both the marker test and the blind test. The presence of long hairs and curled coats, which were successfully predicted by only three markers, indicates a good potential in the category coat structure.

Only the IGF1R marker was utilized to assess body size during testing. The body size of 70% of the dogs was accurately predicted using a basic description of "relatively small" or "relatively tall". Hoopes et al. [49] proposed that the IGF1R nonsynonymous SNP is a causative mutation for small size in dogs. Allele A was found in a majority of the small breeds, albeit not in all of them, according to their analysis. This suggests that incorporating additional markers linked with body size could potentially mitigate any potential bias particular to certain breeds. The presence of breed-specific genes could potentially explain the occurrence of inaccurate tail length predictions in three out of the ten dogs that were examined. Certain breeds, such as English bulldogs and Boston Terriers, possess bobtails that are not caused by a mutation in the T-Box gene [48]. This could potentially account for the observed disparity in samples AT0056 and AT0062, which pertain to their respective breeds.

The marker with the lowest explanatory power proved to be IGF2BP2_BICFPJ1062878 which was selected to differentiate between drop ears and non-drop ears. Particularly, the heterozygous state, which was established in 60% of the tested dogs, did not allow for firm conclusions.

To evaluate the practical efficacy of our method, we conducted a blind test including samples from nine canines, with the aim of determining its potential applicability in forensic investigations. To showcase the comprehensive outcome of the 21-marker set, a visual representation of each dog was generated using the observed genotypes, incorporating all attributes deduced from the genetic data. The accurate physical appearance was unveiled through the utilization of reference photographs subsequent to the completion of the sketches. Figure 2 illustrates a substantial influence on recognition when directly comparing the sketches and the images. The blind test results exhibited remarkable accuracy in predicting coat color, coat pattern, and coat structure, aligning closely with the findings of the marker test. The discrepancies identified in the remaining traits can be attributed to the restricted utilization of genetic markers for these attributes, particularly for ear shape, body size, and tail length. Moreover, the effect of cosmetic modification was exemplified by the erroneous anticipation of dog D4925's tail length (a long tail), which occurred as a consequence of tail cropping. Although tail docking is prohibited in specific regions, it cannot be completely eradicated. The practice of ear cropping, which is also commonly observed, adheres to the same underlying premise. One should take into account the unpredictable characteristics of artificially altered body components when converting genetic information into a physical manifestation.

5. SUMMARY

This proof of concept study introduces a novel experimental method to forecast externally observable characteristics in dogs based on DNA, specifically for forensic applications. We employed six trait categories that were chosen based on the discernibility of an untrained individual, similar to that of an eyewitness. The trials yielded positive results for most of the chosen markers, and the projected attributes provided an accurate representation of the overall physical characteristics of the canines under examination. These encouraging findings motivate further investigation that necessitates a larger array of indicators and participants. The comprehensive phenotypical documentation of the individuals under study is essential for accurately interpreting the expected features. Ultimately, we propose the creation of molecular genetic tools that provide a streamlined laboratory workflow that is compatible with forensic quality sample types.

The prevalence of dogs as human companions elucidates the reason why these creatures frequently become the subject of scrutiny in forensic cases, such as incidents involving bite attacks or accidents. Canine evidence, such as dog hairs, can serve as a connection between the victim and suspect in a criminal investigation due to the intimate interaction between dogs and their owners. Dog individualization from crime scene evidence mostly relies on the study of short tandem repeat (STR) markers, similar to the identification of human DNA. Nevertheless, in cases where the DNA profile does not correspond to a reference, further data regarding the physical characteristics of the dog can offer significant informational worth.

The dog's physical characteristics, such as its body size and coat color, are easily identifiable and can be described to others who are not experts in dogs, including investigators and eyewitnesses. Hence, it is logical to supplement the statements of eyewitnesses with externally observable characteristics that can be deduced from canine DNA samples. This study examines the viability and appropriateness of using canine DNA phenotyping as a proof of concept. In order to get the most accurate prediction of the general physical characteristics of an unfamiliar dog based on its DNA, six specific attributes were selected: (1) coat color, (2) coat pattern, (3) coat structure, (4) body size, (5) ear shape, and (6) tail length. From previously published datasets, a selection of 21 genetic markers with good predictive values for these qualities was made. This selection includes 15 single nucleotide polymorphisms (SNPs) and six insertions/deletions (INDELS). Three of these were associated with SINE insertions. The tests were structured into three distinct phases. During the initial two phases, the markers' effectiveness was assessed using DNA samples obtained from dogs of various breeds, each with thoroughly documented physical attributes. In the conclusive blind test, which involved dogs whose appearance information was initially kept secret, it was found that most of the chosen markers enabled the creation of composite artworks that accurately portrayed the tested canines. This study represents the initial endeavor to assess the potential and constraints of forensic canine DNA phenotyping.

REFERENCES

1. Kayser, M. Forensic DNA Phenotyping: Predicting human appearance from crime scene material for investigative purposes. Forensic Sci. Int. Genet. **2015**, 18, 33–48. **[Google Scholar] [CrossRef] [PubMed]**

2. Kayser, M.; de Knijff, P. Improving human forensics through advances in genetics, genomics and molecular biology. Nat. Rev. Genet. **2011**, 12, 179–192. **[Google Scholar] [CrossRef]**

3. Grimes, E.A.; Noake, P.J.; Dixon, L.; Urquhart, A. Sequence polymorphism in the human melanocortin 1 receptor gene as an indicator of the red hair phenotype. Forensic Sci. Int. **2001**, 122, 124–129. **[Google Scholar] [CrossRef]**

4. Chaitanya, L.; Breslin, K.; Zuniga, S.; Wirken, L.; Pospiech, E.; Kukla-Bartoszek, M.; Sijen, T.; Knijff, P.; Liu, F.; Branicki, W.; et al. The HIrisPlex-S system for eye, hair and skin colour prediction from DNA: Introduction and forensic developmental validation. Forensic Sci. Int. Genet. **2018**, 35, 123–135. **[Google Scholar] [CrossRef] [PubMed] [Green Version]**

5. Walsh, S.; Chaitanya, L.; Clarisse, L.; Wirken, L.; Draus-Barini, J.; Kovatsi, L.; Maeda, H.; Ishikawa, T.; Sijen, T.; de Knijff, P.; et al. Developmental validation of the HIrisPlex system: DNA-based eye and hair colour prediction for forensic

and anthropological usage. Forensic Sci. Int. Genet. **2014**, 9, 150–161. **[Google Scholar] [CrossRef] [PubMed]**

6. Walsh, S.; Kayser, M. A Practical Guide to the HIrisPlex System: Simultaneous Prediction of Eye and Hair Color from DNA. In Forensic DNA Typing Protocols. Methods Mol Biol. **2016**, 1420, 213–231. **[Google Scholar] [CrossRef]**
7. Walsh, S.; Lindenbergh, A.; Zuniga, S.B.; Sijen, T.; de Knijff, P.; Kayser, M.; Ballantyne, K.N. Developmental validation of the IrisPlex system: Determination of blue and brown iris colour for forensic intelligence. Forensic Sci. Int. Genet. **2011**, 5, 464–471. **[Google Scholar] [CrossRef]**
8. Walsh, S.; Liu, F.; Ballantyne, K.N.; van Oven, M.; Lao, O.; Kayser, M. IrisPlex: A sensitive DNA tool for accurate prediction of blue and brown eye colour in the absence of ancestry information. Forensic Sci. Int. Genet. **2011**, 5, 170–180. **[Google Scholar] [CrossRef]**
9. Schneider, P.M.; Prainsack, B.; Kayser, M. The Use of Forensic DNA Phenotyping in Predicting Appearance and Biogeographic Ancestry. Dtsch. Ärzteblatt Int. **2019**, 116, 873–880. **[Google Scholar] [CrossRef]**
10. Ostrander, E.A.; Wayne, R.K.; Freedman, A.H.; Davis, B.W. Demographic history, selection and functional diversity of the canine genome. Nat. Rev. Genet. **2017**, 18, 705–720. **[Google Scholar] [CrossRef]**
11. Freedman, A.H.; Gronau, I.; Schweizer, R.M.; Ortega-Del Vecchyo, D.; Han, E.; Silva, P.M.; Galaverni, M.; Fan, Z.; Marx, P.; Lorente-Galdos, B.; et al. Genome sequencing highlights the dynamic early history of dogs. PLoS Genet. **2014**, 10, e1004016. **[Google Scholar] [CrossRef] [Green Version]**
12. Freedman, A.H.; Wayne, R.K. Deciphering the Origin of Dogs: From Fossils to Genomes. Annu. Rev. Anim. Biosci. **2017**, 5, 281–307. **[Google Scholar] [CrossRef]**
13. Thalmann, O.; Shapiro, B.; Cui, P.; Schuenemann, V.J.; Sawyer, S.K.; Greenfield, D.L.; Germonpre, M.B.; Sablin, M.V.; Lopez-Giraldez, F.; Domingo-Roura, X.; et al. Complete mitochondrial genomes of ancient canids suggest a European origin of domestic dogs. Science **2013**, 342, 871–874. **[Google Scholar] [CrossRef] [PubMed] [Green Version]**
14. Frantz, L.A.; Mullin, V.E.; Pionnier-Capitan, M.; Lebrasseur, O.; Ollivier, M.; Perri, A.; Linderholm, A.; Mattiangeli, V.; Teasdale, M.D.; Dimopoulos, E.A.; et al. Genomic and archaeological evidence suggest a dual origin of domestic dogs. Science **2016**, 352, 1228–1231. **[Google Scholar] [CrossRef] [PubMed]**
15. Perri, A.R.; Feuerborn, T.R.; Frantz, L.A.F.; Larson, G.; Malhi, R.S.; Meltzer, D.J.; Witt, K.E. Dog domestication and the dual dispersal of people and dogs

into the Americas. Proc. Natl. Acad. Sci. USA **2021**, 118, 6. **[Google Scholar]** **[CrossRef]** **[PubMed]**

16. Vilà, C.; Leonard, J.A. Canid Phylogeny and Origin of the Domestic Dog. In The Genetics of the Dog; Ostrander, E.A., Ruvinsky, A., Eds.; CABI: Wallingford, UK, 2012. **[Google Scholar]**
17. Perri, A. A wolf in dog's clothing: Initial dog domestication and Pleistocene wolf variation. J. Archaeol. Sci. **2016**, 68, 1–4. **[Google Scholar]** **[CrossRef]**
18. Baumann, C.; Pfrengle, S.; Munzel, S.C.; Molak, M.; Feuerborn, T.R.; Breidenstein, A.; Reiter, E.; Albrecht, G.; Kind, C.J.; Verjux, C.; et al. A refined proposal for the origin of dogs: The case study of Gnirshohle, a Magdalenian cave site. Sci. Rep. **2021**, 11, 5137. **[Google Scholar]** **[CrossRef]**
19. Botigue, L.R.; Song, S.; Scheu, A.; Gopalan, S.; Pendleton, A.L.; Oetjens, M.; Taravella, A.M.; Seregely, T.; Zeeb-Lanz, A.; Arbogast, R.M.; et al. Ancient European dog genomes reveal continuity since the Early Neolithic. Nat. Commun. **2017**, 8, 16082. **[Google Scholar]** **[CrossRef]**
20. Bergstrom, A.; Frantz, L.; Schmidt, R.; Ersmark, E.; Lebrasseur, O.; Girdland-Flink, L.; Lin, A.T.; Stora, J.; Sjogren, K.G.; Anthony, D.; et al. Origins and genetic legacy of prehistoric dogs. Science **2020**, 370, 557–564. **[Google Scholar]** **[CrossRef]**
21. Skoglund, P.; Ersmark, E.; Palkopoulou, E.; Dalen, L. Ancient wolf genome reveals an early divergence of domestic dog ancestors and admixture into high-latitude breeds. Curr. Biol. **2015**, 25, 1515–1519. **[Google Scholar]** **[CrossRef]** **[Green Version]**
22. Parker, H.G.; Gilbert, S.F. From caveman companion to medical innovator: Genomic insights into the origin and evolution of domestic dogs. Adv. Genom. Genet. **2015**, 5, 239–255. **[Google Scholar]** **[CrossRef]** **[Green Version]**
23. Moody, J.A.; Clark, L.A.; Murphy, K.E. Working Dogs: History and Applications. In The Dog and Its Genome; Ostrander, E., Giger, U., Lindblad-Toh, E., Eds.; Cold Springer Harbor Laboratory Press: New York, NY, USA, 2006; pp. 1–18. **[Google Scholar]**
24. Lindblad-Toh, K.; Wade, C.M.; Mikkelsen, T.S.; Karlsson, E.K.; Jaffe, D.B.; Kamal, M.; Clamp, M.; Chang, J.L.; Kulbokas, E.J., 3rd; Zody, M.C.; et al. Genome sequence, comparative analysis and haplotype structure of the domestic dog. Nature **2005**, 438, 803–819. **[Google Scholar]** **[CrossRef]**
25. Parker, H.G. Genomic analyses of modern dog breeds. Mamm. Genome **2012**, 23, 19–27. **[Google Scholar]** **[CrossRef]** **[Green Version]**

26. Parker, H.G.; Dreger, D.L.; Rimbault, M.; Davis, B.W.; Mullen, A.B.; Carpintero-Ramirez, G.; Ostrander, E.A. Genomic Analyses Reveal the Influence of Geographic Origin, Migration, and Hybridization on Modern Dog Breed Development. Cell Rep. **2017**, 19, 697–708. **[Google Scholar] [CrossRef]**

27. Berryere, T.G.; Kerns, J.A.; Barsh, G.S.; Schmutz, S.M. Association of an Agouti allele with fawn or sable coat color in domestic dogs. Mamm. Genome **2005**, 16, 262–272. **[Google Scholar] [CrossRef]**

28. Candille, S.I.; Kaelin, C.B.; Cattanach, B.M.; Yu, B.; Thompson, D.A.; Nix, M.A.; Kerns, J.A.; Schmutz, S.M.; Millhauser, G.L.; Barsh, G.S. A β-defensin mutation causes black coat color in domestic dogs. Science **2007**, 318, 1418–1423. **[Google Scholar] [CrossRef] [Green Version]**

29. Dreger, D.L.; Schmutz, S.M. A SINE insertion causes the black-and-tan and saddle tan phenotypes in domestic dogs. J. Hered. **2011**, 102, S11–S18. **[Google Scholar] [CrossRef] [PubMed]**

30. Philipp, U.; Hamann, H.; Mecklenburg, L.; Nishino, S.; Mignot, E.; Gunzel-Apel, A.R.; Schmutz, S.M.; Leeb, T. Polymorphisms within the canine MLPH gene are associated with dilute coat color in dogs. BMC Genet. **2005**, 6, 34. **[Google Scholar] [CrossRef] [PubMed] [Green Version]**

31. Schmutz, S.M.; Berryere, T.G. The genetics of cream coat color in dogs. J. Hered. **2007**, 98, 544–548. **[Google Scholar] [CrossRef] [Green Version]**

32. Schmutz, S.M.; Berryere, T.G.; Ellinwood, N.M.; Kerns, J.A.; Barsh, G.S. MC1R studies in dogs with melanistic mask or brindle patterns. J. Hered. **2003**, 94, 69–73. **[Google Scholar] [CrossRef] [PubMed] [Green Version]**

33. Schmutz, S.M.; Berryere, T.G.; Goldfinch, A.D. TYRP1 and MC1R genotypes and their effects on coat color in dogs. Mamm. Genome **2002**, 13, 380–387. **[Google Scholar] [CrossRef]**

34. Newton, J.M.; Wilkie, A.L.; He, L.; Jordan, S.A.; Metallinos, D.L.; Holmes, N.G.; Jackson, I.J.; Barsh, G.S. Melanocortin 1 receptor variation in the domestic dog. Mamm. Genome **2000**, 11, 24–30. **[Google Scholar] [CrossRef]**

35. Clark, L.A.; Starr, A.N.; Tsai, K.L.; Murphy, K.E. Genome-wide linkage scan localizes the harlequin locus in the Great Dane to chromosome 9. Gene **2008**, 418, 49–52. **[Google Scholar] [CrossRef] [PubMed]**

36. Cadieu, E.; Neff, M.W.; Quignon, P.; Walsh, K.; Chase, K.; Parker, H.G.; Vonholdt, B.M.; Rhue, A.; Boyko, A.; Byers, A.; et al. coat variation in the domestic dog is governed by variants in three genes. Science **2009**, 326, 150–153. **[Google Scholar] [CrossRef] [Green Version]**

37. Clark, L.A.; Tsai, K.L.; Starr, A.N.; Nowend, K.L.; Murphy, K.E. A missense mutation in the 20S proteasome beta2 subunit of Great Danes having harlequin coat patterning. Genomics **2011**, 97, 244–248. **[Google Scholar] [CrossRef] [Green Version]**

38. Kaelin, C.B.; Barsh, G.S. Genetics of pigmentation in dogs and cats. Annu. Rev. Anim. Biosci. **2013**, 1, 125–156. **[Google Scholar] [CrossRef] [PubMed]**

39. Murphy, S.C.; Evans, J.M.; Tsai, K.L.; Clarke, L.A. Length variations within the Merle retrotransposon of canine PMEL: Correlating genotype with phenotype. Mob. DNA **2018**, 9, 1. **[Google Scholar] [CrossRef] [PubMed]**

40. Saif, R.; Iftekhar, A.; Asif, F.; Alghanem, M.S. Dog Coat Colour Genetics: A Review. Adv. Life Sci. **2020**, 7, 215–224. **[Google Scholar]**

41. Varga, L.; Lenart, X.; Zenke, P.; Orban, L.; Hudak, P.; Ninausz, N.; Pelles, Z.; Szoke, A. Being Merle: The Molecular Genetic Background of the Canine Merle Mutation. Genes **2020**, 11, 660. **[Google Scholar] [CrossRef] [PubMed]**

42. Vaysse, A.; Ratnakumar, A.; Derrien, T.; Axelsson, E.; Rosengren Pielberg, G.; Sigurdsson, S.; Fall, T.; Seppala, E.H.; Hansen, M.S.; Lawley, C.T.; et al. Identification of genomic regions associated with phenotypic variation between dog breeds using selection mapping. PLoS Genet. **2011**, 7, e1002316. **[Google Scholar] [CrossRef] [Green Version]**

43. Boyko, A.R. The domestic dog: Man's best friend in the genomic era. Genome Biol. **2011**, 12, 216. **[Google Scholar] [CrossRef]**

44. Boyko, A.R.; Quignon, P.; Li, L.; Schoenebeck, J.J.; Degenhardt, J.D.; Lohmueller, K.E.; Zhao, K.; Brisbin, A.; Parker, H.G.; vonHoldt, B.M.; et al. A simple genetic architecture underlies morphological variation in dogs. PLoS Biol. **2010**, 8, e1000451. **[Google Scholar] [CrossRef] [Green Version]**

45. Shearin, A.L.; Ostrander, E.A. Canine morphology: Hunting for genes and tracking mutations. PLoS Biol. **2010**, 8, e1000310. **[Google Scholar] [CrossRef] [PubMed] [Green Version]**

46. Clark, L.A.; Wahl, J.M.; Rees, C.A.; Murphy, K.E. Retrotransposon insertion in SILV is responsible for merle patterning of the domestic dog. Proc. Natl. Acad. Sci. USA **2006**, 103, 1376–1381. **[Google Scholar] [CrossRef] [Green Version]**

47. Leegwater, P.A.; van Hagen, M.A.; van Oost, B.A. Localization of white spotting locus in boxer dogs on CFA20 by genome-wide linkage analysis with 1500 SNPs. J. Hered. **2007**, 98, 549–552. **[Google Scholar] [CrossRef] [PubMed] [Green Version]**

48. Hytonen, M.K.; Grall, A.; Hedan, B.; Dreano, S.; Seguin, S.J.; Delattre, D.; Thomas, A.; Galibert, F.; Paulin, L.; Lohi, H.; et al. Ancestral T-Box Mutation Is Present in Many, but Not All, Short-Tailed Dog Breeds. J. Hered. **2009**, 100, 236–240. **[Google Scholar] [CrossRef] [Green Version]**

49. Hoopes, B.C.; Rimbault, M.; Liebers, D.; Ostrander, E.A.; Sutter, N.B. The insulin-like growth factor 1 receptor (IGF1R) contributes to reduced size in dogs. Mamm. Genome **2012**, 23, 780–790. **[Google Scholar] [CrossRef] [PubMed] [Green Version]**

50. Karlsson, E.K.; Baranowska, I.; Wade, C.M.; Salmon Hillbertz, N.H.C.; Zody, M.C.; Anderson, N.; Biagi, T.M.; Patterson, N.; Pielberg, G.R.; Kulbokas, E.J.; et al. Efficient mapping of mendelian traits in dogs through genome-wide association. Nat. Genet. **2007**, 39, 1321–1328. **[Google Scholar] [CrossRef]**

51. Thomas, R.; Duke, S.E.; Karlsson, E.K.; Evans, A.; Ellis, P.; Lindblad-Toh, K.; Langford, C.F.; Breen, M. A genome assembly-integrated dog 1 Mb BAC microarray: A cytogenetic resource for canine cancer studies and comparative genomic analysis. Cytogenet. Genome Res. **2008**, 122, 110–121. **[Google Scholar] [CrossRef] [Green Version]**

52. Sutter, N.B.; Bustamante, C.D.; Chase, K.; Gray, M.M.; Zhao, K.Y.; Zhu, L.; Padhukasahasram, B.; Karlins, E.; Davis, S.; Jones, P.G.; et al. A single IGF1 allele is a major determinant of small size in dogs. Science **2007**, 316, 112–115. **[Google Scholar] [CrossRef] [Green Version]**

53. Parker, H.G.; VonHoldt, B.M.; Quignon, P.; Margulies, E.H.; Shao, S.; Mosher, D.S.; Spady, T.C.; Elkahloun, A.; Cargill, M.; Jones, P.G.; et al. An Expressed Fgf4 Retrogene Is Associated with Breed-Defining Chondrodysplasia in Domestic Dogs. Science **2009**, 325, 995–998. **[Google Scholar] [CrossRef] [Green Version]**

54. Haworth, K.; Putt, W.; Cattanach, B.; Breen, M.; Binns, M.; Lingaas, F.; Edwards, Y.H. Canine homolog of the T-box transcription factor T; failure of the protein to bind to its DNA target leads to a short-tail phenotype. Mamm. Genome **2001**, 12, 212–218. **[Google Scholar] [CrossRef] [PubMed]**

55. Schmutz, S.M.; Berryere, T.G. Genes affecting coat colour and pattern in domestic dogs: A review. Anim. Genet. **2007**, 38, 539–549. **[Google Scholar] [CrossRef]**

56. Welle, M.; Philipp, U.; Rufenacht, S.; Roosje, P.; Scharfenstein, M.; Schutz, E.; Brenig, B.; Linek, M.; Mecklenburg, L.; Grest, P.; et al. MLPH Genotype-Melanin Phenotype Correlation in Dilute Dogs. J. Hered. **2009**, 100, S75–S79. **[Google Scholar] [CrossRef] [Green Version]**

57. Sykes, N.; Beirne, P.; Horowitz, A.; Jones, I.; Kalof, L.; Karlsson, E.; King, T.; Litwak, H.; McDonald, R.A.; Murphy, L.J.; et al. Humanity's Best Friend: A Dog-Centric Approach to Addressing Global Challenges. Animals **2020**, 10, 502. **[Google Scholar] [CrossRef] [PubMed] [Green Version]**

58. Hughes, J.; Macdonald, D.W. A review of the interactions between free-roaming domestic dogs and wildlife. Biol. Conserv. **2013**, 157, 341–351. **[Google Scholar] [CrossRef]**

59. Sarenbo, S.; Svensson, P.A. Bitten or struck by dog: A rising number of fatalities in Europe, 1995–2016. Forensic Sci. Int. **2021**, 318, 110592. **[Google Scholar] [CrossRef]**

60. Berger, B.; Berger, C.; Hecht, W.; Hellmann, A.; Rohleder, U.; Schleenbecker, U.; Parson, W. Validation of two canine STR multiplex-assays following the ISFG recommendations for non-human DNA analysis. Forensic Sci. Int. Genet. **2014**, 8, 90–100. **[Google Scholar] [CrossRef]**

61. Berger, B.; Berger, C.; Heinrich, J.; Niederstätter, H.; Hecht, W.; Hellmann, A.; Rohleder, U.; Schleenbecker, U.; Morf, N.; Freire-Aradas, A.; et al. Dog breed affiliation with a forensically validated canine STR set. Forensic Sci. Int. Genet. **2018**, 37, 126–134. **[Google Scholar] [CrossRef]**

62. Eichmann, C.; Berger, B.; Parson, W. A proposed nomenclature for 15 canine-specific polymorphic STR loci for forensic purposes. Int. J. Leg. Med. **2004**, 118, 249–266. **[Google Scholar] [CrossRef]**

63. Wictum, E.; Kun, T.; Lindquist, C.; Malvick, J.; Vankan, D.; Sacks, B. Developmental validation of DogFiler, a novel multiplex for canine DNA profiling in forensic casework. Forensic Sci. Int. Genet. **2013**, 7, 82–91. **[Google Scholar] [CrossRef] [PubMed]**

64. Van Asch, B.; Pereira, F. State-of-the-Art and Future Prospects of Canine STR-Based Genotyping. Open Forensic Sci. J. **2010**, 3, 45–52. **[Google Scholar] [CrossRef]**

65. Kanthaswamy, S.; Oldt, R.F.; Montes, M.; Falak, A. Comparing two commercial domestic dog (Canis familiaris) STR genotyping kits for forensic identity calculations in a mixed-breed dog population sample. Anim. Genet. **2019**, 50, 105–111. **[Google Scholar] [CrossRef] [Green Version]**

66. Kanthaswamy, S.; Tom, B.K.; Mattila, A.-M.; Johnston, E.; Dayton, M.; Kinaga, J.; Erickson, B.J.-A.; Halverson, J.; Fantin, D.; DeNise, S.; et al. Canine population data generated from a multiplex STR kit for use in forensic casework. J. Forensic Sci. **2009**, 54, 829–840. **[Google Scholar] [CrossRef]**

67. Hellmann, A.P.; Rohleder, U.; Eichmann, C.; Pfeiffer, I.; Parson, W.; Schleenbecker, U. A Proposal for Standardization in Forensic Canine DNA Typing: Allele Nomenclature of Six Canine-Specific STR Loci. J. Forensic Sci. **2006**, 51, 274–281. **[Google Scholar] [CrossRef]**

68. Van Asch, B.; Alves, C.; Gusmao, L.; Pereira, V.; Pereira, F.; Amorim, A. A new autosomal STR nineplex for canine identification and parentage testing. Electrophoresis **2009**, 30, 417–423. **[Google Scholar] [CrossRef]**

69. Budowle, B.; Garofano, P.; Hellman, A.; Ketchum, M.; Kanthaswamy, S.; Parson, W.; van Haeringen, W.; Fain, S.; Broad, T. Recommendations for animal DNA forensic and identity testing. Int. J. Leg. Med. **2005**, 119, 295–302. **[Google Scholar] [CrossRef]**

70. Linacre, A.; Gusmao, L.; Hecht, W.; Hellmann, A.P.; Mayr, W.R.; Parson, W.; Prinz, M.; Schneider, P.M.; Morling, N. ISFG: Recommendations regarding the use of non-human (animal) DNA in forensic genetic investigations. Forensic Sci. Int. Genet. **2011**, 5, 501–505. **[Google Scholar] [CrossRef]**

71. Safer, M.A.; Murphy, R.P.; Wise, R.A.; Bussey, L.; Millett, C.; Holfeld, B. Educating jurors about eyewitness testimony in criminal cases with circumstantial and forensic evidence. Int. J. Law Psychiatry **2016**, 47, 86–92. **[Google Scholar] [CrossRef]**

72. Albright, T.D. Why eyewitnesses fail. Proc. Natl. Acad. Sci. USA **2017**, 114, 7758–7764. **[Google Scholar] [CrossRef] [Green Version]**

73. Wise, R.A.; Kehn, A. Can the effectiveness of eyewitness expert testimony be improved? Psychiatry Psychol. Law **2020**, 27, 315–330. **[Google Scholar] [CrossRef] [PubMed]**

74. Wixted, J.T.; Wells, G.L. The Relationship between Eyewitness Confidence and Identification Accuracy: A New Synthesis. Psychol. Sci. Public Interest **2017**, 18, 10–65. **[Google Scholar] [CrossRef]**

75. Berger, B.; Heinrich, J.; Niederstatter, H.; Hecht, W.; Morf, N.; Hellmann, A.; Rohleder, U.; Schleenbecker, U.; Berger, C.; Parson, W.; et al. Forensic characterization and statistical considerations of the CaDNAP 13-STR panel in 1184 domestic dogs from Germany, Austria, and Switzerland. Forensic Sci. Int. Genet. **2019**, 42, 90–98. **[Google Scholar] [CrossRef]**

76. Evans, J.J.; Wictum, E.J.; Penedo, M.C.; Kanthaswamy, S. Real-time polymerase chain reaction quantification of canine DNA. J. Forensic Sci. **2007**, 52, 93–96. **[Google Scholar] [CrossRef]**

77. Little, C.C. The Inheritance of Coat Color in Dogs; Comstock: Ithaca, NY, USA, 1957; Volume 118, p. 572. **[Google Scholar]**

78. Schmutz, S.M.; Melekhovets, Y. Coat color DNA testing in dogs: Theory meets practice. Mol. Cell. Probes **2012**, 26, 238–242. **[Google Scholar] [CrossRef]**

79. Kaelin, C.B.; Barsh, G.S. Molecular genetics of coat colour, texture and length in the dog. In The Genetics of the Dog; Ostrander, E.A., Ruvinsky, A., Eds.; CABI: Wallingford, UK, 2012; pp. 57–82. **[Google Scholar]**

80. Kerns, J.A.; Cargill, E.J.; Clark, L.A.; Candille, S.I.; Berryere, T.G.; Olivier, M.; Lust, G.; Todhunter, R.J.; Schmutz, S.M.; Murphy, K.E.; et al. Linkage and segregation analysis of black and brindle coat color in domestic dogs. Genetics **2007**, 176, 1679–1689. **[Google Scholar] [CrossRef] [Green Version]**

81. Kerns, J.A.; Newton, J.; Berryere, T.G.; Rubin, E.M.; Cheng, J.F.; Schmutz, S.M.; Barsh, G.S. Characterization of the dog Agouti gene and a nonagoutimutation in German Shepherd Dogs. Mamm. Genome **2004**, 15, 798–808. **[Google Scholar] [CrossRef]**

82. Dreger, D.L.; Hooser, B.N.; Hughes, A.M.; Ganesan, B.; Donner, J.; Anderson, H.; Holtvoigt, L.; Ekenstedt, K.J. True Colors: Commercially-acquired morphological genotypes reveal hidden allele variation among dog breeds, informing both trait ancestry and breed potential. PLoS ONE **2019**, 14, e0223995. **[Google Scholar]**

83. Schmutz, S.M.; Berryere, T.G.; Barta, J.L.; Reddick, K.D.; Schmutz, J.K. Agouti sequence polymorphisms in coyotes, wolves and dogs suggest hybridization. J. Hered. **2007**, 98, 351–355. **[Google Scholar] [CrossRef] [Green Version]**

84. Philipp, U.; Quignon, P.; Scott, A.; Andre, C.; Breen, M.; Leeb, T. Chromosomal assignment of the canine melanophilin gene (MLPH): A candidate gene for coat color dilution in Pinschers. J. Hered. **2005**, 96, 774–776. **[Google Scholar] [CrossRef] [Green Version]**

85. Schmutz, S.M.; Berryere, T.G.; Dreger, D.L. MITF and White Spotting in Dogs: A Population Study. J. Hered. **2009**, 100, S66–S74. **[Google Scholar] [CrossRef] [Green Version]**

86. Langevin, M.; Synkova, H.; Jancuskova, T.; Pekova, S. Merle phenotypes in dogs-SILV SINE insertions from Mc to Mh. PLoS ONE **2018**, 13, e0198536. **[Google Scholar]**

87. Parker, H.G.; Shearin, A.L.; Ostrander, E.A. Man's best friend becomes biology's best in show: Genome analyses in the domestic dog. Annu. Rev. Genet. **2010**, 44, 309–336. **[Google Scholar] [CrossRef] [Green Version]**

88. Indrebo, A.; Langeland, M.; Juul, H.M.; Skogmo, H.K.; Rengmark, A.H.; Lingaas, F. A study of inherited short tail and taillessness in Pembroke Welsh corgi. J. Small Anim. Pract. **2008**, 49, 220–224. **[Google Scholar] [CrossRef]**

89. Jones, P.; Chase, K.; Martin, A.; Davern, P.; Ostrander, E.A.; Lark, K.G. Single-nucleotide-polymorphism-based association mapping of dog stereotypes. Genetics **2008**, 179, 1033–1044. **[Google Scholar] [CrossRef] [Green Version]**

90. Bannasch, D.; Young, A.; Myers, J.; Truve, K.; Dickinson, P.; Gregg, J.; Davis, R.; Bongcam-Rudloff, E.; Webster, M.T.; Lindblad-Toh, K.; et al. Localization of canine brachycephaly using an across breed mapping approach. PLoS ONE **2010**, 5, e9632. **[Google Scholar] [CrossRef] [Green Version]**

91. Schoenebeck, J.J.; Hutchinson, S.A.; Byers, A.; Beale, H.C.; Carrington, B.; Faden, D.L.; Rimbault, M.; Decker, B.; Kidd, J.M.; Sood, R.; et al. Variation of BMP3 Contributes to Dog Breed Skull Diversity. PLoS Genet. **2012**, 8, e1002849. **[Google Scholar] [CrossRef] [Green Version]**

92. Schoenebeck, J.J.; Ostrander, E.A. The genetics of canine skull shape variation. Genetics **2013**, 193, 317–325. **[Google Scholar] [CrossRef] [Green Version]**

93. Rimbault, M.; Ostrander, E.A. So many doggone traits: Mapping genetics of multiple phenotypes in the domestic dog. Hum. Mol. Genet. **2012**, 21, R52–R57. **[Google Scholar] [CrossRef] [Green Version]**

94. Dreger, D.L.; Parker, H.G.; Ostrander, E.A.; Schmutz, S.M. Identification of a Mutation that Is Associated with the Saddle Tan and Black-and-Tan Phenotypes in Basset Hounds and Pembroke Welsh Corgis. J. Hered. **2013**, 104, 399–406. **[Google Scholar] [CrossRef] [Green Version]**

95. Wang, C.; Wallerman, O.; Arendt, M.L.; Sundstrom, E.; Karlsson, A.; Nordin, J.; Makelainen, S.; Pielberg, G.R.; Hanson, J.; Ohlsson, A.; et al. A novel canine reference genome resolves genomic architecture and uncovers transcript complexity. Commun. Biol. **2021**, 4, 185. **[Google Scholar] [CrossRef]**

96. Hoeppner, M.P.; Lundquist, A.; Pirun, M.; Meadows, J.R.; Zamani, N.; Johnson, J.; Sundstrom, G.; Cook, A.; FitzGerald, M.G.; Swofford, R.; et al. An improved canine genome and a comprehensive catalogue of coding genes and non-coding transcripts. PLoS ONE **2014**, 9, e91172. **[Google Scholar] [CrossRef] [PubMed]**

97. Schoenebeck, J.J.; Ostrander, E.A. Insights into morphology and disease from the dog genome project. Annu. Rev. Cell. Dev. Biol. **2014**, 30, 535–560. **[Google Scholar] [CrossRef] [PubMed] [Green Version]**

98. Donner, J.; Anderson, H.; Davison, S.; Hughes, A.M.; Bouirmane, J.; Lindqvist, J.; Lytle, K.M.; Ganesan, B.; Ottka, C.; Ruotanen, P.; et al. Frequency and distribution of 152 genetic disease variants in over 100,000 mixed breed and purebred dogs. PLoS Genet. **2018**, 14, e1007361. **[Google Scholar] [CrossRef]**

99. Anderson, H.; Honkanen, L.; Ruotanen, P.; Mathlin, J.; Donner, J. Comprehensive genetic testing combined with citizen science reveals a recently characterized ancient MC1R mutation associated with partial recessive red phenotypes in dog. Canine Med. Genet. **2020**, 7, 16. **[Google Scholar]** **[CrossRef]** **[PubMed]**

100. Grubwieser, P.; Muhlmann, R.; Berger, B.; Niederstatter, H.; Pavlic, M.; Parson, W. A new "miniSTR-multiplex" displaying reduced amplicon lengths for the analysis of degraded DNA. Int. J. Leg. Med. **2006**, 120, 115–120. **[Google Scholar]** **[CrossRef]** **[PubMed]**

101. Grubwieser, P.; Muhlmann, R.; Parson, W. New sensitive amplification primers for the STR locus D2S1338 for degraded casework DNA. Int. J. Leg. Med. **2003**, 117, 185–188. **[Google Scholar]** **[CrossRef]**

102. Hughes-Stamm, S.R.; Ashton, K.J.; van Daal, A. Assessment of DNA degradation and the genotyping success of highly degraded samples. Int. J. Leg. Med. **2011**, 125, 341–348. **[Google Scholar]** **[CrossRef]**

03 AN EVALUATION OF PROBABILISTIC GENOTYPING SYSTEMS: EUROFORMIX, DNASTATISTX AND STRMIX™

1. INTRODUCTION: AN OVERVIEW

Software is commonly employed within the forensic biology profession to assess DNA profile evidence. Software tools have been utilized since the late 1990s to apply statistical assessment models to observed DNA profile data. Currently, there are more than twelve distinct software solutions that perform this activity. These systems can be categorized as 'probabilistic genotyping' (PG) systems. All DNA profile data is assessed using a probabilistic framework and a likelihood ratio (LR) is generated to quantify the strength of the evidence. The likelihood ratio (LR) represents the probability of the observed DNA profile data, given two competing propositions. More precisely, when assessing DNA profile data in this context, the likelihood ratio (LR) is the ratio of the total weighted genotype sets that are relevant to each proposition.

Section 2 covers many software-independent aspects of PG. We provide a comprehensive analysis of the existing PG software and the specific modeling techniques utilized by each for conducting evaluations. The sensitivity of the LR to both the data used for modeling and the choice of model, as well as the underlying assumptions, is a crucial factor in any evaluation. Ideally, the learning rate (LR) should be consistent regardless of the decisions made inside or between software, and consequently, between models. Software validations have been conducted both on an individual basis and in a comparative manner between laboratories employing the same software, as well as between different software packages (as stated in Section 2.4 and Section 3.6). User inputs are crucial for addressing ambiguity regarding the number of contributors to a DNA profile and for establishing propositions that are best suited for assessing the evidential value.

Sections 3 and 4 provide a comprehensive analysis of three software applications: EuroForMix, DNAStatistX (which share the same underlying idea but were developed separately), and STRmix™. These methods are often employed in numerous forensic biology laboratories worldwide. These software tools employ several models to depict the behavior of DNA profiles and have acquired specialized skills. In addition, there are other support products outlined in Section 3 and Section 4. These products enhance the user's experience by providing extra analysis capabilities or presenting results in a more interactive and user-friendly way.

2. PROBABILISTIC GENOTYPING IN GENERAL

2.1. Probabilistic Genotyping Software

The recommended method for evaluation of DNA profile data in the forensic field is the LR [**1,2,3**]. It is assumed that autosomal markers are independent and in Hardy–Weinberg equilibrium. The LR seeks to determine the probability of obtaining some observed data (O) given a pair of competing propositions (H_1 and H_2), and any background information (I) about the framework of circumstances of the case that is relevant to the evaluation. Formulaically, the LR is expressed as:

$$LR = \frac{Pr(O|H_1, I)}{Pr(O|H_2, I)} \quad (1)$$

From this point on we omit the background information term, I, for visual clarity but note that it is ever present in the evaluation of any data. To calculate the LR, as shown in Equation (1), a number of nuisance parameters must be considered. The most fundamental of these (universal to any method of LR assignment) is the set of genotypes, S, that could belong to individuals whose DNA is present in the profile. Incorporating the J possible genotype sets into the LR from Equation (1) gives:

$$LR = \frac{\sum_{j=1}^{J} Pr(O|S_j)Pr(S_j|H_1)}{\sum_{j=1}^{J} Pr(O|S_j)Pr(S_j|H_2)} \quad (2)$$

The terms $P(Sj|Hx)$, $x \in \{1,2\}$, refer to the prior probability of observing the genotype set given a proposition. If the proposition specifies the presence of a particular individual, then any genotype set that does not contain the genotype corresponding to that individual (and depending on the model, the genotype of that individual in a specific component of the evidence profile) necessarily has a probability of 0. Any other genotype set has a prior probability that is assigned based on population genetic models and allele frequency databases. The terms $Pr(O|Sj)$ in Equation (2) are the probability of obtaining the observed data given a particular genotype set. These are often referred to as weights (and given the short-hand nomenclature of wj and are independent of propositions. The assignment of weights in the LR has been fundamental to much of the advancement that has occurred in probabilistic genotyping software used to interpret mixtures can be divided into three different groups;

- Binary models
- Qualitative, discrete or semi-continuous models
- Quantitative, or continuous models

In the initial binary models, drop-out and drop-in were not taken into account. In these models, weights were assigned values of either 0 or 1, depending on whether the genotype set explained the observed peaks (unconstrained combinatorial). Additionally, the weights could also be based on whether the peak balances were deemed acceptable (constrained combinatorial). Binary models essentially employ yes/no decisions to establish associations between genotypes and contributions, as outlined in the Clayton recommendations [4]. These initial prototypes served as the predecessors of more advanced techniques that were used in subsequent years. Although they utilize probabilistic methods for calculations, these systems are not inherently probabilistic genotyping systems since they do not handle DNA profile information in a probabilistic manner beyond determining whether genotypes are feasible or impossible.

Subsequent versions, known as qualitative (sometimes called 'discrete' or 'semi-continuous') models [5,6,7,8,9,10], determined weights by combining probabilities of drop-out and drop-in. These weights were based on the genotype set being analyzed and were used to describe the observed data. The qualitative models did not directly use peak heights, but they could utilize them to determine the nuisance parameter for the chance of drop-out. Additionally, these models could infer the genotype of a large donor by applying varying drop-out probabilities for each contributor [11]. Qualitative models do not directly utilize peak heights. However, these methods are an improvement over binary models as they can consider numerous contributors, low-template DNA, and duplicated samples.

Quantitative models, also known as continuous models, are considered the most comprehensive as they utilize peak height information to provide numerical values to the weights. This is supported by references [12,13,14,15,16,17,18]. These quantitative systems employ statistical models to predict the peak behavior in DNA profiles. They incorporate nuisance parameters that correspond to real-world aspects like DNA quantity and degradation.

2.2. Investigative vs. Evaluative Forensic Genetics

The forensic scientist assumes a dual function as both an investigator and an evaluator [3]. In traditional casework, the process involves identifying a suspect, reviewing the case conditions, and formulating alternative arguments. This constitutes the foundation of the court case for which the scientist will offer testimony. The individual is said to be in a state of "evaluative mode" and the principles of interpretation, as outlined in the ENFSI guideline [19], are applicable.

In contrast, it is possible to obtain a piece of evidence from a crime scene without having an available suspect. In this case, the scientists will operate in a state of "investigation mode". In order to discover possible individuals for additional investigation, a commonly employed method is to do a search of a national DNA database.

Typically, traditional database searches are limited to searching for the person of interest (POI) based on a crime-stain profile that has been analyzed and separated into its components. This technique is enough for individual profiles and combinations of major and minor components, where the person of interest is present in the individual profiles. However, in cases when allele dropout has been place and there are several donors, it is possible that the person of interest (POI) cannot be definitively identified. The search gets increasingly challenging due to the larger pool of potential candidates, making it less probable to locate 'true-donor' possibilities and more likely to generate a lengthy list of incidental matches.

Probabilistic genotyping offers a much more complete way to search large databases. With a database of N individuals, each is considered as a possible candidate that is compared to the crime stain O. Consequently, a likelihood ratio can be generated for every individual in the database, where the propositions are:

- H_1: Candidate n is a contributor to the evidence profile O
- H_2: An unknown person is a contributor to the evidence profile O

Where all contributors to the profile not being considered as the candidate are designated as unknown and unrelated to the candidate. Consequently, for a well-represented DNA profile, the majority of candidates will return a low LR < 1, which means that they will be eliminated from the investigation; one or more may return LR > 1, and they are forwarded to the prosecuting authorities for further investigation. If the crime-stain is a low-template mixture of several contributors, the LRs will be lower and there may be numerous potential candidates, especially with searches of large databases of several million individuals. A list, ranked according to high→low LR, can be provided to investigators, but the extent of the investigation will be dependent upon the resources available. Lists may be shortened by prioritising candidates from a geographical location, or with known modus operandi. Once suspects are identified, they may become defendants and the scientist returns to evaluative mode reporting.

With complex cases, it may be of interest to identify individuals that may have contributed to multiple crime-stains. STRmix™ utilises the semi-continuous method of Slooten [**20**] to compare the alternative propositions:

- The DNA profiles have a common contributor
- The DNA profiles do not have any common contributors (it is assumed that contributors are unrelated)
- The method does not depend upon a database search or direct reference profile comparison.

CaseSolver [21] is derived from EuroForMix and is specifically developed to handle intricate cases involving numerous reference samples and crime-stains. In this context, mixtures are exclusively compared to reference samples. However, it is possible to deconvolve mixtures in order to compare unknown contributors identified in other samples. SmartRank [22,23] is employed for qualitative searches in huge databases, while DNAmatch2 [24] is used for quantitative searches. Both tools can also be utilized for contamination searches.

2.3. *Utilizing Probabilistic Genotyping for the Identification of Contamination Incidents*

Investigative searches extend to comparisons of samples to detect potential contamination events [**25**,**26**] that may be propagated either by:

- Contamination of reagents or consumables by laboratory staff or other laboratory employees, or at the crime scene, or in the examination room by investigators.
- Sample to sample cross contamination during processing.
- Type 1 contamination may be detected if each sample/mixture is compared to an elimination database of, e.g., crime scene investigators and laboratory staff.

Type 2 cross contamination, e.g., between capillary electrophoresis (CE) plates may occur. An extreme example is illustrated by the case of "wrongful arrest of Adam Scott" [**27**] pp. 21–31, where CE plates were accidentally reused by the laboratory. However, the biggest risk is with accidental carry-over of DNA on reusable tips or by capillary carry-over, where PCR products injected by a capillary are not completely removed during the cleaning process [**25**].

The advancements in PG systems have not only enhanced the capability to detect individuals who contribute DNA to crime scene profiles, but also improved the ability to identify instances of contamination. Furthermore, in order to achieve high-throughput capabilities, numerous contamination detection procedures in PG systems are automated, integrated into the laboratory's information management system, or capable of being executed in large quantities with minimal human intervention. For further details about investigative searches with STRmixTM refer to **Section 4.5**. CaseSolver, DNAmatch2 and SmartRank are described in **Section 3.4.**

2.4. Inter and Intra-Laboratory Studies

The ultimate objective of a forensic biology evaluation is to provide evidence that can be submitted in a court of law. There is a general expectation that information provided should be trustworthy. One way to establish the trustworthiness of PG systems is to conduct studies on their practical application in real-life cases. These studies can give a comprehensive analysis of the overall performance of the PG systems, including specific data outlined in Section 2.7. Additionally, they assess the uniformity of their utilization across several laboratories and by multiple individuals. Inter- and intra-laboratory studies entail the dissemination of mixes containing established ground truth, typically in the form of electronic files, among forensic scientists inside a laboratory or across many laboratories. The combined results provide a quantification of the variability in performance both within and between laboratories [28,29,30,31,32,33,34,35,36,37]. Two studies, including the GHEP-ISFG research and NIST studies, have gained attention in courtroom discussions because to the diverse range of outcomes observed.

The GHEP-ISFG study utilizes many probabilistic genotyping software programs to analyze the same mixture and has been deliberated in hearings over its acceptability. The outcomes obtained by the utilization of LRmix ranged from 2.6 × 103 to 3.2 × 1014. The diversity mostly stems from human decision-making and interpretation, such as the selection of drop-in probability, drop-out probability, and population correction for sub-structuring. The situation is worsened by the existence of three sets of unresolved peaks. The variation is not inherent to the software but underscores the fact that achieving great reproducibility requires careful consideration of the human aspect. It is worth mentioning that a significant portion of the diversity in human decision making stems from various conservative acts. The results obtained from other research utilizing LRmix, such as the one mentioned in reference [40], are similar in nature.

The NIST studies predate PG but have been subsequently reworked [**41**] using STRmix™, EuroForMix v1.10.0, EuroForMix v1.11.4, Lab Retriever, LRmix, and RMP (random match probability) [**42**]. The quantitative software, STRmix and EuroForMix (both versions), produced similar results with the exception of ref 5C for case 5. The qualitative software, Lab Retriever and LRmix, also produced results similar to each other. RMP was given as a benchmark.

Alladio et al. [43] compared Lab Retriever, LRmix Studio, DNA-VIEW®, EuroForMix, and STRmixTM. In general, the quantitative software DNA-VIEW®, EuroForMix, and STRmixTM performed similarly and the qualitative software Lab Retriever and LRmix Studio also performed similarly to each other, but differed from the quantitative methods. Alladio et al. concluded "results provided by fully-continuous models proved similar and convergent to one another, with slightly higher within-software differences (i.e., approximatively 3–4 degrees of magnitude)". Iyer [44] has appealed to the community not to overlook the differences between software of the order of 3–4 orders of magnitude even in a pattern of overall similarity arguing that in some circumstances such differences could be crucial.

Alladio et al. suggested the use of a "statistic consensus approach [45]" which "consists in comparing likelihood ratio values provided by different software and, only if results turn out to be convergent, the most conservative likelihood ratio value is finally reported. On the contrary, if likelihood ratio results are not convergent, DNA interpretation is considered inconclusive." In the paper, convergent (a) and non-convergent (b) are defined as the two results both having (a) $LR > 1$ or $LR < 1$ and (b) one result $LR > 1$ and the other is $LR < 1$. Using such an approach would deem ref 5C for case 5 of the NIST study inconclusive using EuroForMix (LR about 10^3–10^6) and STRmix (LR about 0). The ground truth is that ref 5C is a non-donor, although it was an artificial construct based on resampling alleles from the profile [41] and consequently represents an outcome that would be rarely observed in actual case-work. However, from a recent collaborative study [46] we note that STRmix is more likely to report lower LRs when the alternative contributor has a high degree of shared alleles (as in cases of relatedness). In a much-discussed case in upstate New York (NY v Hillary) the result would also have been reported as inconclusive (STRmix LR about 10^5, TrueAllele LR not known but plausibly slightly less than 1). The ground truth in NY v Hillary is, of course, not known. Taylor et al. [47] take up the subject of the "statistic consensus approach" pointing out that either two quantitative or two qualitative systems should be used (this plausibly is also Alladio et al.'s view) and averaging might be better than taking the lowest. Furthermore, there is no particular reason to choose $LR = 1$ as a value to use in the definition of non-convergent. In fact, an LR that is the inverse of the, unknown, prior odds is more crucial from a decision theory perspective. To illustrate, suppose that the prior odds are 1:X, then it is not until the LR reaches X:1 that the posterior odds will begin to support a proposition that is potentially different from that supported by the prior odds. From a decision theory perspective, this is a threshold at which a switch may occur between two possible actions when making a decision.

Swaminathan et al. [48] create four variants of their CEESIt software and note some large differences in the resulting LR. This is relatively unsurprising as the underlying differences between their four versions are quite substantial and they analyse very low peak heights. For example, one large LR difference is driven by a peak at 6 rfu.

Whilst the "statistic consensus approach" is a rational approach to lack of consistency between different software we would add that it is vital to increase efforts to diagnose, and hopefully remedy, the inconsistency. It is a great pity that much larger efforts have not been made in this regard. Some of the authors are currently involved in such an exercise and results are already greatly promising.

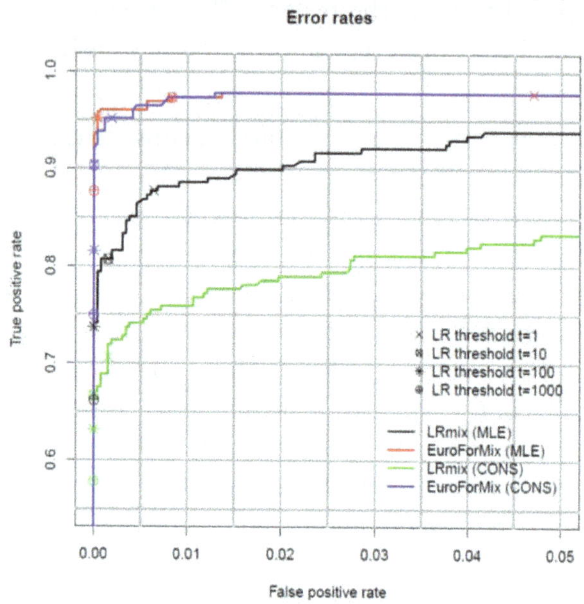

Figure 1. Receiver operating characteristic (ROC) plot where the rate of false positive support (FP) (horizontal axis) and true positives support (TP) (vertical axis) are plotted as a function of LR thresholds. The plot shows the results for the maximum likelihood estimation method (MLE) and the conservative method (CONS) for both LRmix and EuroForMix. The points on the curves show the FP and TP rates for different LR thresholds. Note that with this dataset, approximately 5% of samples were very low-level mixtures so that the POI was undetectable This caused the number of contributors to be underestimated, leading to very low (exclusionary) LRs. Therefore, the true positive rate does not reach 1.0 with the MLE method. Reprinted from [50].

ROC charts [49] are a valuable tool for quantifying and comparing the performance of models. These graphs illustrate the relationship between the rates of false positive support and false negative support in relation to the observed likelihood ratio (Figure 1). An effective model aims to reduce both false positive and false negative rates while maintaining low values of LR. Figure 1 demonstrates that the LRmix maximum likelihood estimation (MLE) and conservative qualitative models exhibit lower rates of correctly identifying positive cases compared to the quantitative EuroForMix MLE and conservative models. However, the rates of incorrectly identifying positive cases are equal for both models. This demonstrates the superior efficiency of the examined quantitative models. As mentioned in the preceding paragraph, this finding does not endorse a consensus approach between distinct categories of models, namely quantitative and qualitative. ROC charts are valuable for comparing the performance of several models while analyzing a specific dataset.

You and Balding [51] conducted a ROC analysis to compare EuroForMix with LikeLTD. Both of these models are γ models, although they have different modelling assumptions. However, the overall conclusions were similar. The LikeLTD model shown improvement in predicting forward n + 1 and complicated n - 2 stutters. However, this improvement was only detected with certain low template samples, as the version of EuroForMix used did not support these types of stutters. In their study, Manabe et al. [52] conducted a comparison between Kongoh and EuroForMix, both of which are γ models. They discovered significant similarities between the two.

The first interlaboratory study with STRmix was reported by Cooper et al. [**33**]. In a subsequent enlargement of this exercise [**53**] two samples were examined. For one sample 176 responses were received with LRs ranging from $10^{28.3}$ to $10^{29.4}$. The bottom and top values were obtained by variation in human judgement elements such as dropping a locus (lowest LR) and a laboratory procedure that used a bespoke artefact handling process (top LR). For the 173 responses to the other sample, nine false exclusions were obtained by assigning numbers of contributors (NOC) as one fewer than the number used in construction of the sample. The remaining LRs reported varied from $10^{4.3}$ to $10^{6.6}$ with most of the variation attributable to GeneMapper® ID-X analysis settings used.

McNevin et al. [54] characterize this fluctuation as "extreme sensitivity" and anticipate a far higher level of reproducibility in the given statistic. This aligns with the recommendation, made by the UK Forensic Science Regulator (personal communication), to achieve consistent outcomes irrespective of the laboratory to which the case is referred. The outcome would rely on human variables, laboratory policies, external elements, and the theory and execution of the program.

Non-Contributor Tests and Calibration of the LR

Ramos and Gonzalez-Rodriguez [**55**] introduced the concept of "calibration of the likelihood ratio". Their purpose was to: "highlight that some desirable behaviour of LR values happens if they are well calibrated", meaning that the behaviour of the software is consistent with the expectations of a predefined model. Calibration applies a much more rigorous criterion than Turing expectation: the rate of non-contributor inclusionary support is at most the reciprocal of the LR, i.e., $\Pr(LR > x|H_2) \leq 1/x$ [**56**]. Calibration tests that LRs of any given magnitude are occurring at the expected rate. It has been applied to STRmix™ and EuroForMix [**57,58**]. Testing larger LRs gets progressively challenging due to the excessively huge number of samples required. Importance testing is proposed as a solution for this issue [59,60].

2.5. Number of Contributors (NOC)

The number of contributors in casework is uncertain. This also applies to numerous simulated samples, particularly in cases where at least one contributor has not produced any discernible signal. When a parameter's value is not known, it is highly advantageous to consider it as a bothersome parameter. We will examine several recently devised techniques that rely on this principle.

The NOC attributed to a DNA profile has traditionally been determined by using the maximum allele count (MAC) method, which is often adjusted based on a visual assessment of peak heights. This method utilizes the locus that displays the highest number of alleles at a specific location. The number is divided by two and rounded up to the nearest whole number, as stated in references [4,61], [62] (chapter 7), and the SWGDAM interpretation guidelines [63]. This method establishes a direct correlation between the NOC and the minimum number of contributors. The accurate determination of the true NOC (Number of Contributors) is uncertain when using this particular method, particularly in cases involving complex mixtures with three or more contributors and/or low levels of DNA [64,65,66]. Referring to the true NOC, even in simulated samples, can be challenging. However, for the purpose of this discussion, we will define it as the count of donors who have exhibited a detectable signal above the analytical threshold.

Misjudging the NOC, whether by underestimating or overestimating it, can have an impact on the strength of evidence [67] when using qualitative models [35,68,69].

Quantitative models often result in false negative support for the lowest template contributor when underestimation occurs, although this is not always the case. Overestimation often leads to inaccurate positive endorsements for individuals who do not donate, typically with low likelihood ratios. The larger template donors exhibit greater stability in relation to various NOC [70,71,72,73].

There are instances where it is solely feasible to determine the primary contributor(s) of the DNA combination. If small contributors are not of interest, the NOC can be based just on the forme.There are situations where it is solely feasible to determine the primary contributor(s) of the DNA combination. If the inclusion of minor contributors is not relevant, the NOC can be established based on the former, hence streamlining the model [72,74].Furthermore, this aids in streamlining the model [72,74]. The utilization of a greater number of loci, particularly those with a higher capacity for differentiation, or the application of massively parallel sequencing (MPS) data on STR loci, led to a reduced occurrence of misinterpretations in the NOC as compared to the MAC approach [75,76,77,78].

Alternative approaches, such as utilizing the total number of alleles (total allele count, TAC), analyzing the distribution of allele counts across the loci, examining the genotype frequencies within the population, considering peak heights (PH), incorporating replicates, accounting for the probability of allelic drop-out and stutter, or employing a Bayesian network approach, have been demonstrated to produce more accurate estimates of the number of contributors (NOC) [68,79,80,81,82,83,84,85,86,87,88,89].

Machine learning algorithms are now being used to improve the estimation of the NOC by making the best possible use of the available profile information. So far, a limited number of models have been created specifically for application in forensic DNA casework [37,90,91,92]. These models utilize additional information compared to the previously proposed algorithms as they are trained on a distinct ground truth dataset. One major advantage of machine learning systems is that they can quickly estimate the NOC (Number of Components) in a matter of seconds. This is particularly valuable in situations when fast analyses are needed. Refer to Section 3.1.3 for an elucidation of the NOC-tool employed in DNAxs. The limitations of machine learning methods include the need for extensive datasets that are tailored to the laboratory that produced the data, as well as a lack of transparency in the prediction process. To effectively handle the assignment of the NOC for weight of evidence computations, it is best to treat it as a nuisance parameter [71,92,93,94,95,96,97,98].

In an elegant mathematical development Slooten and Caliebe [**94**], making a few reasonable assumptions, show that the LR considering a reasonable range of NOC is the weighted average of the LR for each separate NOC. Specifically: $LR{=}\sum iLRiwi$ where

$$LR_i = \frac{Pr(O_c, O_p | H_1, NOC = i)}{Pr(O_c, O_p | H_2, NOC = i)}$$

where $wi{=}Pr(NOC{=}i|H2{,}Oc{,}Op)$ terms the weights, and Oc and Op are the genotype of the crime profile and the POI, respectively. The weights are the probability of the number of contributors given the profile and assuming the POI is not a donor. This is the term that has been assessed subjectively for many years and can now be assigned as a probability distribution, sometimes with the assistance of software.

In an alternative approach, used with EuroForMix, the effective NOC is decided by maximizing the likelihood adjusted by application of the 'Akaike information criterion' (AIC) [**99**], which favours simpler models to explain the evidence. The smallest number of unknown contributors needed to explain the evidence usually maximises the respective likelihoods.

These approaches can be very useful since it is not necessary to define an absolute NOC and the field should move this way, though most of the current probabilistic genotyping systems still require that the user specifies the NOC [**100**]. STRmix™ v2.6 and higher treat NOC as a nuisance parameter but is currently only validated for taking into account two consecutive NOC values (say NOC = 3 or 4).

2.6. Proposition Setting/Hierarchy of Propositions

Applying Bayes' rule in odds form necessitates a minimum of two propositions, typically selected to support the prosecution's viewpoint, taking into account the specific facts of the case, as well as a plausible alternative. The alternative will be determined by the specific facts of the case, primarily relying on material provided by the defense. Consequently, this option is commonly referred to as the defense argument in the literature.

There are at least two perspectives on how the alternative should be established:

- The scientist representing the defense should propose this idea. If there is no meaningful discussion with the defense, the scientist advising the prosecution should propose a reasonable alternative that aligns with the strongest defense proposition and is comprehensive.
- The concept of the hierarchy of propositions is well established [**101,102**]. Gittelson et al. [**103**] discussed this concept more recently; the ISFG DNA commission provides an extensive review [**3**], with recommendations for practitioners.
- Propositions are classified into four levels: offence, activity, source, and sub-source.
- Offence level propositions describe the issue for the fact finder which is one of guilt or innocence. This is a decision of the court; the forensic scientist does not offer opinions at this level.
- Activity level propositions describe the activity that deposited the DNA. Provided that there is sufficient information, the forensic scientist may assist the court.
- Source level refers to the origin of the body fluid or cell type examined. This is relatively straightforward if there is sufficient body fluid to test but may be challenging to address if there are low level mixtures of body-fluids.
- Sub-source level refers to the origin of the DNA (i.e., donor).
- It has proven useful to use a fifth level.

- Sub-sub-source refers to the origin of part of the DNA, for example the major donor [**104,105**].

Probabilistic genotyping offers data exclusively at the sub-source and sub-sub-source levels. To derive conclusions at both the source and activity levels, distinct computations are necessary. Inadequate explanation of the differentiation between levels in the hierarchy might result in the transfer of legal reasoning from one level to another, thereby resulting in miscarriages of justice [3,27,106,107].

2.7. Validation of PG Systems

There are several publications that address 'validation' from scientific societies; for example: SWGDAM [**108**], ISFG [**109**], the AAFS Standards Board [**110**] and the UK Forensic Science Regulator [**111**]. Some laboratories have published validation studies—see Coble and Bright [**100**] for an excellent review and other guidance [**108,109,112,113,114,115,116,117**].

The purpose of validation is to define the scope and limitations of software. This is described in detail for STRmix (**Section 4.6**) and EuroForMix/DNAStatistX (**Section 3.6**).

George Box (a British statistician) famously stated: "Essentially, all models are wrong, but some are useful" [**118**]. All models are "wrong" in the sense that they are approximations of some unknown reality. However, so long as models demonstrate an empirical behaviour that conforms to expectations of a given reality, then they are "useful". The question that follows in relation to different PG software is whether models that are based upon different theories and assumptions are "equally reliable" or "equally useful"?

The terms "right" or "wrong" are two extremes. Probability is a numerical description, somewhere between 0 and 1, which describes how likely it is that an event will occur. Importantly, probability represents a personal belief about uncertainty, that is informed by available data. Provided scientists use the same or similar datasets and the same methods of analysis, then their personal beliefs should coincide. We never know if something is true or not, but probability is always conditioned upon some hypothesis/ proposition being true.

As an example, consider the probability assigned for an allele that has never been seen before in the population sample (hereafter "rare allele"), but is observed in this case. We can say for certain that the "true" probability of this allele is not 0, but we are uncertain exactly what it is. Whenever something is unknown and uncertain it is best to model the uncertainty with a probability density function. A workable option may be to insert a reasonable point estimate. Further, in forensic science, some aspects of utility are usually confounded into the probability assignment by deliberately biassing the assignment in a direction thought to be conservative. However, in mixture evaluation the conservative direction is very uncertain. For example, it is typically conservative to raise the sample allele probability for the alleles that correspond with the person of interest (POI), but for any other alleles the effect may be neutral or may vary either way. The use of a point estimate biased upwards (for example 5/2N or 3/2N where N is the number of alleles in the sample) is plausibly conservative on average, although we are unaware of any systematic investigation of this assumption. The use of a probability density distribution and resampling may enable the choice of a conservative quantile but requires assignment of a distribution. It would be very difficult, and be a matter of subjective judgement, to choose which of these methods is appropriately conservative.

In the context of PG software, where two software may implement two different models for the same process we can assess how well the models describe the empirical data, then we can have confidence in the result. This can readily be supplemented by varying the model within reasonable limits dictated by the data and thus creating a range of plausible outcomes. We are left with the uncertainty that small modelling and inferential errors accrue, or that the training data for the models are inappropriate.

There are various phases to a validation programme, originally described by Rykiel [**119**] in relation to ecological models:

- Conceptual validation: verification of the mathematical formulae used in the software are correct.
- Software validation: Verification and testing of the code, e.g., by running test scripts.
- Operational validation: The output of the model is tested against a wide range of evidence types, representing a typical case, as well as extreme examples.
- A validation programme can address the following:
- Sensitivity (demonstrate the range of LRs that can be expected for true contributors)
- Specificity (demonstrate the range of LRs that can be expected for non-contributors)
- Precision (variation in LRs from repeated software analyses of the same input data)

Accuracy of statistical calculations and other results (comparison to an alternate statistical model or software program) Determination of the limits of the software (either computational or conceptual, regarding for instance the number of unknown contributors or types of DNA profiles)

Steps towards internal validation, to enable a laboratory to adopt a given procedure, was described by **[115]** as an "accumulation of representative test data within the laboratory to demonstrate that the established parameters, software settings, formulae, algorithms and functions perform as expected"

In real casework, we do not know the ground truth. In validation, the model is tested against samples where the ground truth is usually known. This enables two kinds of tests to be carried out using the standard likelihood ratio formula: $LR = Pr(O|H_1)/Pr(O|H_2)$

- H_1 = true: where we know the POI is a contributor.
- H_2 = true: where we know that the POI is not a contributor

As a small word of caution: the ground truth is not known even for mock samples for very low level contributors. For these it can be unclear whether they are, in reality, a donor at all.

3. EVOLUTION OF EUROFORMIX AND DNASTATISTX

3.1. Evolution

An outline of the development and evolution of the software EuroForMix and DNAStatistX, including its predecessors and related modules is shown in **Figure 2**. These software will be discussed in the next sections.

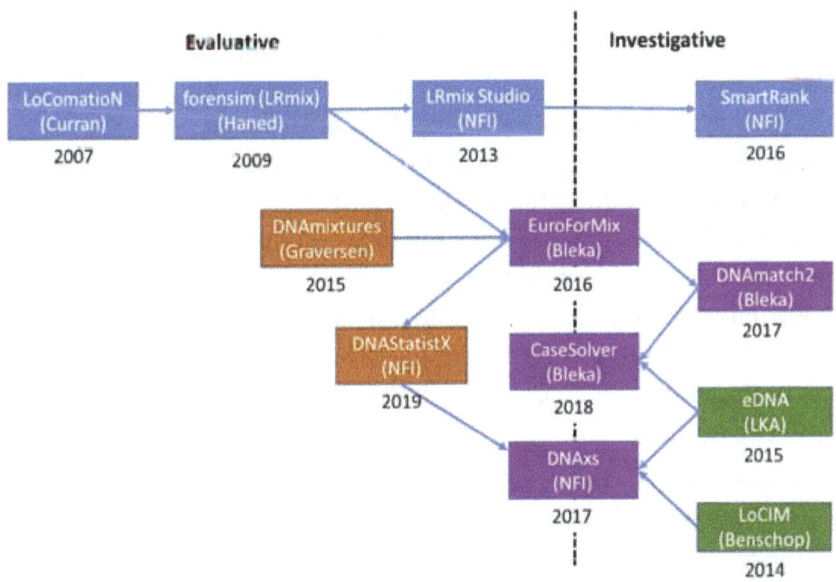

Figure 2. A diagram showing the evolution of probabilistic genotyping software developed by the NFI and Oslo University Hospital. Blue and orange boxes indicate qualitative and quantitative (γ) models, respectively. Green boxes are binary methods and purple boxes indicate software that include multiple types of methods.

3.1.1. Qualitative Software

The development of probabilistic genotyping undertaken by the authors began in 2007 with the development of qualitative software (discrete or semi-continuous) which took account of allele drop-out and drop-in, but peak heights were not modelled. The first software was the introduction of LoComatioN by James Curran [**120**], whilst at the Forensic Science Service (UK). The model was re-programmed by Hinda Haned [**121,122**], as part of her PhD at the University of Lyon: LRmix is written in R and the module is found in the forensim package: **https://forensim.r-forge.r-project.org/** accessed on 28 September 2021. Four years later, in 2013, the Netherlands Forensic Institute (NFI) adopted LRmix, rewriting the code into Java and rebranding it as LRmix Studio: **https://github.com/smartrank/lrmixstudio** accessed on 28 September 2021. This software has been widely adopted in Europe and elsewhere. LRmix Studio was further developed by NFI to provide SmartRank: **https://github.com/smartrank/smartrank** accessed on 28 September 2021, a database search engine [**23**] which was shown to be more efficacious than the CODIS search engine [**22**]; it is still widely used by caseworkers (see collaborative study of Prieto et al. [**40**]).

3.1.2. Quantitative Software

Early models designed to explain variation in peak area observations were described in 1998 by Evett et al. [**123**] who defined an underlying normal distribution and in 2007 by Cowell et al. [**18,124**] who also defined a γ distribution (the γ model).

In 2013, Cowell, Graversen and colleagues released DNAmixtures which was based on the γ model [**125,126**]: **http://dnamixtures.r-forge.r-project.org/** accessed on 28 September 2021, written in R code as open-source, but requires HUGIN (commercial software) to run it. Supported by the EU-funded EuroForGen-Network- of-Excellence: **https://www.euroforgen.eu/** accessed on 28 September 2021, the γ model was re-written in R and C++ by Øyvind Bleka as EuroForMix: **http://www.euroformix.com/** accessed on 28 September 2021. This program had enhanced capabilities compared to DNAmixtures, including degradation parameterisation and "theta-correction" (Fst).

EuroForMix was further utilized to provide the database search tool DNAmatch2, which also incorporated the forensimLRmix module, in order to carry out searches of large national DNA databases. Later, the same modules were integrated into a more user-friendly expert system called CaseSolver which is integrated into casework for analysing complex cases where there are multiple suspects and case-stains. CaseSolver includes many useful features for caseworkers: Visualization, automated comparison, deconvolution, weight-of-evidence evaluation and reporting (discussed in **Section 3.4**).

In 2019, the NFI implemented DNAStatistX, the statistical module based on the EuroForMix code which is further elucidated in **Section 3.3.1.** DNAStatistX can be used as a stand-alone application or within the DNA eXpert System, DNAxs. DNAxs is a software suite that was developed by the NFI, for the data management and (probabilistic) interpretation of DNA profiles. It was implemented in forensic casework in 2017 and is under continuous development to further advance the software, to improve the process of DNA casework and to broaden the scope of application. Further information on the DNAxs functionalities is provided in the following section.

3.1.3. DNAxs and Related Modules

Increased complexity of DNA profile comparisons and interpretation demands fast and automated software tools to assist DNA experts in routine casework. eDNA is one such application [**127**], whose functionalities were an inspiration for the development of CaseSolver [**21**] and the DNA eXpert System DNAxs [**128**].

Within DNAxs, profile comparisons can be achieved at various levels:

- By aggregating replicate profiles into one composite view (bar graphs)
- By viewing the trace profile as bar graphs underneath which alleles of reference profiles are comparedThrough the match matrix option
- By sending a DNA profile for a SmartRank search against the DNA database
- By calculating LRs using DNAStatistX for a comparison of a person of interest to a trace DNA profile [**128**]

DNAxs imports (pre-analyzed) DNA profiling data which is shown as the original electropherogram and is graphically represented as bar graphs with a color coding for reproduced and non-reproduced alleles in case of PCR replicates, and a color coding for alleles of the major component of a mixture through the LoCIM method (Locus Classification and Inference of the Major) [**29**]. This LoCIM method can be applied to one amplification of a DNA extract or to replicate DNA profiles. In the latter case, LoCIM first generates a consensus profile that includes alleles that are observed in at least half of the replicates [**86**]. Next, LoCIM classifies each locus as type I, II or III based on thresholds for peak height; ratio of major to minor contributors; and heterozygote balance. A Type I locus fulfils the most stringent criteria and will most likely be correctly inferred. Type II loci may have lower peak heights or a smaller difference in peak heights compared to minor donors. Type III loci do not meet one or more of the Type II criteria and are the most complex to infer a major contributor's genotype. Lastly, thresholds are used per locus type to infer the major component's alleles. It has been demonstrated that the LoCIM approach is successful regardless of the laboratory's STR typing kit and PCR and

CE settings and the method is easy to implement (one only needs to specify the laboratory's stochastic threshold) [**29,37**].

The major contributor's genotype predicted by the deconvolution method of EuroForMix described in **Section 3.3.4** (on loci with a probability that was at least twice as large as the second likeliest genotype possibility) was compared to that of LoCIM (on type I and II loci). Both methods are able to perform deconvolution by utilizing the peak height information, though LoCIM is threshold based while EuroForMix applies a statistical model which consists of a set of parameters which are inferred by maximizing the likelihood function [**50**]. EuroForMix applies a more comprehensive statistical model which calculates the uncertainty of different suggested genotype profiles extracted from the inferred uncertainty of the whole evidence profile. Therefore, these calculations are much more computationally intensive compared to the extremely fast LoCIM method. At the locus level, and as expected, the EuroForMix deconvolution showed improved performance compared to LoCIM [**50**]. Regardless, since LoCIM is extremely fast and was regarded useful to many cases, this approach was implemented in DNAxs [**62**], chapter 10 and [**37**].

DNAxs provides summary statistics for its comparisons, such as the number of mismatches or unseen alleles, and to help estimating the NOC- such as the maximum allele count (MAC) and the total allele count (TAC). Furthermore, DNAxs includes NOC tools based on a machine learning approach. These are designated as the RFC19 model that is specific to PowerPlex Fusion 6C (PPF6C) data as generated within NFI [**89**] and the generic RFC11 model which is laboratory independent [**37**]. The RFC19 model outperformed the MAC method and an in-house developed tool that utilised the TAC [**89,91**]. A drawback of such models is that it requires a large dataset for development and is specific to a laboratory's data. To that end, the generic model was developed, which only involves features of the 12 European Standard Set and U.S. core loci, and does not include features holding information on peak heights or fragment lengths. The generic RFC11 model overall showed improved NOC estimates for data of different laboratories when compared to the MAC method but performed less efficiently when compared to the PPF6C specific RFC19 model, since it uses less of the available information. However, in absence of a data specific machine learning NOC model, or in absence of data or too limited resources to develop such model, the generic RFC11 model was found to be a useful alternative that can serve as an addition to the reporting officer's toolbox to interpret mixed DNA profiles [**37**]. Another drawback of machine learning models is their lack of transparency; the model outputs a prediction but not how it obtained to the particular result. Therefore, in a study of Veldhuis et al. [**129**], eXplainable artificial intelligence (XAI) was introduced to help users understand why such predictions are made.

Lastly, through web APIs (Application Programming Interfaces) DNAxs can communicate with, for instance, CODIS, LIMS systems, SmartRank, and Bonaparte [**128**]. Additionally, as previously mentioned, for weight of evidence calculations, DNAxs implements DNAStatistX, which, alike EuroForMix, uses the γ distribution to model peak heights.

3.2. The γ Model

The model adopted by the authors is known as the "γ model" which was first described by Cowell et al. [**124,130**].

The γ distribution is defined by two parameters known as shape α and scale β. There is a different shape parameter per contributor in the EuroForMix model, but there is only one (universal) scale parameter that is applied. The observed peak height is given as y.

The probability density function of the γ distribution is:

$$f(y|\alpha,\beta) = \frac{1}{\beta^{\alpha}\Gamma(\alpha)} y^{\alpha-1} \exp(-\frac{y}{\beta}) = gamma(y|\alpha,\beta) \tag{3}$$

where α and β are the shape and scale parameters, respectively, and (x) is the γ function. The density function given in Equation (3) and provides the 'weightings' in EuroForMix and DNAStatistX.

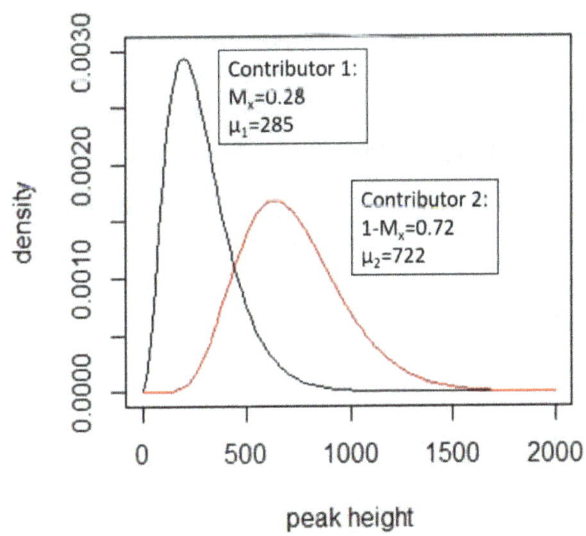

Figure 3. γ distributions for a simple case, where shape parameters = 3.312 and 8.381, respectively and the scale parameter is 86.2. The peak height expectation (μ) and Mx are shown for each contributor. The probability density function for the individual peak height contributions are derived from these curves. Reprinted from [62], chapter 7, Copyright (2020) with permission from Elsevier.

The shape and scale parameters are calculated based on the following model parameters (for two donors):

- Mx: the mixture proportion for contributor 1 and 1-Mx, the mixture proportion for contributor 2
- μ: the peak height expectation (close to the average peak heights)
- ω: the coefficient of peak height variation (indicates variability)
- An example is provided in **Figure 3.**

The complexity of the γ model is increased by additional parameters: degradation, forward and backward stutter.

3.3. An Outline of the γ Model Incorporated into Euroformix and DNAStatistX

The aim is to quantify the value of evidence if a POI is a contributor to a crime-scene profile O. Two alternative propositions are specified and the likelihood ratio (LR) evaluates how many more times likely it is to observe the evidence given that H_1 is true compared to the alternative that H_2 is true.

3.3.1. Model Features

EuroForMix and DNAStatistX support multiple contributors, can condition upon any number of reference profiles and can specify any number of unknown individuals, although there is a practical limit of c. 4 due to computational time.

- The software accommodates degradation, allele drop-out, allele drop-in, 'n - 1' and 'n + 1' stutters and sub-population structure (Fst correction). Note that stutters are not accommodated in the current version of DNAStatistX, but is under development for a future version.
- Replicated samples can be analysed. Consensus or composite profiles, a feature of pre-PG software, are not used.
- The model assumes same contributors and the same peak height properties for each replicate.

Optional Locus specific settings (DNAStatistX from v1, EuroForMix v3 onwards) are as follows:

- Analytical threshold
- Drop-in model
- Fst correction

Although EuroForMix and DNAStatistX are based upon the same model, there are some differences. The software are programmed in different languages (EuroForMix in R and C++ and DNAStatistX in Java) and therefore not all of the numerical libraries EuroForMix uses were available when developing DNAStatistX. As a result, alternative methods for function optimization were explored and selected. Despite the differences in the choice of function optimizer, the two software yield LRs in the same order of magnitude when the same data and model options are used [**128**]. DNAStatistX is implemented within the overall software package, DNAxs, which supports parallel computing that can be delegated to a computer cluster and enables queuing of requested LR calculations. This feature can be extremely useful in a routine casework setting. Both software continue development though functionalities and options can be prioritized differently by their developers and users.

Whereas DNAxs parallelises over independent function optimizations (current version), EuroForMix applies parallelisation within the inner part of the algorithm, where genotype summation is performed (versions before v3 also parallelised over function optimizations).

3.3.2. Exploratory Data Analysis

The reported LR is critically dependent upon the assumptions applied in the model. The parameters that are fixed include: the population database including allele frequencies, the level of Fst and the drop-in parameters used to specify the drop-in model.

The variable parameters are mixture proportions (Mx), peak height variation (coefficient-of-variation), peak height expectation and the NOC. Decisions are needed whether to use a stutter and/or a degradation model: Real case examples typically employ degraded DNA causing a reduction in observed peak heights when the molecular fragment lengths increase. The stutter models are important to apply when stutter filters are not applied—nevertheless there may still be alleles present in the profile which could be explained as stutters. In addition, the number of contributors can have an impact—so this must be carefully decided (**Section 2.5**).

Finally, any model that is used for reporting must be a reasonable fit to the γ distribution.

3.3.3. Relatedness

The defence may wish to put forward a proposition that a sibling (or another close relative) was the contributor to the crime stain, hence the defence alternative considered may be H_2: "The DNA is from a sibling of Mr. X".

This folder contains laboratory data from derived samples of three person mixtures using the 'PowerPlex® Fusion 6C' kit and Dutch database frequencies from a study by Benschop et al. [**73**]. To explore whether closely related individuals will give a high LR when Mr X is substituted by a sibling, we specify following propositions:

- H_1: The DNA is from Mr. X
- H_2: The DNA is from an unknown contributor

A total of 100 siblings were simulated. The majority provide a low LR (exclusionary: LR < 1). A total of six LRs were greater than 100, with two approximating $\log_{10}LR \approx 6$. However, if the propositions are altered to:

- H_1: The DNA is from Mr. X
- H_2: The DNA is from a sibling of Mr. X,

both LRs returned values less than one, favouring H_2. This exercise illustrated that (a) close relatives can occasionally provide high LRs when tested against the proposition of unrelatedness, but (b) if the proposition is altered to ask the question of relatedness, then the evidence can support H_2. This illustrates the importance of asking the right questions based upon the case-circumstances, i.e., when propositions are formulated, they must be reasonable and they must above all be based upon a clear understanding of the case circumstances.

3.3.4. Deconvolution

Deconvolution is used to predict the genotype of an 'unknown' contributor to a crime stain and it is typically undertaken to extract a profile in order to search a national DNA database. There are several different ways to represent the data. The most common usage is to provide the 'top marginal' where the most likely genotype (for the unknown component) is extracted. Each genotype (per locus) is accompanied by 'the ratio to next genotype' which is the ratio of the top probability to the second highest probability. The larger the ratio, the greater the confidence in the genotype selected [**50,131**].

3.4. Investigative Forensic Genetics

Probabilistic Genotyping to Carry out Searches of National DNA Databases : SmartRank is based upon LRmix Studio [**22,23**], but was modified to enable searches of very large national DNA databases. A validation study [**22**] tested anonymised parts of the national DNA databases of Belgium, the Netherlands, Italy, France and Spain, along with a simulated DNA database. To each of the databases, 44 reference profiles were added. A total of 343 mixed DNA profiles were prepared from the reference samples, to act as the test set of data. Finally, the data were searched with both SmartRank and CODIS software.

Searches are most successfully employed when the mixtures are simple (major/minor) coupled with low levels of dropout. CODIS works by applying simple allele matching criteria whereas SmartRank takes account of allele drop-out, and was shown to be a more effective method to identify contributors for mixed profiles with low to moderate drop-out. SmartRank can be downloaded from **https://github.com/smartrank/smartrank** accessed on 28 September 2021 along with user guides; exercises are available at: **https://www.dropbox.com/home/Book/Data%20for%20website/Chapter%2011/SmartRank_Exercises** and chapter accessed on 28 September 2021 [**62**].

DNAmatch2 and CaseSolver are search engines which also adopt the quantitative model from EuroForMix [**21,24**]. A stepwise strategy is employed to search for matches, since a search using EuroForMix alone would be time-consuming. Consequently, the comparisons are filtered in a stepwise procedure. First, a simple matching allele count is carried out where for example, samples exceeding a defined drop-out level are rejected. The remaining comparisons are then searched using the qualitative LRmix model from forensim (similar to SmartRank). This step is very fast: samples providing LRs above a certain threshold are then re-tested using the quantitative EuroForMix model to provide a final list of ranked LRs. Studies show that quantitative models out-perform qualitative models [**50,132**]. DNAmatch2 is used both as a database search engine as well as providing a platform to carry out contamination searches during routine casework, whereas CaseSolver is mainly used for profile comparisons in casework. Importantly, both CaseSolver and EuroForMix can conduct (reference to evidence) database searches; with the main difference that CaseSolver can perform this with many evidence items at the same time, and it provides a more flexible interface for data integration.

Casesolver contains more functionalities than DNAmatch2, with the focus of being an effective and simple-to-use comparison tool for case officers (similar as DNAxs). This software is especially designed to cope with complex cases which have a large number of evidence profiles and multiple reference samples. An example with 119 evidence profiles and three references is described by Bleka et al. [**21**]. CaseSolver compares each reference sample with each evidence profile, identifying potential 'matches' qualified by an LR. The second step carries out cross-comparisons between case-stains to identify unknown contributors. These can be deconvolved and used in further searches as required. If it is known that contributors may be related to each other, then simple relatedness searches can also be carried out. CaseSolver offers various ways to visualise or export the data, even to a comprehensive report; for example, an informative graphical network can be displayed that summarises the connections between the case samples (**Figure 4**). The latest version of CaseSolver (v1.8) provides a weight-of-evidence module which offers conservative corrections of LR for evaluative purposes, and automated report generation.

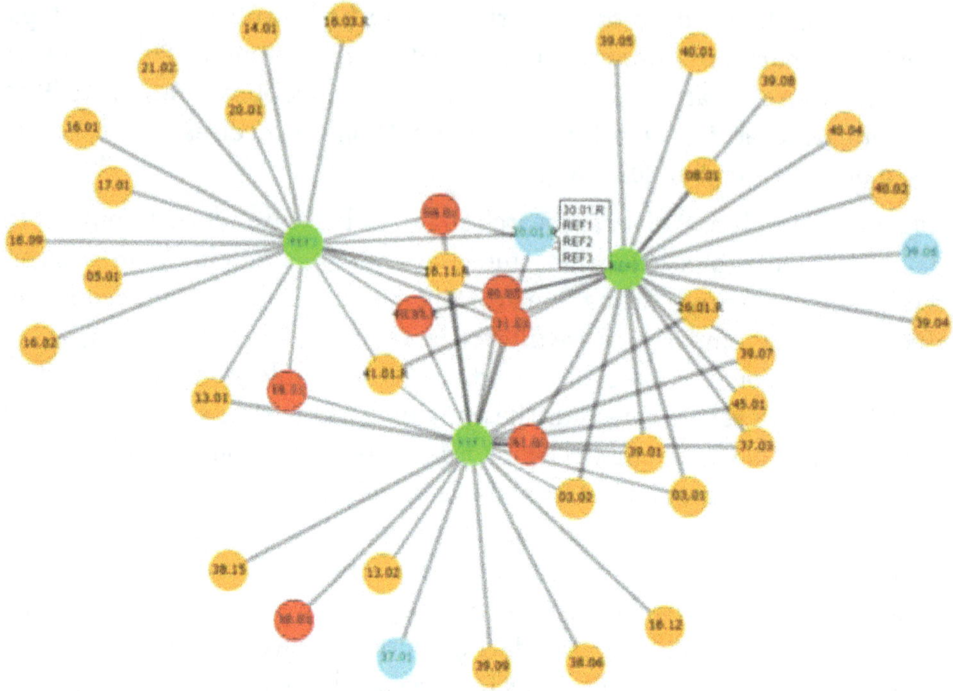

Figure 4. Graphical network summarizing the connections between case samples through LR calculations. The references are the green nodes. Single contributor evidences are in cyan; two contributors are in orange and three or more contributors are in red. If the 'plotly' function in R is used then the mouse can be hovered over a node and this displays a list of the matches, as shown for sample 30.01. The thickness of the edges between the nodes is inversely proportional to the size of the LR on a log10 scale. Reprinted from [62], chapter 11, Copyright (2020) with permission from Elsevier.

CaseSolver is available at: **http://www.euroformix.com/casesolver** accessed on 28 September 2021. Data and presentations are available at **https://sites.google.com/view/dnabook/chapter-11?authuser=0** accessed on 28 September 2021.

3.5. Massively Parallel Sequencing (MPS)

Massive Parallel sequencing (MPS) is becoming increasingly used throughout the forensic community and may eventually supersede classic capillary gel (CE) methods [**133**]. MPS returns the entire sequence of a locus, not only the repeat region, but the flanking sequence as well; there is much more information to deal with compared to the standard repeat unit count used in classic CE. The main advantage of MPS is the potential to combine many more loci in multiplexes compared to CE. This results in much higher discriminating power. Shorter amplicon lengths should mean that more highly degraded DNA may be detected, but this will increase the potential to detect background DNA, as well as contamination. An additional challenge is that interpretation systems must be able to deal with profiles that are complicated by the presence of complex stutters.

Just and Irwin [**134**] developed a method of nomenclature of MPS-STRs that was based upon the longest uninterrupted sequence (LUS) and they used LRmix Studio to analyse mixtures. Later, the LUS nomenclature was extended to LUS+ [**135**], which is similar to that of Vilsen et al. [**136**], in order to identify as many different sequences as possible. They were able to identify 1050 out of 1059 sequences alleles. This system was adopted by Bleka et al. [**137,138,139**] who extended the analysis to the quantitative EuroForMix model. Instead of peak height (rfu), coverage (reads) are used to quantify allelic sequences. CE and MPS stutters are comparable [**140**]; 'n - 1' stutters are the most common to be found, but 'n - 1' and 'n + 2' forms are also observed, though the latter have much lower coverage and can be removed by filtering. Stutters can arise from different blocks of sequences within the same allele. Software packages such as FDSTools [**141**] are able to predict stutters, both simple and complex, based upon the allelic sequence.

The EuroForMix implementation of MPS-STR interpretation is described by [**138,139**] and both 'n - 1' and 'n + 1' stutters are accommodated from version 3. In order to obtain data in LUS/LUS+ format, the R program seq2lus can be used to convert raw sequence data derived from the ForenSeqVerogen Universal Analysis (UAS) software: **https://verogen.com/wp-content/uploads/2018/08/ForenSeq-Univ-Analysis-SW-Guide-VD2018007-A.pdf** accessed on 28 September 2021. Once the nomenclature conversions are made, the analysis can proceed. The tool and updated look-up files, together with a tutorial is provided at: **http://euroformix.com/seq2lus** accessed on 28 September 2021. A more general tool called lusSTR, written in python, has been developed to avoid the need of a lookup table (available at: **https://github.com/bioforensics/lusSTR** accessed on 28 September 2021).

Bleka et al. [**138**] explored the information gain, i.e., the LR increase, of the LUS vs. standard repeat unit (RU) nomenclature. Full profiles with the RU nomenclature provided an average log10LR = 37.04 whereas the LUS nomenclature returned log10LR = 43.3; the ratio is the theoretical information gain TIGRU→LUS = 1.17. However, the LRs are massive, and represent redundant information. Huge likelihood ratios have no benefit when presented in court. In practice any log10LR > 9 may be considered as providing redundant information because a greater LR has no impact upon a jury decision. Some jurisdictions e.g., UK have a reporting limit, upper threshold of 1 billion.

Therefore, the main benefit of MPS-STR is related to the analysis of low-level DNA profiles that may be highly degraded, so that the probability of successful amplification is low. If the number of loci is increased, then the chance of successful amplification of a given locus is also increased and this will be reflected in an expected increased LR (provided that H_1 is true). Doubling the number of loci from 27 loci to 54 loci will have an approximate proportionate doubling effect on the LR (log-scale). E.g., if log10LR = 2 for the former, it will return log10LR = 4 for the latter; if 128 loci are utilised then log10LR = 8, i.e., the more loci that are analysed, the more likely it is that reportable profiles can be achieved. We can summarise that the main advantage of MPS is the possibility to greatly increase the number of loci in the multiplex, the increased discrimination power per locus is secondary to this.

In addition, Benschop et al. [**142**] examined allele detection and LRs obtained from STR profiles generated by two different MPS systems that were analyzed with different settings. The LR results for the over 2000 sets of propositions were affected by the variation for the number of markers and analysis settings used in the three approaches tested. Nevertheless, trends for true and non-contributors, effects of replicates, assigned number of contributors, and model validation results were comparable for the different MPS approaches and were similar to the trends observed in CE data.

Even though sequence information from MPS technology provides higher data resolution, there is still a limitation in how mixture profiles, including major/minor components, are exported from MPS software. Two papers [**138,142**] point out that default analysis settings such as dynamic threshold potentially removes useful information forwarded for interpretation, weakening the ability to detect low-template components.

The above mentioned studies [**142**] demonstrate that probabilistic interpretation of MPS-STR data using the γ model in EuroForMix and DNAStatistX is fit for forensic DNA casework.

Probabilistic genotyping is not restricted to STRs, SNPs are also amenable [**143,144**]. Whereas STRs are multi-allelic, SNPs are generally di-allelic. This represents a particular challenge to assess the numbers of contributors because, with a maximum of two alleles in a population, we cannot use allele counting methods to ascertain this value.

Using a panel of 134 SNPs from Life Technologies' HID-Ion AmpliSeq™ Identity Panel v2.2: **https://www.thermofisher.com/content/dam/LifeTech/Documents/PDFs/HID-Ion-AmpliSeq-Identity-Panel-Flyer.pdf** accessed on 28 September 2021, Bleka et al. [**143**] compared the LRmix model with EuroForMix showing that the latter was much more efficient especially when there are more than two contributors. The effective NOC is decided by following exploratory data analysis, outlined for STRs in **Section 2.5**, where the likelihood is maximised under H_2. LRs obtained from overestimation of the actual NOC showed concordance with results compared to the actual NOC (from simulations up to six contributors). With the SNP panel tested, there is a limitation of that the mixture proportion (Mx) of the POI must exceed 0.2 in order to achieve an LR > 100, although this restriction would be removed with much larger SNP panels. More recently, the performance of EuroForMix was compared to machine learning approaches [**145**].

The data used in the MPS SNP and STR publications cited, along with presentations available online: **https://sites.google.com/view/dnabook/chapter-13?authuser=0** accessed on 28 September 2021.

3.6. Best Practice Guidelines, and Quality Assurance

Developmental and internal validation of the probabilistic genotyping software LRmix, LRmix Studio, SmartRank, EuroForMix, CaseSolver, DNAmatch2, and DNAxs/DNAStatistX is described in internal validation documents; much information has been published [**22,23,62,113,128**]. Furthermore, there has been much research effort to gain insights into trends and to characterize the various models, as well as to inform guidelines for best practice.

Using the qualitative model LRmix Studio research was carried out to show the effects of over- or under-assigning the NOC; the number of PCR replicates; the amount of DNA; and the drop-in rate [**68,69,146,147,148**].

The SmartRank output was compared to that of LRmix Studio in order to gain insight into the effects of model adaptations that enabled fast and efficient searching of voluminous databases [**23**]. In addition, the software was characterized in terms of the retrieval of true and non-donors; the effects of the size and composition of the DNA database; the number of contributors; the number of markers; and the level of drop-out [**22,23**]. As expected, positive effects on the retrieval of true donors were observed with: (1) a higher number of loci, (2) fewer contributors, (3) lower drop-out rates and/or (4) a higher discriminatory power. Retrieval of true donors was not influenced by the size of the DNA-databases used in this study (37,000–1.55 million). The size of the DNA-database, however, can have an effect on the retrieval of non-donors because of adventitious matches.

LRs generated from EuroForMix and LRmix were compared for true and non-donors to two- or three-person NGM DNA profiles [**50**] and to two- to four-person PPF6C DNA profiles [**73**]. This research demonstrated the effects of the NOC, over- or under-assigning the NOC; the number of PCR replicates; the amount of DNA; the level of unseen alleles for the person of interest; and the effect of increased PCR cycles. H_1-true tests and H_2-true tests were utilised. In the H_2-true tests, non-contributors were selected deliberately to a have large overlap with the alleles within the mixture and worst-case scenarios were examined where a simulated relative of one of the true donors was considered as the person of interest under the prosecution hypothesis [**73**]. A somewhat similar study was performed to compare MPS with CE-based DNA profiling data [**142**]. It was observed that the MPS read counts behaved in a similar manner to CE peak heights, and therefore similar results were obtained.

To summarize, the following overall trends were observed for CE and MPS profiles (note that exceptions can occur):

- The lower the NOC and the lower the drop-out rate for the POI, the more often larger LRs were obtained.
- The more donors and the more drop-out for the person of interest, the more often false-negative support was observed.
- Using a lower NOC than designed yielded either equal results (predominantly with a true major donor as POI) or lower LRs.
- Over assigning the NOC hardly affected LRs for true major donors.
- An over-assigned NOC for H_2-true tests can have the effect of increasing the LR to around neutral evidence.
- False-positive support, LR > 1, was observed more often and with larger LRs when the POI was a (simulated) relative of a true donor rather than if the POI was an unrelated non-donor to the DNA mixture.
- The use of multiple, instead of one PCR replicate, often increased the LR for true minor donors and decreased the LR for non-donors.

Based on the outcomes of the above-mentioned research studies, guidelines for best practice in forensic casework were developed. For LRmix (Studio) this included the exploratory data analysis approach, in which the effect of model parameters (such as the probability of drop-out) on the LR is examined. Non-contributor tests provide an indication of the range of LRs obtained if H_2 is true. Although it is not mandatory, laboratories may find this a useful feature that can help to explain results in court. For EuroForMix and DNAStatistX, it is advised to perform model selection, to examine the model validation ('pp-plots') and iteration results and to report the LR only if defined criteria are met. Furthermore, for reasons of quality, efficiency and usefulness of performing weight of evidence calculations, guidelines for application of the LR models were developed by NFI. For EuroForMix/DNAStatistX these are presented in [**128**]; for instance there is an upper limit on the number of unseen alleles that a person of interest can have before an LR calculation is advised. Another quality aspect that relates to the use of the DNAxs/DNAStatistX software is the audit trail which automatically keeps track of who performed which action and when.

Apart from software validation, guidelines for best practice and an audit trail, NFI invests in (automated) software testing during development, prior to release and during validation. This is important to ensure that the software is robust and behaves as designed. With a growing number of features, software testing becomes a very time-consuming task if performed manually. To save time, improve the test coverage, increase ad hoc and exploratory testing, and, in the end, reduce costs and maintenance, automated tests were designed and built for DNAxs. In the first three years after implementation of the DNAxs software suite, a total of 521 bugs were reported by the software engineers during development, by testers during validation, by users in casework, or by users performing research. Software bugs are errors, flaws or faults causing the software to produce an incorrect or an unexpected result, or to behave in unintended ways. The majority of bugs were solved in major or minor software releases that were planned and a minority required the release of a bug fix version or occurred during the development of these version. This shows that bug detection and debugging is part of the developmental and validation process, but also occurs in validated and released software versions. The reported bugs are viewed from a software perspective and relate to the use of the software or functionalities thereof. The observed bugs did not have effects on the DNA profile interpretation and/or reported conclusions. Further information on code coverage by testing, bug detection and debugging, but also information on the use of DNAxs (including DNAStatistX and SmartRank) and post-analytical errors in forensic casework can be found in [**149**].

4. STRMIX™

4.1. History of STRmix™ Creation

STRmix™ is an Australian and New Zealand initiative that was jointly developed by Duncan Taylor from Forensic Science SA (FSSA) in Australia and John Buckleton and Jo-Anne Bright from the Institute of Environmental Science and Research (ESR) in New Zealand. STRmix™ was first introduced into casework at FSSA and ESR in August 2012, however the events that lead to its development occurred three years prior.

Prior to 2010 there was no focussed effort to drive standardisation in forensic biology between laboratories in Australasia (Australia and New Zealand). Each laboratory had accrued knowledge and developed policies in a siloed manner, which meant that in one state Random Man Not Excluded (RMNE) also known as Cumulative Probability of Inclusion (CPI) was being used, in others likelihood ratios (LR), and amongst those there was a variety of implementations. In 2009 the Victoria Police Forensic Science Laboratory (VPFSL) in Melbourne had been using a software program called DNAmix [**150,151**] for calculating LRs in situations where unresolvable mixtures were obtained. DNAmix had been created as a result of DNA profile evaluations in the OJ Simpson trial, and the models within DNAmix required that no dropout-out had occurred. The VPFSL came to realise that this assumption was not being met in the evaluations being carried out, which resulted in the DNA profile evaluations in a number of cases being redone and reports reissued. One result in particular, which shifted an LR from 550 billion to 3, concerned Victoria's police chief Simon Overland who ordered all DNA evidence be banned from court proceedings.

Following the laboratory shutdown, crisis talks were held with members of government forensic laboratories from across Australia and New Zealand. One of the outcomes was to form an Australasian forensic biology statistics working group in 2010 (with members from all government forensic laboratories from across Australia and New Zealand) with the overarching remit of standardisation across Australasia through the adoption of world leading evaluation and statistical practices. In this group were John Buckleton and Duncan Taylor, who started working on the ideas that would eventually become STRmix™ (Taylor and Buckleton thankfully acknowledge the technical input of David Balding and the vision of Ross Vining, Linzi Wilson-Wilde and Keith Bedford). In 2011 Buckleton and Taylor presented the idea of STRmix™ (initially to be called DyNAmix) to their member organisations, and the National Institute of Forensic Sciences (NIFS), and development was supported. Jo-Anne Bright joined the development team and by 2012 Taylor, Buckleton and Bright had completed development and validation on version 1.0 of STRmix™.

4.2. Probabilistic Genotyping and STRmix™

STRmix™ considers parameters that describe some observed fluorescent peak collectively as 'mass parameters', M. In essence probability of the observed data, given a genotype, treats these mass parameters as nuisance variables that are integrated across:

$$w_j = Pr(O|S_j) = \int p(O, M|S_j)p(M)dM$$

In STRmix™ this integration is carried out using Markov Chain Monte Carlo (MCMC) sampling. The equation above applies across the whole profile. The locus terms (a superscript 'l') are a product within the integral, across all loci in the profile with data. The model of STRmix™ then makes the assumption that the profile weight is approximated by the product of the integrals at each locus:

$$w_j = \int \prod_l p(O^l, M|S_j^l)p(M)dM = \prod_l \int p(O^l, M|S_j^l)p(M)dM$$

When tested, this assumption appears reasonable (see Figure 2 of [**15**]). As well as using weights to calculate the LR, having the weights themselves allows probing of the DNA profile data in powerful investigative ways, which we describe later.

Assumption 1 fulfils Slooten's [**152**] requirement that "we will assume that the model ... parameters are chosen independently of the hypotheses." This allows the statement that the "model cannot overstate the evidence very strongly very often for actual contributors: it cannot, averaged over all mixtures and contributors, happen with probability more than 1/t that the evidence is overstated by a factor t."

We round out this claim by repeating Slooten's [**152**] statement in his Equation (5.2), which has a pedigree back to Turing (quoted in Good [**153**]), that the probability of obtaining an LR ≥≥ t from a non-donor is ≤1*t*≤1.

4.3. Capabilities of STRmix™

4.3.1. Deconvolution

The process of deconvolution is the assignment of weights to genotype sets. In other words, combinations of genotypes that could describe a profile(s) are considered, and a probability is assigned to them, proportional to how well they explain the observed peaks. In STRmix™ this is achieved by integrating across a set of mass parameters using MCMC. The base model for STRmix™ was described by Taylor et al. [**15**] and included parameters:

- A template amount for each of the n contributors,
- A degradation (described in [**154**]) which models the decay with respect to molecular weight (m) in the template for each of the contributors,
- Amplification efficiency at each locus to allow for the observed amplification levels of each locus,
- Replicate multipliers, which scales all peaks up or down between PCR replicates.

Later, Taylor et al. [**155**] extended the model to not only consider PCR replicates produced under the same system, but also DNA profiles from the sample produced under different conditions, i.e.,

Using the same DNA profiling kit, but with different laboratory processes (such as different PCR cycles or different models of laboratory hardware), Using two different DNA profiling kits which require the addition of mass parameter(s): Kit multipliers, which scale all peaks in all replicates up or down between kits.

The extension of the model to numerous kits/processes enabled the incorporation of different parameter variations among profiles generated by distinct procedures. STRmix™ proved particularly valuable in cold-case investigations, where it facilitated the integration of original profiling efforts with more recent ones. This was especially beneficial in cases where technology had advanced over multiple generations of profiling kits, and the DNA sample itself may have shown varying degradation patterns between the two profiles.

Using a chosen set of values for the mass parameters allows the calculation of Total Allelic Product (TAP) [**156**], the total amount of fluorescence expected resulting from the amplification of an allele present in a DNA extract. As the PCR occurs, some of the fluorescence that was destined for the allele will shift to stutter positions on the EPG. The amount of the TAP that is expected to become stutter is based on the expected stutter ratios for each allele at each locus, either measured directly or regressed using the longest uninterrupted sequence (LUS) [**156**], or incorporating multiple repeat sequences of an interrupted STR in a multi-LUS model [**136,157**]. In reality, there are a number of stutter types that can occur, but the original STRmix™ model (described in [**15**]) only included back stutter. This was later extended to include forward stutter (with modelling of forward stutter described in [**157,158**]), and then generalised so that any number of stutters (and with any size-based relationship to the parent peak), applied to any combination of specific loci, could be added by users with the mathematical framework automatically extending to incorporate them (generalised stutter modelling is described in [**155**]). The height of coincident peaks (either from multiple allele donations, or allele and stutter) are added [**159,160**] to produce the final expected peak heights.

The computation of anticipated allele and stutter (in any combination) pinnacle magnitudes utilizing a collection of mass parameters and projected stutter ratios ultimately yields a collection of projected peaks and their magnitudes, for each locus, in each PCR replication, and for each procedure or kit in which they have been produced. The extent to which the mass parameter values accurately account for the observed peak heights, specifically the probability of the observed data given the mass parameter values, is contingent upon the degree of alignment between the observed and expected peak heights.

Differences between an observed (O) and an expected (E) peak height are assigned a probability based on empirical models. These models take account of the magnitude of the difference and use a proxy for template to assess how tolerable such differences are. In order to determine how much to penalise stochastic effects in different types of fluorescence (i.e., allele, or stutter, or a combination), peak height variability models are used. An observed peak comprising a single fluorescence type, with peak height variability parameter value c^2 is modelled by a log-Normal distribution with mean and variance parameters:

$$O \sim LN\left(ln(E), \frac{c^2}{f(E)}\right) \text{ where } f(E) = \frac{b}{E} + E$$

and b is a constant that typically takes values around 1000. The variance is inversely proportional to the function of expected peak height (which is approximately equal to E when E is large), which describes the well-known phenomenon that the relative size of stochastic peak height imbalance tends to increase as peak height decrease. The function f(E), deals with the fact that as the expected height decreases to very low levels the peak height variability starts to contract (see [**161**]). The constant b can be altered by the user from 0 (which turns off this low-level peak height variability contraction effect) to any arbitrarily high value.

A range of distributions were investigated for modelling stutter in Bright et al. [**162**]. The log-normal appeared to fit the empirical data adequately.

When a peak comprises different fluorescence types, the sum of log-normal random variables is approximated by a shifted-log-normal distribution using moment matching.

If a peak has an expected height, but is not observed, then it is modelled as a drop-out peak and a probability is used that is based on the integral of the probability of observing a peak between baseline and AT for a peak at expected height E. If a peak is not expected, but observed in the profile then it is modelled as a drop-in and a probability applied, based on the model of Puch-Solis [**13**].

The above process describes the generation of a set of expected peak heights and the probability for deviations of the expected heights from observed heights. The constant, 'b' in the variance term and the prior distribution parameters for c^2 are set during model calibration in a tool called 'Model Maker' (described in **Section 4.4**). The MCMC process within STRmix™ starts by assigning starting positions for all mass parameters, and randomly assigning genotype sets to each locus. This is the current set of parameters. Then, iteratively

- Choose a locus at random and propose a genotype set at that locus.
- Choose new values for all mass parameters by stepping a small distance from the values in the current set (known as a random walk, and with step size dictated by a Gaussian distribution). Propose these values.
- Calculate the expected peak heights using the proposed sample values.
- Calculate the likelihood value of the proposed sample values.
- Use a Metropolis-Hastings algorithm to accept or reject the proposed sample. If the proposed sample is accepted, then the proposed set of parameter values becomes the current set. If the proposed sample is rejected, then the proposal is discarded.

- Repeat steps 1 to 6 until a defined number of proposal accepts have been attained.

The first iterations of the MCMC are considered burn-in (the number of steps is set by the user) and discarded. After the burn-in the proportion of total iterations that a genotype set was the focus of the MCMC (called residence time) is the weight assigned to that genotype set.

A contributor that is assumed to be present under both H_1 and H_2 is described as a conditioning contributor. It is highly desirable to include as many contributors as possible as conditioning profiles. This is for practical reasons such as improving run time, but also for the much more important reason that any correctly assumed donor improves the ability of the system to differentiate between true and false donors [**163**]. Historically the use of conditioning contributors has been restricted to those situations where a donor is certain to correctly assumed, largely intimate samples. This underutilises the tool and is not in the interests of an innocent person accused of being a donor [**95**]. We recommend the extension of the use of conditioning to other evidential items such as assuming the presence of the habitual wearer of clothing and to any co-accused with a very high LR, especially if the POI is related to these persons [**95,96**]. Within a deconvolution, any number (up to the NOC from which the profile is designated as having originated) can be assumed as a conditioning profile, which during MCMC, locks their genotypes (known from their references) into any genotype set being considered.

Starting from STRmix™ V2.6, the analysis of a profile no longer requires a specific single number to be supplied, as STRmix™ can now take a range of contributions as the user input [164]. If the user finds it difficult to provide a single value to the profile due to its complexity or quality, or if different parties require different numbers to have their most plausible explanations for the profile(s) [95,97], a variety of contributors might be selected. This approach operates by doing a deconvolution of the evidence profile(s) for each NOC within the specified range. It then calculates the Bayes Factor, using a method proposed by Weinberg et al. [165,166], to enable the combination or comparison of the deconvolution results. This presents a different approach to the recent strategy outlined by Slooten et al. [94], but produces identical outcomes based on the same assumptions [71].

4.3.2. LR Calculation

Given the weights from a deconvolution, the calculation of an LR in STRmix™ is achieved by taking the ratio of the weighted sum of genotype set probabilities given two competing propositions. One or more references (some of which can have been assumed at the point deconvolution) are compared to the evidence profile(s) using propositions that are aligned with prosecution and a sensible alternative, in a way that best represents the strength of the evidence given the framework of circumstances of the case (see [**3,71,95,103,167**] for guidance documents on proposition setting). STRmix™ can compare individuals to specific combinations of contributor positions within the evidence profile(s), generating an LR considering sub-sub-source level propositions [**104**], or to the mixture as a whole (i.e., all components and all combinations) to generate an LR that considers sub-source level propositions. When considering sources of DNA under the H_2, STRmix™ can consider these to be unrelated to the POI or related to the POI [**168**] in various relationship types.

Following Balding [**169,170**] the different potential relationship types that the alternate donor could be to the POI can be assembled into one statistic. Writing $wj=P(O|Sj)$ and introducing the different relationship types Ri, i = 1, r, where is the number of relationship types considered we obtain

$$LR = \frac{\sum_{j=1}^{J} w_j Pr(S_j|H_1)}{\sum_{i=1}^{r} Pr(R_i|H_2) \sum_{j=1}^{J} w_j Pr(S_j|H_2, R_i)}$$

The terms, $Pr(Ri|H2)$, represent the prior probability that a person related to the POI by relationship Ri is the donor (given that the POI is not, H_2). The expected prior proportions that different relative types can make up in the population, $Pr(Ri|H2)$, can either be set manually in STRmix™ or estimated using the number of individuals in the population and the average number of children per family in that population [**171**].

STRmix™ uses the sub-population model of Balding et al. [**172**], although the co-ancestry coefficient (FST, θ) can be set to 0 by the user if desired in order to revert the calculation to using the 'product rule'.

When assigning probabilities for an allele in the population the value is set using a Dirichlet distribution with a uniform prior. The posterior means of the allele probabilities are then obtained by updating the prior with the counts of alleles in a database (using a similar method as described in [**173**]). For allele 'A', the probability of occurrence in the population, given it has been seen xA times out of N

$$Pr(A) = \frac{x_A + k^{-1}}{N+1} \text{ in early } STRmix \text{ versions or } Pr(A) = \frac{x_A + (k+1)^{-1}}{N+1} \text{ in V2.8 and higher}$$

alleles is calculated by: where k^{-1} is the prior allele probability [**174**], and k is the number of different allele states that have been observed in the population.

Multiple populations can be set up in STRmix™, each with their own allele frequency file, θ and population proportion in the local geographical region. This allows STRmix™ to calculate an LR considering the contributors to be from any of the set populations individually, or anyone in the local geographical region, by stratifying across all populations [**175**].

In addition to the point estimate LR STRmix™ also provides a credible interval [**176**] using the highest posterior density (HPD) method. While there has been justified debate over the provision of intervals for LRs [**177,178,179,180,181,182,183,184**], it is the preference for most practising forensic DNA laboratories to report a lower bound interval on the LR value. Within STRmix™ the HPD interval optionally takes into account any combination of:

- Sampling variation in allele frequency database
- Sampling variation in the iterations of the MCMC leading to the assignment of weights
- Uncertainty in the value of θ

The second of these factors intends to capture the amount of variability in the LR resulting from Monte Carlo resampling inherent within MCMC processes. More recently this process has been found to have variable coverage [**185**] although taken collectively with other aspects of conservative behaviours the coverage is good [**186**] The third of these factors is achieved by STRmix™ being able to take a point value for θ or a distribution described by a β distribution (see [**187,188,189**] for examples of θ distribution models).

The result of an LR calculation on STRmix™ is that the user can be provided with the LRs for the:

- Sub-sub-source proposition pair,
    - The sub-source proposition pair considering the alternate DNA donor as
    - Unrelated,
    - Sibling,
    - Half-sibling,
    - Parent/child,
    - Aunt/uncle/niece/nephew,
    - Grandparent,
    - Cousin, or
    - Unified across all relationship types,
- All of the above for:
    - Each ethnic population in the local geographical region, and
    - Stratified across all populations,

- All of the above for:
  - Each NOC in a chosen range, and
  - Stratified across the range (or with bespoke NOC choice for proposition),

and all with an associated HPD interval to account for uncertainty in allele frequencies, weights and θ. As well as generating LRs for the comparison of a reference to a deconvolution, STRmix™ can also compare a list of references in a database. Using an LR threshold provides a search capability [**190**]. This is not restricted to resolved genotypes of a single individual, but rather can be applied to any profile (single source or mixtures, resolved or unresolved). Using the LR calculation feature than considers a relative of a POI as a source of DNA, allows STRmix™ to carry out familial searches against any profile (again from complete single source to complex and unresolved mixtures) [**168**]. This lead to Australia's first conviction resulting from a familial search [**191**]. The ability to search any DNA profile against a database is also commonly used as a Quality Assurance tool to screen evidence profiles for potential contamination or assist in environmental monitoring [**192**].

STRmix™ has a profile sampling tool that can be used to generate profiles from a population and calculate LRs by comparison to a deconvolution. These profiles can either be generated using probabilities based on their probability of occurrence in a population [**59**] or using importance sampling [**60**] in order to build distributions of 'H_2 true' LRs and determine exceedance probabilities. Exceedance probabilities (sometimes called non-contributor performance tests [**9**]) provide the probability of randomly selecting someone from the population who would provide a particular level of support (typically for their inclusion to the profile, and typically the level of interest is that yielded by a POI). These probabilities, however, are fundamentally different from LRs and should not be confused with, or substituted for LRs in evaluations [**193**]. The LR itself provides an upper bound on exceedance probabilities (a simple proof was provided in [**59**] so that if LR_{POI} is produced by the comparison of a POI to an evidence profile the statement can be made:

The probability of observing a likelihood ratio of LR_{POI} or larger from an unrelated non-donor is less than or equal to 1 in LR_{POI}. Another database searching tool available in STRmix™ is to carry out a top-down analysis [**74**] in which only the main contributors to a highly complex profile are compared. In concept, a top-down analysis is similar to carrying out an evaluation on a major 'cluster' of peaks in a profile [**194**]. The process works by carrying out deconvolutions in steps, where in each step the AT is altered (on a per-locus basis) and only the peak information that meets or exceed the step-AT is used. Each deconvolution considers the profile as originating from N individuals (where N here represents the top N contributors in which you are interested, to the profile and not the total number of contributors to the profile). At the conclusion of each step's deconvolution the result is searched against a database and individuals that yield an LR that exceed a pre-determined LR threshold are flagged. The first step raises the AT (on a per-locus basis) to the height of the highest peaks and each step lowers the ATs by a proportion of the distance from the highest peak to the standard AT used.

The stages cease when the profile can no longer be characterized by N people, as a result of an excessive number of peaks that cannot be accounted for as allele, stutter, or drop-in occurrences. The ultimate database search report provides a list of individuals who were flagged at any stage, together with the highest likelihood ratio achieved throughout all stages in which they were flagged. This approach has been applied to the quantitative model of STRmix™ and has been tested on a collection of intricate mixtures (including 5 or more contributors) from the no-suspect workflow of a forensic laboratory. The results revealed an 80% correlation rate with an individual in the local database [195].

4.4. Implementation of STRmix™

STRmix™ employs universal models to explain the behavior of DNA profiles. For instance, it acknowledges that as peak heights decrease, there is an increase in variability in peak height. It also recognizes that loci can differ in their amplification efficiencies based on the PCR micro-environment. Additionally, it expects stutters to occur at a specific size relative to their parent peak size and at a height that depends on their parent peak height. Each of these models possesses parameters that can be adjusted to match the performance of DNA profile production in a specific laboratory or procedure. The primary goal of a DNA profile analysis is to utilize calibrated models and observed data to derive weights. Figure 5 illustrates these three features in a diagram, with each component interconnected with the other two.

By utilizing this correlation, if the weights are already determined for a given set of observed profiles, this data can be employed to fine-tune the models. STRmix™ has a feature called Model Maker [196], which uses sets of single source input profiles (with known donor references) to adjust parameters in the STRmix™ models. The overall procedure involves using a component-wise Markov Chain Monte Carlo (MCMC) method. This method consists of iteratively sampling mass parameters for each profile, followed by sampling variance parameters for the entire dataset. This process continues until a steady-state is reached for all parameters in the dataset. The variance parameter values are adjusted to align with the characteristics of profiles generated under the tested conditions and can be established as the default values for casework application in STRmix™.

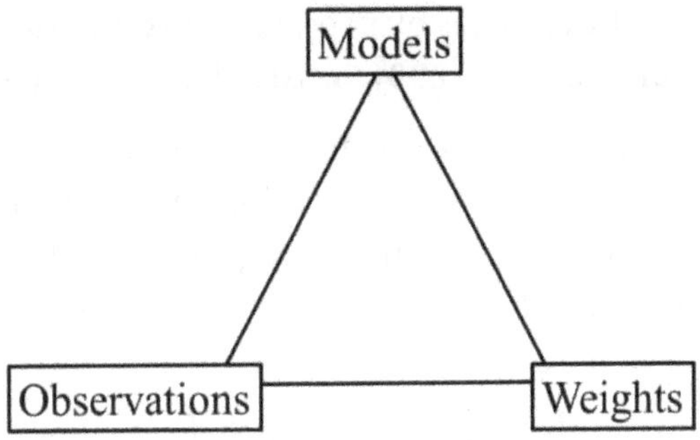

Figure 5. Representation of the components involved in the analysis of a DNA profile.

Some, parameters such as expected stutter ratios have been shown to be robust to laboratory effects [**197**], while others are more sensitive [**196**]. The most important factors for peak height variability have been found to be the number of PCR cycles carried out during amplification, the PCR kit used and the models of electrophoresis instrumentation [**196**]. The use of prior distributions rather than point values for parameters such as variances with the calibration setting the hyper-parameters of the prior distribution (using hierarchical Bayesian modelling) has shown that general settings can be applied and are robust to a wide range of factors [**198**]. Despite this robustness, it is standard practice (and the recommendation of the STRmix™ group, the SWGDAM 2015 [**108**] and the ASB guidelines (Standards for Validation Studies of DNA Mixtures, and Development and Verification of a Laboratory's Mixture Interpretation Protocol: **http://asb.aafs.org/** accessed on 28 September 2021)) that each laboratory implementing STRmix™ undertakes a calibration prior to use on casework samples. In part this ensures the best alignment of the prior distributions for the input parameters to the validation data.

4.5. DBLR—A Companion Product to STRmix™

STRmix™ has closely aligned companion product DBLR (which stands for DataBase Likelihood Ratio, **https://www.strmix.com/dblr/** accessed on 28 September 2021), which can take the results of a deconvolution and carry out interrogations of the results. An overview and developmental validation is given by Kelly at el [**199**]. It also has the flexibility and power to construct propositions that consider aspects of relatedness of contributors within a sample or between samples (including common DNA donorship). DBLR has databasing properties that allow automated, and auditable searching of deconvoluted mixtures against a reference DNA database.

The investigative properties of DBLR allow the user to probe the deconvolution to see what DNA profiles are the most supported by the data, to gauge the discrimination power of the analysis by producing distributions of LRs expected for contributor and non-contributors [**200**], or to calculate exceedance probabilities.

Two mixtures can be compared using DBLR in order to determine whether there is support for a common DNA donor, using the method described by Slooten [**20**]. Studies into this feature have found a high efficacy for identifying common donors [**159**]. The process has been shown to have use as a Quality Assurance tool to identify potential sample to sample contamination events [**25**].

Recently DBLR has implemented a general framework for the comparison of deconvoluted profiles or references. This general framework allows multiple deconvolutions, from different evidence samples that are believed to possess a common DNA donor, to be considered together in order to obtain better resolution in the genotypes of the donors to any (or multiple) of the profiles [**201**]. The distribution of probabilities across a number of potential genotypes (or genotype sets) can be thought of in similar ways whether considering a mixture deconvolution, or a kinship calculation [**152**]. Using this idea, the general framework in DBLR allows the setting-up of competing pedigrees within the evaluation [**202**]. The pedigrees can be linked to components of mixtures so that bespoke propositions can be set up to consider issues such as:

- How many common donors are in a mixture?
- Are any donors of the multiple mixtures related (see [**203**] for an investigation into the effect of not recognising relatedness in mixtures)?
- If I assume a relative of a POI to one mixture does that assist in resolving the other components?
- If I use multiple mixed samples from a disaster victim identification (DVI) together in a single analysis will that help to better resolve the genotypes of the donors?

The range of potential propositions is practically infinite. These types of questioning and subsequent evaluations are applicable not just to ordinary casework, but also to DVI investigations, which involve serial offenders or offenses that involve several family members.

4.6. Validation of STRmix™

When STRmix™ was first implemented into active casework in 2012, probabilistic genotyping was not as prevalent as it is in 2021. There were not yet the standards developed as there are now for the validation or use of such software [**108,109,204**]. In these guidance documents there are outlined various requirements for the development, validation, and implementation of probabilistic genotyping systems. One of the criteria mentioned is that the statistical and biological models used be published or otherwise generally accessible. In **Table 1** we provide a list of publications that detail the models used within STRmix™.

Table 1. Publications of conceptual components of STRmix™ modelling.

Algorithms, Scientific Principles and Methods	Version Introduced	Reference
Allele and stutter peak height variability as separate constants within the MCMC	V2.0	[15]
Peak height variability as random variables within the MCMC	V2.3	[196]
Model for calibrating laboratory peak height variability	V2.0	[196]
Application of a Gaussian random walk to the MCMC process	V2.3	[205]
Modelling of back stutter by regressing stutter ratio against allelic designation	V2.0	[156,197,206,207]
Modelling of back stutter by regressing stutter ratio against LUS	V2.3	[156,162,206,207]
Modelling of forward stutter	V2.4	[157]
Modelling of allelic drop-in using a simple exponential or uniform distribution	V2.0	[15]
Modelling of allelic drop-in using a γ distribution	V2.3	[13]
Modelling of degradation and dropout	V2.0	[154]
Modelling of the uncertainties in the allele frequencies using the HPD	V2.0	[208]
Modelling of the uncertainties in the MCMC	V2.3	[171,208,209]
Database searching of mixed DNA profiles	V2.0	[190]
Familial searching of mixed DNA profiles	V2.3	[168]
Relatives as alternate contributors under the defence proposition	V2.3	[168]
Modelling expected stutter peak heights in saturated data	V2.3	[157]
Taking into account the 'factor of two' in *LR* calculations	V2.3	[104]
Model for incorporating prior beliefs in mixture proportions	V2.3	[210]
Combining DNA profiles produced under different conditions into a single analysis	V2.5	[155]
Assigning a range for the number of contributors to a DNA profile	V2.6	[164]
Mixture-to-mixture comparison to identify common DNA donors	V2.7	[20]
A top-down DNA search approach	V2.8	[74]
The diagnostic outputs of *STRmix™*	V2.3	[211]

All the articles regarding STRmix™ models, including some preliminary validation work, were originally documented in the publication by Taylor et al. titled "The interpretation of single source and mixed DNA profiles" [15]. Subsequent to that initial article, there have been ongoing advancements in models, which have consequently been featured in multiple subsequent publications. The STRmix™ instructions contain comprehensive details on modelling and validation. These materials are given to software users and can be accessed by the defense through a non-disclosure agreement.

In addition to explaining the inner workings of the models, it is necessary to evaluate their performance on data in order to demonstrate both their fundamental validity and their applicability. We have compiled a list of published validations of the performance of STRmix™ modeling, both in part and as a whole. This list may be found in Table 2. A significant number of these validations have been prompted by the developers and, more recently, users of STRmix™ who seek to assess the effectiveness of the models. However, some validations have been conducted in response to criticisms raised in published evaluations of validation efforts, such as the report by the President's Council of Advisors on Science and Technology [117].

Table 2. Publications of validation of STRmix™ models.

Focus of Validation	Reference
Ability of *STRmix*™ to deconvolute profiles and assign *LR*s that comport to manual interpretation and human expectation	[15]
Ability of *STRmix*™ to discriminate between donors and non-donors in database searches	[190]
Behaviour of *STRmix*™ to assign *LR*s when dealing with multiple replicates, different number of contributors, and assumed contributors	[163]
Sensitivity of *LR* produced by *STRmix*™ to different factors of uncertainty such as theta, relatedness of alternate DNA source and length of MCMC analysis	[171]
Tests to be performed when validating probabilistic genotyping, using *STRmix*™ as an example	[112]
Ability of individuals from different laboratories to standardise evaluations when using *STRmix*™	[33,53]
Ability of *STRmix*™ to reliably use peak height information in very low intensity profiles	[56,132,210]
Ability of *STRmix*™ to discriminate between donors and non-donors in large-scale Hd true tests, or using importance sampling	[59,60,190,200,212,213]
Sensitivity of *STRmix*™ model parameters to laboratory factors	[196,198]
Ability of *STRmix*™ to utilise information from profiles produced under different laboratory conditions within a single analysis	[155]

Focus of Validation	Reference
Effect of mixture complexity, allele sharing and contributor proportions on the ability *STRmix*™ to distinguish contributors from non-contributors	[54]
The ability of *STRmix*™ to identify common DNA donors in mixed samples	[25,159]
The sensitivity of *LR*s produced in *STRmix*™ to the choice of the number of contributors	[71,72,97]
Ability to use *STRmix*™ to resolve major components of mixtures	[72]
Testing the assumption of additivity of peak heights in *STRmix*™ models	[159,160]
Performance of the degradation model within *STRmix*™	[214]
The effect of relatedness of contributors to the *STRmix*™ analysis	[203,215]
Testing the calibration of *LR*s produced in *STRmix*™	[58]
Validation overviews of *STRmix*™	[205,216]
Comparison of *STRmix*™ to other probabilistic genotyping software	[41,43,112,217]

In a brief summary STRmix™ publications on validation work from **Table 2** include data from profiling kits; Profiler Plus, Identifiler Plus, Fusion (5C, 6C), NGM SElect, GlobalFiler, PowerPlex (21, ESI17 Pro, 16 HS, ESI17 Fast), SGMPlus and MiniFiler (we are also aware of numerous other profiling kits that have been validated for use in casework, but do not have the work published). There have been hundreds of millions of 'H_2 true' tests, spanning over 3000 laboratory-produced profiles under a range of conditions (from 26 to 34 PCR cycles, and on multiple models of thermocycler or electrophoresis instrument) and of complexity spanning single source to six person mixtures.

4.7. Growth of STRmix™

Since its introduction in 2012 in ESR and FSSA, STRmix™ has now been adopted throughout Australia and New Zealand and currently over 60 DNA forensic laboratories throughout the world, including the US army and the Federal Bureau of Investigation (FBI). **Figure 6** shows the growth of STRmix™ between 2012 and 2020.

When last tallied, STRmix™ is believed to have been used in over 220,000 cases worldwide, available online: **https://www.strmix.com/news/survey-shows-strmix-has-been-used-in-220000-cases-worldwide/** accessed 28 September 2021. For the past 6 years, users in the USA have organised a yearly STRmix™ workshop/conference, that had over 750 attending online presentations in 2020.

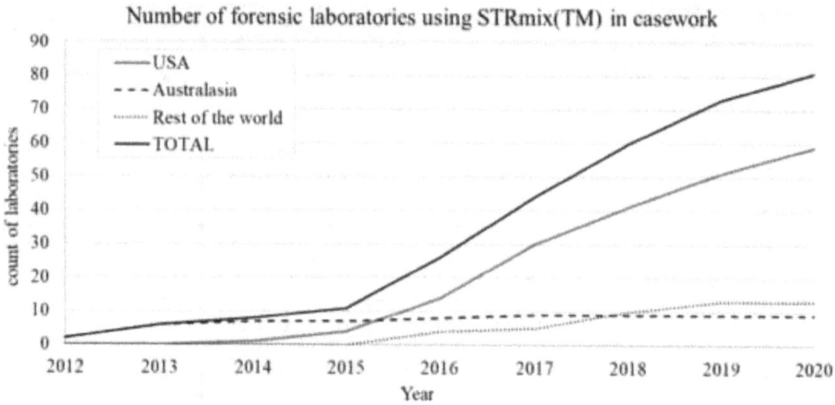

Figure 6. Growth of STRmix™ use over eight years.

The STRmix™ team has grown from an original three developers to employing over 20 individuals who work in training, support, validation, research and development, programming and quality assurance.

4.8. Admissibility Experiences with STRmix™

The STRmix™ group's experience with court and admissibility is mainly in the USA and Australia. In the, at least, 83 admissibility hearings to which STRmix™ has been subjected (as of 1 January 2021), a very wide range of issues have been raised but there are a few that recur. These can be divided into those specifically aimed at STRmix™, those aimed at PG in general, and those that relate more broadly to the use of LRs and especially understandability and the verbal scale. See information available online: **https://johnbuckleton.wordpress.com/strmix/** accessed 28 September 2021, for a non-exhaustive list of admissibility hearings, most with attached rulings or transcripts

Recurrent issues that have been raised regarding STRmix™ include independence of validation, run to run variability, code access, code quality, and validation.

4.8.1. Independence of Validation

Perhaps the most recurrent complaint refers to the established fact that most publications on STRmix include one or more of the original developers. This is exemplified by two comments in the PCAST [**117**] report. PCAST @ pg 79 give: "Appropriate evaluation of the proposed methods should consist of studies by multiple groups, not associated with the software developers, that investigate the performance and define the limitations of programs by testing them on a wide range of mixtures with different properties." PCAST @ pg 81 give: "As noted above, such studies should be performed by or should include independent research groups not connected with the developers of the methods and with no stake in the outcome."

This argument has been taken further to suggest that even those labs separate from the developers but who have purchased STRmix™ have a vested interest and hence their publications should not be trusted.

Whilst we reject the suggestion that we, and the many professional collaborators that we have worked with, would distort our publications because of self-interest we acknowledge the desire to have further distance between the validators and the developers. The National Institute of Standards and Technology (NIST) is often suggested as a suitable organization for this purpose [**218**]. NIST has had STRmix since March 2014 initially as an evaluation copy but subsequently purchased. There is one publication from NIST [**217**] that represents a comparison of STRmix™ and EuroForMix and both software perform well. There is desire for more independent work to be done and the developers would like to assist, at an appropriate distance, any efforts at independent validation.

4.8.2. Run to Run Variability

One complaint is that the MCMC means that the exact value reported for the LR could be different if the process were rerun. The argument is that the existence of variability raises doubts about whether any of the results should be accepted. This raises very significant questions about precision and accuracy that we will touch on briefly later. However, a full treatment is beyond the scope of this work. Here we simply note that STRmix™ includes a partially successful attempt to give a lower bound to the MCMC variability [**185**]. In conjunction with other conservancies, it is almost certain that the LR is understated in the overwhelming majority of cases [**186**].

4.8.3. Code Access

The code for open source software is freely available on the internet. STRmix's code is not open source but is available under an non-disclosure agreement (NDA) [**219**] This meets the ISFG guidelines [**109**] requirement "However, if requested by the legal system, the code should be made available subject to the software provider's legitimate copyright or commercial interests being safeguarded. Supervised access to the code under a "no copy" policy is acceptable." Objections to the use of an NDA have included that inconvenience of supervision and the risk presented by the sanctions agreed to in the NDA if the NDA is contravened.

4.8.4. Code Quality

The STRmix™ code has been inspected three times by the same independent analyst under NDA. The comments made centre around coding practice, documentation, and adherence to software engineering standards [**220**]. At no stage has a coding fault been identified that affects the accuracy of the output although comments have been made that certain coding practices might increase the risk of, as yet undiscovered, miscodes. The STRmix™ team maintain regularly updated specifications documentation, risk analysis, and a gap analysis. This latter specifies any gaps between current STRmix practice and various guidance documents. In summary STRmix™ complies or very nearly complies with the SWGDAM [**108**], ISFG [**109**], Forensic Science Regulator [**116**] and IEEE requirements [**221**]. The STRmix™ group is accredited to ISO 9001 standard.

4.8.5. Validation

Courts have questioned several elements of STRmix™ validity since 2012.The primary obstacles involved the conceptual validation of the models utilized by STRmix™, as well as the inhouse validation of the program to demonstrate its excellent performance. Subsequent difficulties arose in relation to the meticulousness of developmental validation, the conformity of developmental validation to established norms, and the validation of computer coding (distinct from the validation of the outcomes generated by the computer code). The aforementioned aspect was the central theme of a prolonged legal fight against STRmix™ in the case of R v Tuite [222] in Australia.

5. SUMMARY

The adoption of probabilistic genotyping has become extensive. EuroForMix and DNAStatistX employ maximum likelihood estimation with a γ model, while STRmix™ utilizes a Bayesian technique that defines prior distributions for the unknown model parameters. This article is a comprehensive summary of the historical progression of probabilistic genotyping. The text describes several fundamental concepts of interpretation, such as the differentiation between investigative and evaluative reporting, identification of contamination events, conducting research inside and between laboratories, determining the number of contributors, establishing propositions, and validating software and its performance. Subsequently, the text provides information regarding the development, usefulness, implementation, and acceptance of the software under consideration.

REFERENCES

1. Gill, P.; Brenner, C.; Buckleton, J.; Carracedo, A.; Krawczak, M.; Mayr, W.; Morling, N.; Prinz, M.; Schneider, P.M.; Weir, B. DNA commission of the International Society of Forensic Genetics: Recommendations on the interpretation of mixtures. Forensic Sci. Int. **2006**, 160, 90–101. [**Google Scholar**] [**CrossRef**]

2. Gill, P.; Gusmão, L.; Haned, H.; Mayr, W.; Morling, N.; Parson, W.; Prieto, L.; Prinz, M.; Schneider, H.; Schneider, P.; et al. DNA commission of the

International Society of Forensic Genetics: Recommendations on the evaluation of STR typing results that may include drop-out and/or drop-in using probabilistic methods. Forensic Sci. Int. Genet. **2012**, 6, 679–688. **[Google Scholar] [CrossRef] [Green Version]**

3. Gill, P.; Hicks, T.; Butler, J.M.; Connolly, E.; Gusmão, L.; Kokshoorn, B.; Morling, N.; van Oorschot, R.A.; Parson, W.; Prinz, M.; et al. DNA commission of the International society for forensic genetics: Assessing the value of forensic biological evidence—Guidelines highlighting the importance of propositions. Forensic Sci. Int. Genet. **2018**, 36, 189–202. **[Google Scholar] [CrossRef] [PubMed] [Green Version]**
4. Clayton, T.; Whitaker, J.; Sparkes, R.; Gill, P. Analysis and interpretation of mixed forensic stains using DNA STR profiling. Forensic Sci. Int. **1998**, 91, 55–70. **[Google Scholar] [CrossRef]**
5. Gill, P.; Whitaker, J.; Flaxman, C.; Brown, N.; Buckleton, J. An investigation of the rigor of interpretation rules for STRs derived from less than 100 pg of DNA. Forensic Sci. Int. **2000**, 112, 17–40. **[Google Scholar] [CrossRef]**
6. Balding, D. Evaluation of mixed-source, low-template DNA profiles in forensic science. Proc. Natl. Acad. Sci. USA **2013**, 110, 12241–12246. **[Google Scholar] [CrossRef] [Green Version]**
7. Balding, J.D.; Buckleton, J. Interpreting low template DNA profiles. Forensic Sci. Int. Genet. **2009**, 4, 1–10. **[Google Scholar] [CrossRef]**
8. Puch-Solis, R.; Clayton, T. Evidential evaluation of DNA profiles using a discrete statistical model implemented in the DNA LiRa software. Forensic Sci. Int. Genet. **2014**, 11, 220–228. **[Google Scholar] [CrossRef]**
9. Gill, P.; Haned, H. A new methodological framework to interpret complex DNA profiles using likelihood ratios. Forensic Sci. Int. Genet. **2013**, 7, 251–263. **[Google Scholar] [CrossRef]**
10. Curran, J.; Gill, P.; Bill, M. Interpretation of repeat measurement DNA evidence allowing for multiple contributors and population substructure. Forensic Sci. Int. **2005**, 148, 47–53. **[Google Scholar] [CrossRef]**
11. Slooten, K. Accurate assessment of the weight of evidence for DNA mixtures by integrating the likelihood ratio. Forensic Sci. Int. Genet. **2017**, 27, 1–16. **[Google Scholar] [CrossRef]**
12. Puch-Solis, R.; Rodgers, L.; Mazumder, A.; Pope, S.; Evett, I.; Curran, J.; Balding, D. Evaluating forensic DNA profiles using peak heights, allowing for multiple donors, allelic dropout and stutters. Forensic Sci. Int. Genet. **2013**, 7, 555–563. **[Google Scholar] [CrossRef]**

13. Puch-Solis, R. A dropin peak height model. Forensic Sci. Int. Genet. **2014**, 11, 80–84. **[Google Scholar] [CrossRef] [PubMed]**

14. Perlin, M.W.; Legler, M.W.; Spencer, C.E.; Smith, J.L.; Allan, W.P.; Belrose, J.L.; Duceman, B.W. Validating TrueAllele® DNA mixture interpretation. J. Forensic Sci. **2011**, 56, 1430–1447. **[Google Scholar] [CrossRef] [PubMed]**

15. Taylor, D.; Bright, J.-A.; Buckleton, J. The interpretation of single source and mixed DNA profiles. Forensic Sci. Int. Genet. **2013**, 7, 516–528. **[Google Scholar] [CrossRef] [PubMed]**

16. Robert, G.C. Validation of an STR peak area model. Forensic Sci. Int. Genet. **2009**, 3, 193–199. **[Google Scholar]**

17. Bleka, Ø.; Storvik, G.O.; Gill, P. EuroForMix: An open source software based on a continuous model to evaluate STR DNA profiles from a mixture of contributors with artefacts. Forensic Sci. Int. Genet. **2016**, 21, 35–44. **[Google Scholar] [CrossRef] [Green Version]**

18. Cowell, R.; Lauritzen, S.; Mortera, J. Probabilistic expert systems for handling artifacts in complex DNA mixtures. Forensic Sci. Int. Genet. **2011**, 5, 202–209. **[Google Scholar] [CrossRef] [Green Version]**

19. ENFSI Guideline for Evaluative Reporting in Forensic Science. European Network of Forensic Science Institutes. 2015. Available online: **https://enfsi.eu/wp-content/uploads/2016/09/m1_guideline.pdf** (accessed on 28 September 2021).

20. Slooten, K. Identifying common donors in DNA mixtures, with applications to database searches. Forensic Sci. Int. Genet. **2017**, 26, 40–47. **[Google Scholar] [CrossRef]**

21. Bleka, Ø.; Prieto, L.; Gill, P. CaseSolver: An investigative open source expert system based on EuroForMix. Forensic Sci. Int. Genet. **2019**, 41, 83–92. **[Google Scholar] [CrossRef]**

22. Benschop, C.C.; van de Merwe, L.; de Jong, J.; Vanvooren, V.; Kempenaers, M.; van der Beek, C.; Barni, F.; Reyes, E.L.; Moulin, L.; Pene, L.; et al. Validation of SmartRank: A likelihood ratio software for searching national DNA databases with complex DNA profiles. Forensic Sci. Int. Genet. **2017**, 29, 145–153. **[Google Scholar] [CrossRef]**

23. Benschop, C.; Jong, J.; Merwe, L.; Haned, H. Adapting a likelihood ratio model to enable searching DNA databases with complex STR DNA profiles. In Proceedings of the 2016 27th International Symposium on Human Identification, Nagoya, Japan, 28–30 November 2016; Available online: **https://promega.media/-/media/files/products-and-services/genetic-identity/ishi-27-oral-abstracts/4-benschop.pdf** (accessed on 28 September 2021).

24. Bleka, Ø.; Bouzga, M.; Fonneløp, A.; Gill, P. dnamatch2: An open source software to carry out large scale database searches of mixtures using qualitative and quantitative models. Forensic Sci. Int. Genet. Suppl. Ser. **2017**, 6, e404–e406. **[Google Scholar] [CrossRef] [Green Version]**

25. Taylor, D.; Rowe, E.; Kruijver, M.; Abarno, D.; Bright, J.-A.; Buckleton, J. Inter-sample contamination detection using mixture deconvolution comparison. Forensic Sci. Int. Genet. **2019**, 40, 160–167. **[Google Scholar] [CrossRef] [Green Version]**

26. Kloosterman, A.; Sjerps, M.; Quak, A. Error rates in forensic DNA analysis: Definition, numbers, impact and communication. Forensic Sci. Int. Genet. **2014**, 12, 77–85. **[Google Scholar] [CrossRef] [PubMed]**

27. Gill, P. Misleading DNA Evidence: Reasons for Miscarriages of Justice. Int. Comment. Évid. **2012**, 10, 55–71. **[Google Scholar] [CrossRef]**

28. Duewer, D.L.; Kline, M.C.; Redman, J.W.; Butler, J.M. NIST Mixed Stain Study 3: Signal Intensity Balance in Commercial Short Tandem Repeat Multiplexes. Anal. Chem. **2004**, 76, 6928–6934. **[Google Scholar] [CrossRef] [PubMed]**

29. Benschop, C.C.; Sijen, T. LoCIM-tool: An expert's assistant for inferring the major contributor's alleles in mixed consensus DNA profiles. Forensic Sci. Int. Genet. **2014**, 11, 154–165. **[Google Scholar] [CrossRef] [PubMed]**

30. Butler, J.M. Scientific Working Group on DNA Analysis Methods (SWGDAM) Mixture Interpretation Issues & Insights. 2007. Available online: **https://strbase.nist.gov/pub_pres/SWGDAM_Jan2007_MixtureInterpretation.pdf** (accessed on 28 September 2021).

31. Coble, M.D. MIX13: An Interlaboratory Study on the Present State of DNA Mixture Interpretation in the U.S. In Proceedings of the 5th Annual Prescription for Criminal Justice Forensics, New York, NY, USA, 6 June 2014; Available online: **http://www.cstl.nist.gov/strbase/pub_pres/Coble-ABA2014-MIX13.pdf** (accessed on 28 September 2021).

32. Crespillo, M.; Barrio, P.A.; Luque, J.A.; Alves, C.; Aler, M.; Alessandrini, F.; Andrade, L.; Barretto, R.; Bofarull, A.; Costa, S.; et al. GHEP-ISFG collaborative exercise on mixture profiles of autosomal STRs (GHEP-MIX01, GHEP-MIX02 and GHEP-MIX03): Results and evaluation. Forensic Sci. Int. Genet. **2014**, 10, 64–72. **[Google Scholar] [CrossRef]**

33. Cooper, S.; McGovern, C.; Bright, J.-A.; Taylor, D.; Buckleton, J. Investigating a common approach to DNA profile interpretation using probabilistic software. Forensic Sci. Int. Genet. **2015**, 16, 121–131. **[Google Scholar] [CrossRef]**

34. Torres, Y.; Flores, I.; Prieto, V.; López-Soto, M.; Farfán, M.J.; Carracedo, A.; Sanz, P. DNA mixtures in forensic casework: A 4-year retrospective study. Forensic Sci. Int. **2003**, 134, 180–186. **[Google Scholar] [CrossRef]**

35. Benschop, C.C.; Haned, H.; de Blaeij, T.J.; Meulenbroek, A.J.; Sijen, T. Assessment of mock cases involving complex low template DNA mixtures: A descriptive study. Forensic Sci. Int. Genet. **2012**, 6, 697–707. **[Google Scholar] [CrossRef] [PubMed]**

36. Benschop, C.C.G.; Connolly, E.; Ansell, R.; Kokshoorn, B. Results of an inter and intra laboratory exercise on the assessment of complex autosomal DNA pro-files. Sci. Justice **2017**, 57, 21–27. **[Google Scholar] [CrossRef] [PubMed]**

37. Benschop, C.C.; Hoogenboom, J.; Bargeman, F.; Hovers, P.; Slagter, M.; van der Linden, J.; Parag, R.; Kruise, D.; Drobnic, K.; Klucevsek, G.; et al. Multi-laboratory validation of DNAxs including the statistical library DNAStatistX. Forensic Sci. Int. Genet. **2020**, 49. **[Google Scholar] [CrossRef] [PubMed]**

38. Butler, J.M.; Kline, M.C.; Coble, M.D. NIST Interlaboratory Studies Involving DNA Mixtures (MIX05 and MIX13): Varia-tion Observed and Lessons Learned. Forensic Sci. Int. Genet. **2018**, 37, 81–94. **[Google Scholar] [CrossRef] [PubMed] [Green Version]**

39. Barrio, P.A.; Crespillo, M.; Luque, J.; Aler, M.; Baeza-Richer, C.; Baldassarri, L.; Carnevali, E.; Coufalova, P.; Flores, I.; García, O.; et al. GHEP-ISFG collaborative exercise on mixture profiles (GHEP-MIX06). Reporting conclusions: Results and evaluation. Forensic Sci. Int. Genet. **2018**, 35, 156–163. **[Google Scholar] [CrossRef]**

40. Prieto, L.; Haned, H.; Mosquera, A.; Crespillo, M.; Alemañ, M.; Aler, M.; Álvarez, F.; Baeza-Richer, C.; Dominguez, A.; Doutremepuich, C.; et al. Euroforgen-NoE collaborative exercise on LRmix to demonstrate standardization of the interpretation of complex DNA profiles. Forensic Sci. Int. Genet. **2014**, 9, 47–54. **[Google Scholar] [CrossRef] [PubMed] [Green Version]**

41. Buckleton, J.S.; Bright, J.-A.; Cheng, K.; Budowle, B.; Coble, M.D. NIST interlaboratory studies involving DNA mixtures (MIX13): A modern analysis. Forensic Sci. Int. Genet. **2018**, 37, 172–179. **[Google Scholar] [CrossRef]**

42. Bille, T.; Bright, J.-A.; Buckleton, J. Application of Random Match Probability Calculations to Mixed STR Profiles. J. Forensic Sci. **2013**, 58, 474–485. **[Google Scholar] [CrossRef]**

43. Alladio, E.; Omedei, M.; Cisana, S.; D'Amico, G.; Caneparo, D.; Vincenti, M.; Garofano, P. DNA mixtures interpretation—A proof-of-concept multi-software comparison highlighting different proba-bilistic methods' performances on challenging samples. Forensic Sci. Int. Genet. **2018**, 37, 143–150. **[Google Scholar] [CrossRef]**

44. Iyer, H.K. Validation Principles, Practices, Parameters, Performance Evaluations, and Protocols Reliability Assessment of LR Systems: General Concepts. In Proceedings of the ISHI 2020 Validation Workshop, Baltimore, MD, USA, 18 September 2020; Available online: **https://strbase.nist.gov/pub_pres/5_W10-Hari.pdf** (accessed on 28 September 2021).

45. Garofano, P.; Caneparo, D.; D'Amico, G.; Vincenti, M.; Alladio, E. An alternative application of the consensus method to DNA typing interpretation for Low Tem-plate-DNA mixtures. FSI: Genet. Suppl. Ser. **2015**, 5, e422–e424. **[Google Scholar]**

46. Cheng, K.; Bleka, Ø.; Gill, P.; Curran, J.; Bright, J.; Taylor, D.; Buckleton, J. A comparison of likelihood ratios obtained from EuroForMix and STRmix™. J. Forensic Sci. **2021. [Google Scholar] [CrossRef]**

47. Taylor, D.A.; Buckleton, J.S.; Bright, J.-A. Comment on "DNA mixtures interpretation—A proof-of-concept multi-software comparison highlighting different probabilistic methods' performances on challenging samples" by Alladio et al. Forensic Sci. Int. Genet. **2019**, 40, e248–e251. **[Google Scholar] [CrossRef]**

48. Swaminathan, H.; Qureshi, M.O.; Grgicak, C.M.; Duffy, K.; Lun, D.S. Four model variants within a continuous forensic DNA mixture interpretation framework: Effects on evidential inference and reporting. PLoS ONE **2018**, 13, e0207599. **[Google Scholar] [CrossRef]**

49. Zweig, M.H.; Campbell, A.G. Receiver-operating characteristic (ROC) plots: A fundamental evaluation tool in clinical medi-cine. Clin. Chem. **1993**, 39, 561–577. **[Google Scholar] [CrossRef]**

50. Bleka, Ø.; Benschop, C.C.; Storvik, G.O.; Gill, P. A comparative study of qualitative and quantitative models used to interpret complex STR DNA profiles. Forensic Sci. Int. Genet. **2016**, 25, 85–96. **[Google Scholar] [CrossRef] [Green Version]**

51. You, Y.; Balding, D. A comparison of software for the evaluation of complex DNA profiles. Forensic Sci. Int. Genet. **2019**, 40, 114–119. **[Google Scholar] [CrossRef]**

52. Manabe, S.; Morimoto, C.; Hamano, Y.; Fujimoto, S.; Tamaki, K. Development and validation of open-source software for DNA mixture interpretation based on a quantita-tive continuous model. PLoS ONE **2017**, 12, e0188183. **[Google Scholar] [CrossRef] [Green Version]**

53. Bright, J.-A.; Cheng, K.; Kerr, Z.; McGovern, C.; Kelly, H.; Moretti, T.R.; Smith, M.A.; Bieber, F.R.; Budowle, B.; Coble, M.D.; et al. STRmix™ collaborative exercise on DNA mixture interpretation. Forensic Sci. Int. Genet. **2019**, 40, 1–8. **[Google Scholar] [CrossRef] [PubMed]**

54. Bright, J.-A.; Richards, R.; Kruijver, M.; Kelly, H.; McGovern, C.; Magee, A.; McWhorter, A.; Ciecko, A.; Peck, B.; Baumgartner, C.; et al. Internal validation of STRmix™ – A multi laboratory response to PCAST, Forensic Sci. Int. Genet. **2019**, 34, 11–24. Forensic Sci. Int. Genet. **2019**, 41, e14–e17. **[Google Scholar]**

55. Ramos, D.; Gonzalez-Rodriguez, J. Reliable support: Measuring calibration of likelihood ratios. Forensic Sci. Int. **2013**, 230, 156–169. **[Google Scholar]** **[CrossRef]** **[PubMed]** **[Green Version]**

56. Buckleton, J.S.; Pugh, S.N.; Bright, J.-A.; Taylor, D.A.; Curran, J.M.; Kruijver, M.; Gill, P.; Budowle, B.; Cheng, K. Are low LRs reliable? Forensic Sci. Int. Genet. **2020**, 49, 102350. **[Google Scholar]** **[CrossRef]** **[PubMed]**

57. Hannig, J.; Riman, S.; Iyer, H.; Vallone, P.M. Are reported likelihood ratios well calibrated? Forensic Sci. Int. Genet. Suppl. Ser. **2019**, 7, 572–574. **[Google Scholar]** **[CrossRef]**

58. Bright, J.-A.; Dukes, M.J.; Pugh, S.N.; Evett, I.W.; Buckleton, J.S. Applying calibration to LRs produced by a DNA interpretation software. Aust. J. Forensic Sci. **2019**, 53, 147–153. **[Google Scholar]** **[CrossRef]**

59. Taylor, D.; Buckleton, J.; Evett, I. Testing likelihood ratios produced from complex DNA profiles. Forensic Sci. Int. Genet. **2015**, 16, 165–171. **[Google Scholar]** **[CrossRef]**

60. Taylor, D.; Curran, J.M.; Buckleton, J. Importance sampling allows Hd true tests of highly discriminating DNA profiles. Forensic Sci. Int. Genet. **2017**, 27, 74–81. **[Google Scholar]** **[CrossRef]**

61. Butler, J.M. Advanced Topics in Forensic DNA Typing: Interpretation; Academic Press: Cambridge, MA, USA, 2014. **[Google Scholar]** **[CrossRef]**

62. Gill, P.; Bleka, Ø.; Hansson, O.; Benschop, C.; Haned, H. Forensic Practitioner's Guide to the Interpretation of Complex DNA Profiles; Academic Press: London, UK, 2020. **[Google Scholar]** **[CrossRef]**

63. SWGDAM Interpretation Guidelines for Autosomal STR Typing by Forensic DNA Testing Laboratories. 2010. Available online: **http://www.fbi.gov/about-us/lab/codis/swgdam-interpretation-guidelines** (accessed on 28 September 2021).

64. Buckleton, J.S.; Curran, J.M.; Gill, P. Towards understanding the effect of uncertainty in the number of contributors to DNA stains. Forensic Sci. Int. Genet. **2007**, 1, 20–28. **[Google Scholar]** **[CrossRef]**

65. Paoletti, D.R.; Doom, T.E.; Krane, C.M.; Raymer, M.L.; Krane, D.E. Empirical Analysis of the STR Profiles Resulting from Conceptual Mixtures. J. Forensic Sci. **2005**, 50, 1–6. **[Google Scholar]** **[CrossRef]** **[Green Version]**

66. Norsworthy, S.; Lun, D.S.; Grgicak, C.M. Determining the number of contributors to DNA mixtures in the low-template regime: Exploring the impacts of sampling and detection effects. Leg. Med. **2018**, 32, 1–8. **[Google Scholar] [CrossRef]**

67. Weir, B.S.; Triggs, C.M.; Starling, L.; Stowell, L.I.; Walsh, K.A.; Buckleton, J. Interpreting DNA mixtures. J. Forensic Sci. **1997**, 42, 213–222. **[Google Scholar] [CrossRef] [PubMed]**

68. Benschop, C.C.; Haned, H.; Jeurissen, L.; Gill, P.D.; Sijen, T. The effect of varying the number of contributors on likelihood ratios for complex DNA mixtures. Forensic Sci. Int. Genet. **2015**, 19, 92–99. **[Google Scholar] [CrossRef] [PubMed]**

69. Haned, H.; Benschop, C.C.; Gill, P.D.; Sijen, T. Complex DNA mixture analysis in a forensic context: Evaluating the probative value using a likelihood ratio model. Forensic Sci. Int. Genet. **2015**, 16, 17–25. **[Google Scholar] [CrossRef]**

70. Bright, J.A.; Curran, J.M.; Buckleton, J.S. The effect of the uncertainty in the number of contributors to mixed DNA pro-files on profile interpretation. Forensic Sci. Int. Genet. **2014**, 12, 208–214. **[Google Scholar] [CrossRef] [PubMed]**

71. Buckleton, J.S.; Bright, J.-A.; Cheng, K.; Kelly, H.; Taylor, D.A. The effect of varying the number of contributors in the prosecution and alternate propositions. Forensic Sci. Int. Genet. **2018**, 38, 225–231. **[Google Scholar] [CrossRef] [Green Version]**

72. Bille, T.; Weitz, S.; Buckleton, J.S.; Bright, J.-A. Interpreting a major component from a mixed DNA profile with an unknown number of minor contributors. Forensic Sci. Int. Genet. **2019**, 40, 150–159. **[Google Scholar] [CrossRef] [PubMed]**

73. Benschop, C.C.; Nijveld, A.; Duijs, F.E.; Sijen, T. An assessment of the performance of the probabilistic genotyping software EuroForMix: Trends in likelihood ratios and analysis of Type I & II errors. Forensic Sci. Int. Genet. **2019**, 42, 31–38. **[Google Scholar] [CrossRef] [PubMed]**

74. Slooten, K. A top-down approach to DNA mixtures. Forensic Sci. Int. Genet. **2020**, 46, 102250. **[Google Scholar] [CrossRef] [PubMed]**

75. Coble, M.D.; Bright, J.-A.; Buckleton, J.S.; Curran, J.M. Uncertainty in the number of contributors in the proposed new CODIS set. Forensic Sci. Int. Genet. **2015**, 19, 207–211. **[Google Scholar] [CrossRef]**

76. Curran, J.M.; Buckleton, J. Uncertainty in the number of contributors for the European Standard Set of loci. Forensic Sci. Int. Genet. **2014**, 11, 205–206. **[Google Scholar] [CrossRef]**

77. Dembinski, G.M.; Sobieralski, C.; Picard, C.J. Estimation of the number of contributors of theoretical mixture profiles based on allele counting: Does increasing the number of loci increase success rate of estimates? Forensic Sci. Int. Genet. **2018**, 33, 24–32. **[Google Scholar] [CrossRef] [Green Version]**

78. Young, B.A.; Gettings, K.B.; McCord, B.; Vallone, P.M. Estimating number of contributors in massively parallel sequencing data of STR loci. Forensic Sci. Int. Genet. **2019**, 38, 15–22. **[Google Scholar] [CrossRef]**

79. Haned, H.; Pène, L.; Lobry, J.R.; Dufour, A.B.; Pontier, D. Estimating the Number of Contributors to Forensic DNA Mixtures: Does Maximum Likelihood Perform Better Than Maximum Allele Count? J. Forensic Sci. **2011**, 56, 23–28. **[Google Scholar] [CrossRef] [PubMed]**

80. Haned, H.; Pène, L.; Sauvage, F.; Pontier, D. The predictive value of the maximum likelihood estimator of the number of contributors to a DNA mixture. Forensic Sci. Int. Genet. **2011**, 5, 281–284. **[Google Scholar] [CrossRef]**

81. Biedermann, A.; Bozza, S.; Konis, K.; Taroni, F. Inference about the number of contributors to a DNA mixture: Comparative analyses of a Bayesian network approach and the maximum allele count method. Forensic Sci. Int. Genet. **2012**, 6, 689–696. **[Google Scholar] [CrossRef]**

82. Tvedebrink, T. On the exact distribution of the numbers of alleles in DNA mixtures. Int. J. Leg. Med. **2013**, 128, 427–437. **[Google Scholar] [CrossRef]**

83. Benschop, C.; Haned, H.; Sijen, T. Consensus and pool profiles to assist in the analysis and interpretation of complex low template DNA mixtures. Int. J. Leg. Med. **2011**, 127, 11–23. **[Google Scholar] [CrossRef] [Green Version]**

84. Paoletti, D.R.; Krane, D.E.; Raymer, M.L.; Doom, T.E. Inferring the Number of Contributors to Mixed DNA Profiles. IEEE/ACM Trans. Comput. Biol. Bioinform. **2011**, 9, 113–122. **[Google Scholar] [CrossRef]**

85. Perez, J.; Mitchell, A.A.; Ducasse, N.; Tamariz, J.; Caragine, T. Estimating the number of contributors to two-, three-, and four-person mixtures containing DNA in high template and low template amounts. Croat. Med. J. **2011**, 52, 314–326. **[Google Scholar] [CrossRef] [Green Version]**

86. Benschop, C.C.; van der Beek, C.P.; Meiland, H.C.; van Gorp, A.G.; Westen, A.A.; Sijen, T. Low template STR typing: Effect of replicate number and consensus method on genotyping reliability and DNA database search results. Forensic Sci. Int. Genet. **2011**, 5, 316–328. **[Google Scholar] [CrossRef] [PubMed]**

87. Alfonse, L.; Tejada, G.; Swaminathan, H.; Lun, D.S.; Grgicak, C.M. Inferring the Number of Contributors to Complex DNA Mixtures Using Three Methods: Exploring the Limits of Low-Template DNA Interpretation. J. Forensic Sci. **2016**, 62, 308–316. **[Google Scholar] [CrossRef]**

88. Swaminathan, H.; Grgicak, C.M.; Medard, M.; Lun, D.S. NOCIt: A computational method to infer the number of contributors to DNA samples analyzed by STR genotyping. Forensic Sci. Int. Genet. **2015**, 16, 172–180. **[Google Scholar] [CrossRef] [PubMed]**

89. Benschop, C.; Backx, A.; Sijen, T. Automated estimation of the number of contributors in autosomal STR profiles. Forensic Sci. Int. Genet. Suppl. Ser. **2019**, 7, 7–8. **[Google Scholar] [CrossRef]**

90. Marciano, M.A.; Adelman, J.D. PACE: Probabilistic Assessment for Contributor Estimation—A machine learning-based assessment of the number of contributors in DNA mixtures. Forensic Sci. Int. Genet. **2017**, 27, 82–91. **[Google Scholar] [CrossRef] [PubMed]**

91. Benschop, C.C.; van der Linden, J.; Hoogenboom, J.; Ypma, R.; Haned, H. Automated estimation of the number of contributors in autosomal short tandem repeat profiles using a machine learning approach. Forensic Sci. Int. Genet. **2019**, 43, 102150. **[Google Scholar] [CrossRef] [PubMed]**

92. Kruijver, M.; Kelly, H.; Cheng, K.; Lin, M.-H.; Morawitz, J.; Russell, L.; Buckleton, J.; Bright, J.-A. Estimating the number of contributors to a DNA profile using decision trees. Forensic Sci. Int. Genet. **2020**, 50, 102407. **[Google Scholar] [CrossRef] [PubMed]**

93. Taylor, D.; Bright, J.A.; Buckleton, J. Interpreting forensic DNA profiling evidence without specifying the number of con-tribuors. Forensic Sci. Int. Genet. **2014**, 13, 269–280. **[Google Scholar] [CrossRef]**

94. Slooten, K.; Caliebe, A. Contributors are a nuisance (parameter) for DNA mixture evidence evaluation. Forensic Sci. Int. Genet. **2018**, 37, 116–125. **[Google Scholar] [CrossRef]**

95. Buckleton, J.; Taylor, D.; Bright, J.A.; Hicks, T.; Curran, J. When evaluating DNA evidence within a likelihood ratio framework, should the propositions be exhaustive? Forensic Sci. Int. Genet. **2021**, 50, 102406. **[Google Scholar] [CrossRef]**

96. Hicks, T.; Kerr, Z.; Pugh, S.; Bright, J.-A.; Curran, J.; Taylor, D.; Buckleton, J. Comparing multiple POI to DNA mixtures. Forensic Sci. Int. Genet. **2021**, 52, 102481. **[Google Scholar] [CrossRef]**

97. Kelly, H. The effect of user defined number of contributors within the LR assignment. Aust. J. Forensic Sci. **2021**, 1–14. **[Google Scholar] [CrossRef]**

98. McGovern, C.; Cheng, K.; Kelly, H.; Ciecko, A.; Taylor, D.; Buckleton, J.S.; Bright, J.A. Performance of a method for weighting a range in the number of contributors in probabilistic genotyping. Forensic Sci. Int. Genet. **2020**, 48, 102352. **[Google Scholar] [CrossRef]**

99. Akaike, H. A new look at the statistical model identification. IEEE Trans. Autom. Control. **1974**, 19, 716–723. **[Google Scholar] [CrossRef]**

100. Coble, M.D.; Bright, J.-A. Probabilistic genotyping software: An overview. Forensic Sci. Int. Genet. **2018**, 38, 219–224. **[Google Scholar] [CrossRef]**

101. Cook, R.; Evett, I.; Jackson, G.; Jones, P.; Lambert, J. A hierarchy of propositions: Deciding which level to address in casework. Sci. Justice **1998**, 38, 231–239. **[Google Scholar] [CrossRef]**

102. Evett, I.W.; Jackson, G.; Lambert, J.A. More on the hierarchy of propositions: Exploring the distinction between explana-tions and propositions. Sci. Justice **2000**, 40, 3–10. **[Google Scholar] [CrossRef]**

103. Gittelson, S.; Kalafut, T.; Myers, S.; Taylor, D.; Hicks, T.; Taroni, F.; Buckleton, J. A Practical Guide for the Formulation of Propositions in the Bayesian Approach to DNA Evidence Inter-pretation in an Adversarial Environment. J. Forensic Sci. **2016**, 61, 186–195. **[Google Scholar] [CrossRef] [PubMed]**

104. Taylor, D.A.; Bright, J.-A.; Buckleton, J.S. The 'factor of two' issue in mixed DNA profiles. J. Theor. Biol. **2014**, 363, 300–306. **[Google Scholar] [CrossRef] [PubMed]**

105. Evett, I. On meaningful questions: A two-trace transfer problem. J. Forensic Sci. Soc. **1987**, 27, 375–381. **[Google Scholar] [CrossRef]**

106. Gill, P. Analysis and implications of the miscarriages of justice of Amanda Knox and Raffaele Sollecito. Forensic Sci. Int. Genet. **2016**, 23, 9–18. **[Google Scholar] [CrossRef] [PubMed] [Green Version]**

107. Foreman, L.; Smith, A.F.M.; Evett, I.W.; Aitken, C.G.G.; Taroni, A.F. Comment on Foreman L., Smith A.F.M., Evett I.W., Bayesian analysis of DNA profiling data in forensic identification applications. J. R. Stat. Soc. **1997**, 160, 463. **[Google Scholar] [CrossRef]**

108. Scientific Working Group on DNA Analysis Methods (SWGDAM): Guidelines for the Validation of Probabilistic Genotyping Systems. 2015. Available online: **https://1ecb9588-ea6f-4feb-971a-73265dbf079c.filesusr.com/ugd/4344b0_22776006b67c4a32a5ffc04fe3b56515.pdf** (accessed on 25 September 2021).

109. Coble, M.; Buckleton, J.; Butler, J.; Egeland, T.; Fimmers, R.; Gill, P.; Gusmão, L.; Guttman, B.; Krawczak, M.; Morling, N.; et al. DNA Commission of the International Society for Forensic Genetics: Recommendations on the validation of software programs performing biostatistical calculations for forensic genetics applications. Forensic Sci. Int. Genet. **2016**, 25, 191–197. **[Google Scholar] [CrossRef]**

110. ANSI/ASB Standard 018, First Edition. 2020: Standard for Validation of Probabilistic Genotyping Systems. Available online: **http://www.asbstandardsboard.org/wp-content/uploads/2020/07/018_Std_e1.pdf** (accessed on 28 September 2021).

111. Ballim, A.; Wilks, A.Y. Beliefs, stereotypes and dynamic agent modeling. User Model. User-Adapt. Interact. **1991**, 1, 33–65. **[Google Scholar] [CrossRef]**

112. Bright, J.-A.; Evett, I.W.; Taylor, D.; Curran, J.M.; Buckleton, J. A series of recommended tests when validating probabilistic DNA profile interpretation software. Forensic Sci. Int. Genet. **2015**, 14, 125–131. **[Google Scholar] [CrossRef]**

113. Haned, H.; Gill, P.; Lohmueller, K.; Inman, K.; Rudin, N. Validation of probabilistic genotyping software for use in forensic DNA casework: Definitions and illustra-tions. Sci. Justice **2016**, 56, 104–108. **[Google Scholar] [CrossRef] [PubMed]**

114. Ropero-Miller, J.; Melton, P.; Ferrara, L.; Hall, J. Landscape Study of DNA Mixture Interpretation Software. National Institute of Justice, Forensic Technology Centre of Excellence. 2015. Available online: **https://nij.ojp.gov/library/publications/landscape-study-dna-mixture-interpretation-software** (accessed on 28 September 2021).

115. European Network of Forensic Science Institutes (ENFSI). Best Practice Manual for the Internal Validation of Probabilistic Software to Undertake DNA Mixture Interpretation ENFSI-BPM-DNA-01 issue 001. 17 May 2017. Available online: **https://enfsi.eu/wp-content/uploads/2017/09/Best-Practice-Manual-for-the-internal-validation-of-probabilistic-software-to-undertake-DNA-mixture-interpretation-v1.docx.pdf** (accessed on 28 September 2021).

116. Forensic Science Regulator, Software Validation for DNA Mixture Interpretation, FSR-G-223 (2). 2018. Available online: **https://www.gov.uk/government/publications/software-validation-for-dna-mixture-interpretation-fsr-g-223** (accessed on 28 September 2021).

117. PCAST, Forensic Science in Criminal Courts: Ensuring Scientific Validity of Feature Comparison Methods, US President's Council of Advisors on Science and Technology. 2016. Available online: **https://obamawhitehouse.archives.gov/sites/default/files/microsites/ostp/PCAST/pcast_forensic_science_report_final.pdf** (accessed on 28 September 2021).

118. Box, G.E.P.; Draper, N.R. Empirical Model-Building and Response Surfaces; Wiley: New York, NY, USA, 1987. **[Google Scholar]**

119. Rykiel, E.J., Jr. Testing ecological models: The meaning of validation. Ecol. Model. **1996**, 90, 229–244. **[Google Scholar] [CrossRef]**

120. Gill, P.; Kirkham, A.; Curran, J. LoComatioN: A software tool for the analysis of low copy number DNA profiles. Forensic Sci. Int. **2007**, 166, 128–138. **[Google Scholar] [CrossRef] [PubMed]**

121. Haned, H. Forensim: An open-source initiative for the evaluation of statistical methods in forensic genetics. Forensic Sci. Int. Genet. **2011**, 5, 265–268. **[Google Scholar] [CrossRef]**

122. Haned, H.; Gill, P. Analysis of complex DNA mixtures using the Forensim package. Forensic Sci. Int. Genet. Suppl. Ser. **2011**, 3, e79–e80. **[Google Scholar] [CrossRef]**

123. Evett, I.W.; Gill, P.D.; Lambert, J.A. Taking account of peak areas when interpreting mixed DNA profiles. J. Forensic Sci. **1998**, 43, 62–69. **[Google Scholar] [CrossRef]**

124. Cowell, R.G.; Lauritzen, S.L.; Mortera, J. A γ model for {DNA} mixture analyses. Bayesian Anal. **2007**, 2, 333–348. **[Google Scholar] [CrossRef]**

125. Graversen, T.; Lauritzen, S. Estimation of parameters in DNA mixture analysis. J. Appl. Stat. **2013**, 40, 2423–2436. **[Google Scholar] [CrossRef] [Green Version]**

126. Graversen, T.; Lauritzen, S. Computational aspects of DNA mixture analysis. Stat. Comput. **2014**, 25, 527–541. **[Google Scholar] [CrossRef] [Green Version]**

127. Haldemann, B.; Dornseifer, S.; Heylen, T.; Aelbrecht, C.; Bleka, O.; Larsen, H.J.; Neuhaus-Steinmetz, U. eDNA—An expert software system for comparison and evaluation of DNA profiles in forensic case-work. Forensic Sci. Int. Genet. Suppl. Ser. **2015**, 5, e400–e402. **[Google Scholar] [CrossRef]**

128. Benschop, C.C.; Hoogenboom, J.; Hovers, P.; Slagter, M.; Kruise, D.; Parag, R.; Steensma, K.; Slooten, K.; Nagel, J.H.; Dieltjes, P.; et al. DNAxs/DNAStatistX: Development and validation of a software suite for the data management and probabilistic interpretation of DNA profiles. Forensic Sci. Int. Genet. **2019**, 42, 81–89. **[Google Scholar] [CrossRef] [PubMed]**

129. Veldhuis, M. Explainable artificial intelligence in forensics: Realistic explanations for number of contributor predictions of DNA profiles. Forensic Sci. Int. Genet. **2021**, submitted. **[Google Scholar]**

130. Cowell, R.G.; Graversen, T.; Lauritzen, S.L.; Mortera, J. Analysis of forensic DNA mixtures with artefacts. J. R. Stat. Soc. Ser. C Appl. Stat. **2015**, 64, 1–48. **[Google Scholar] [CrossRef] [Green Version]**

131. Duijs, F.E.; Hoogenboom, J.; Sijen, T.; Benschop, C. Performance of EuroForMix deconvolution on PowerPlex® Fusion 6C profiles. Forensic Sci. Int. Genet. Suppl. Ser. **2019**, 7, 5–6. **[Google Scholar] [CrossRef]**

132. Taylor, D.; Buckleton, J. Do low template DNA profiles have useful quantitative data? Forensic Sci. Int. Genet. **2015**, 16, 13–16. **[Google Scholar] [CrossRef]**

133. Bruijns, B.; Tiggelaar, R.M.; Gardeniers, J. Massively parallel sequencing techniques for forensics: A review. Electrophoresis **2018**, 39, 2642–2654. **[Google Scholar] [CrossRef] [Green Version]**

134. Just, R.S.; Irwin, J.A. Use of the LUS in sequence allele designations to facilitate probabilistic genotyping of NGS-based STR typing results. Forensic Sci. Int. Genet. **2018**, 34, 197–205. **[Google Scholar] [CrossRef] [Green Version]**

135. Just, R.S.; Le, J.; Irwin, J.A. LUS+: Extension of the LUS designator concept to differentiate most sequence alleles for 27 STR loci. Forensic Sci. Int. Rep. **2020**, 2, 100059. **[Google Scholar] [CrossRef]**

136. Vilsen, S.B.; Tvedebrink, T.; Eriksen, P.S.; Bøsting, C.; Hussing, C.; Mogensen, H.S.; Morling, N. Stutter analysis of complex STR MPS data. Forensic Sci. Int. Genet. **2018**, 35, 107–112. **[Google Scholar] [CrossRef]**

137. Bleka, Ø.; Just, R.; Le, J.; Gill, P. Automation of high volume MPS mixture interpretation using CaseSolver. Forensic Sci. Int. Genet. Suppl. Ser. **2019**, 7, 14–15. **[Google Scholar] [CrossRef]**

138. Bleka, Ø.; Just, R.; Le, J.; Gill, P. An examination of STR nomenclatures, filters and models for MPS mixture interpretation. Forensic Sci. Int. Genet. **2020**, 48, 102319. **[Google Scholar] [CrossRef]**

139. Gill, P.; Just, R.; Parson, W.; Phillips, C.; Bleka, Ø. Interpretation of complex DNA profiles generated by Massively Parallel Sequencing. In Forensic Practitioner's Guide to the Interpretation of Complex DNA Profiles; Gill, P., Bleka, O., Hansson, O., Benschop, C., Haned, H., Eds.; Academic Press: Cambridge, MA, USA; Elsevier: Amsterdam, The Netherlands, 2020; pp. 419–451. **[Google Scholar] [CrossRef]**

140. van der Gaag, K.J.; de Leeuw, R.H.; Hoogenboom, J.; Patel, J.; Storts, D.R.; Laros, J.F.; de Knijff, P. Massively parallel sequencing of short tandem re-peats-Population data and mixture analysis results for the PowerSeq system. Forensic Sci. Int. Genet. **2016**, 24, 86–96. **[Google Scholar] [CrossRef] [Green Version]**

141. Hoogenboom, J.; van der Gaag, K.J.; de Leeuw, R.H.; Sijen, T.; de Knijff, P.; Laros, J.F. FDSTools: A software package for analysis of massively parallel sequencing data with the ability to recognise and correct STR stutter and other PCR or sequencing noise. Forensic Sci. Int. Genet. **2016**, 27, 27–40. **[Google Scholar] [CrossRef] [PubMed] [Green Version]**

142. Benschop, C.C.; van der Gaag, K.J.; de Vreede, J.; Backx, A.J.; de Leeuw, R.H.; Zuñiga, S.; Hoogenboom, J.; de Knijff, P.; Sijen, T. Application of a probabilistic genotyping software to MPS mixture STR data is supported by similar trends in LRs compared with CE data. Forensic Sci. Int. Genet. **2021**, 52, 102489. **[Google Scholar] [CrossRef] [PubMed]**

143. Bleka, Ø.; Eduardoff, M.; Santos, C.; Phillips, C.; Parson, W.; Gill, P. Open source software EuroForMix can be used to analyse complex SNP mixtures. Forensic Sci. Int. Genet. **2017**, 31, 105–110. **[Google Scholar] [CrossRef] [PubMed]**

144. Bleka, Ø.; Eduardoff, M.; Santos, C.; Phillips, C.; Parson, W.; Gill, P. Using EuroForMix to analyse complex SNP mixtures, up to six contributors. Forensic Sci. Int. Genet. Suppl. Ser. **2017**, 6, e277–e279. **[Google Scholar] [CrossRef] [Green Version]**

145. Yang, T.-W.; Li, Y.-H.; Chou, C.-F.; Lai, F.-P.; Chien, Y.-H.; Yin, H.-I.; Lee, T.-T.; Hwa, H.-L. DNA mixture interpretation using linear regression and neural networks on massively parallel sequencing data of single nucleotide polymorphisms. Aust. J. Forensic Sci. **2021**, 1–13. **[Google Scholar] [CrossRef]**

146. Benschop, C.C.; Haned, H.; Yoo, S.Y.; Sijen, T. Evaluation of samples comprising minute amounts of DNA. Sci. Justice **2015**, 55, 316–322. **[Google Scholar] [CrossRef] [PubMed]**

147. Benschop, C.C.; Yoo, S.Y.; Sijen, T. Split DNA over replicates or perform one amplification? Forensic Sci. Int. Genet. Suppl. Ser. **2015**, 5, e532–e533. **[Google Scholar] [CrossRef] [Green Version]**

148. Benschop, C.C.; Graaf, E.S.; Sijen, T. Is an increased drop-in rate appropriate with enhanced DNA profiling? Forensic Sci. Int. Genet. Suppl. Ser. **2015**, 5, e71–e72. **[Google Scholar] [CrossRef]**

149. Slagter, M.; Kruise, D.; van Ommen, L.; Hoogenboom, J.; Steensma, K.; de Jong, J.; Hovers, P.; Parag, R.; van der Linden, J.; Kneppers, A.L.; et al. The DNAxs software suite: A three-year retrospective study on the development, architecture, testing and implementation in forensic casework. Forensic Sci. Int. Rep. **2021**, 3, 100212. **[Google Scholar] [CrossRef]**

150. Beecham, G.W.; Weir, B.S. Confidence interval of the likelihood ratio associated with mixed stain DNA evidence. J. Forensic Sci. **2010**, 56, S166–S171. **[Google Scholar] [CrossRef]**

151. Curran, J.M.; Triggs, C.M.; Buckleton, J.; Weir, B.S. Interpreting DNA mixtures in structured populations. J. Forensic Sci. **1999**, 44, 12028J. **[Google Scholar] [CrossRef]**

152. Slooten, K. The analogy between DNA kinship and DNA mixture evaluation, with applications for the interpretation of like-lihood ratios produced by possibly imperfect models. Forensic Sci. Int. Genet. **2021**, 52, 102449. **[Google Scholar] [CrossRef]**

153. Good, I.J. Probability and the Weighing of Evidence; Charles Griffin & Company Limited: London, UK, 1950. **[Google Scholar]**

154. Bright, J.A.; Taylor, D.; Curran, J.M.; Buckleton, J.S. Degradation of forensic DNA profiles. Aust. J. Forensic Sci. **2013**, 45, 445–449. **[Google Scholar] [CrossRef]**

155. Taylor, D.; Bright, J.-A.; Kelly, H.; Lin, M.-H.; Buckleton, J. A fully continuous system of DNA profile evidence evaluation that can utilise STR profile data produced under different conditions within a single analysis. Forensic Sci. Int. Genet. **2017**, 31, 149–154. **[Google Scholar] [CrossRef] [Green Version]**

156. Bright, J.-A.; Taylor, D.; Curran, J.M.; Buckleton, J.S. Developing allelic and stutter peak height models for a continuous method of DNA interpretation. Forensic Sci. Int. Genet. **2013**, 7, 296–304. **[Google Scholar] [CrossRef]**

157. Taylor, D.; Bright, J.-A.; McGovern, C.; Hefford, C.; Kalafut, T.; Buckleton, J. Validating multiplexes for use in conjunction with modern interpretation strategies. Forensic Sci. Int. Genet. **2016**, 20, 6–19. **[Google Scholar] [CrossRef] [Green Version]**

158. Bright, J.-A.; Buckleton, J.S.; Taylor, D.; Fernando, M.A.C.S.S.; Curran, J.M. Modeling forward stutter: Toward increased objectivity in forensic DNA interpretation. Electrophoresis **2014**, 35, 3152–3157. **[Google Scholar] [CrossRef]**

159. Bright, J.-A.; Taylor, D.; Kerr, Z.; Buckleton, J.; Kruijver, M. The efficacy of DNA mixture to mixture matching. Forensic Sci. Int. Genet. **2019**, 41, 64–71. **[Google Scholar] [CrossRef] [Green Version]**

160. Cheng, K.; Bright, J.-A.; Kerr, Z.; Taylor, D.; Ciecko, A.; Curran, J.; Buckleton, J. Examining the additivity of peak heights in forensic DNA profiles. Aust. J. Forensic Sci. **2020**, 1–15. **[Google Scholar] [CrossRef]**

161. Hansson, O.; Egeland, T.; Gill, P. Characterization of degradation and heterozygote balance by simulation of the forensic DNA analysis process. Int. J. Leg. Med. **2016**, 131, 303–317. **[Google Scholar] [CrossRef] [PubMed] [Green Version]**

162. Bright, J.-A.; Curran, J.M.; Buckleton, J.S. Investigation into the performance of different models for predicting stutter. Forensic Sci. Int. Genet. **2013**, 7, 422–427. **[Google Scholar] [CrossRef] [PubMed]**

163. Taylor, D. Using continuous DNA interpretation methods to revisit likelihood ratio behaviour. Forensic Sci. Int. Genet. **2014**, 11, 144–153. **[Google Scholar]** **[CrossRef]** **[PubMed]**

164. Taylor, D.A.; Bright, J.-A.; Buckleton, J.S. The effect of varying the number of contributors in the prosecution and alternate propositions. Forensic Sci. Int. Genet. **2019**, 13, 269–280. **[Google Scholar]** **[CrossRef]** **[PubMed]**

165. Weinberg, M. Computing the Bayes Factor from a Markov Chain Monte Carlo Simulation of the Posterior Distribution. Bayesian Anal. **2012**, 7, 737–770. **[Google Scholar]** **[CrossRef]**

166. Weinberg, M.D.; Yoon, I.; Katz, N. A remarkably simple and accurate method for computing the Bayes Factor from a Markov chain Monte Carlo Simulation of the Posterior Distribution in high dimension. arXiv **2013**, arXiv:1301.3156v1. **[Google Scholar]**

167. Buckleton, J.; Bright, J.-A.; Taylor, D.; Evett, I.; Hicks, T.; Jackson, G.; Curran, J.M. Helping formulate propositions in forensic DNA analysis. Sci. Justice **2014**, 54, 258–261. **[Google Scholar]** **[CrossRef]**

168. Taylor, D.; Bright, J.-A.; Buckleton, J. Considering relatives when assessing the evidential strength of mixed DNA profiles. Forensic Sci. Int. Genet. **2014**, 13, 259–263. **[Google Scholar]** **[CrossRef]**

169. Balding, D.J. Weight-of-Evidence for Forensic DNA Profiles; John Wiley and Sons: Chichester, UK, 2005. **[Google Scholar]**

170. Buckleton, J.; Triggs, C. Relatedness and DNA: Are we taking it seriously enough? Forensic Sci. Int. **2005**, 152, 115–119. **[Google Scholar]** **[CrossRef]** **[PubMed]**

171. Taylor, D.; Bright, J.-A.; Buckleton, J.; Curran, J. An illustration of the effect of various sources of uncertainty on DNA likelihood ratio calculations. Forensic Sci. Int. Genet. **2014**, 11, 56–63. **[Google Scholar]** **[CrossRef]** **[PubMed]**

172. Balding, D.; Nichols, R.A. DNA profile match probability calculation: How to allow for population stratification, relatedness, database selection and single bands. Forensic Sci. Int. **1994**, 64, 125–140. **[Google Scholar]** **[CrossRef]**

173. Balding, D.J. Estimating products in forensic identification using DNA profiles. J. Am. Stat. Assoc. **1995**, 90, 839–844. **[Google Scholar]** **[CrossRef]**

174. Curran, J.M.; Buckleton, J.S. An investigation into the performance of methods for adjusting for sampling uncertainty in DNA likelihood ratio calculations. Forensic Sci. Int. Genet. **2011**, 5, 512–516. **[Google Scholar]** **[CrossRef]** **[PubMed]**

175. Triggs, C.; Harbison, S.; Buckleton, J. The calculation of DNA match probabilities in mixed race populations. Sci. Justice **2000**, 40, 33–38. **[Google Scholar] [CrossRef]**

176. Curran, J.M. An introduction to Bayesian credible intervals for sampling error in DNA profiles. Law Probab. Risk **2005**, 4, 115–126. **[Google Scholar] [CrossRef] [Green Version]**

177. Morrison, G.S. Special issue on measuring and reporting the precision of forensic likelihood ratios: Introduction to the debate. Sci. Justice **2016**, 56, 371–373. **[Google Scholar] [CrossRef] [PubMed]**

178. Morrison, G.; Enzinger, E. What should a forensic practitioner's likelihood ratio be? Sci. Justice **2016**, 5, 374–379. **[Google Scholar] [CrossRef]**

179. Curran, J.M. Admitting to uncertainty in the LR. Sci. Justice **2016**, 56, 380–382. **[Google Scholar] [CrossRef]**

180. Ommen, D.M.; Saunders, C.P.; Neumann, C. An argument against presenting interval quantifications as a surrogate for the value of evidence. Sci. Justice **2016**, 56, 383–387. **[Google Scholar] [CrossRef]**

181. Berger, C.E.; Slooten, K. The LR does not exist. Sci. Justice **2016**, 56, 388–391. **[Google Scholar] [CrossRef] [PubMed]**

182. Biedermann, A.; Bozza, S.; Taroni, F.; Aitken, C. Reframing the debate: A question of probability, not of likelihood ratio. Sci. Justice **2016**, 56, 392–396. **[Google Scholar] [CrossRef] [PubMed] [Green Version]**

183. Hout, A.v.d.; Alberink, I. Posterior distribution for likelihood ratios in forensic science. Sci. Justice **2016**, 5, 397–401. **[Google Scholar] [CrossRef] [PubMed]**

184. Taylor, D.; Hicks, T.; Champod, C. Using sensitivity analyses in Bayesian networks to highlight the impact of data pauci-ty and direct future analyses: A contribution to the debate on measuring and reporting the precision of likelihood ratios. Sci. Justice **2016**, 56, 402–410. **[Google Scholar] [CrossRef] [PubMed]**

185. Bright, J.-A. Testing Methods for Quantifying Monte Carlo Variation for Categorical Variables in Probabilistic Genotyping; Report; Institute of Environmental Science and Research: Wellington, New Zealand, 2020. **[Google Scholar] [CrossRef]**

186. Bright, J.-A. Revisiting the STRmix™ Likelihood Ratio Probability Interval Coverage Considering Multiple Factors; Report; Institute of Environmental Science and Research: Wellington, New Zealand, 2021. **[Google Scholar]**

187. Buckleton, J.; Curran, J.; Goudet, J.; Taylor, D.; Thiery, A.; Weir, B.S. Population-specific FST values for forensic STR markers: A worldwide survey. Forensic Sci. Int. Genet. **2016**, 23, 126–133. **[Google Scholar]**

188. Steele, C.D.; Court, D.S.; Balding, D.J. Worldwide F(ST) estimates relative to five continental-scale populations. Ann. Hum. Genet. **2014**, 78, 468–477. **[Google Scholar] [CrossRef] [Green Version]**

189. Weir, B.S.; Cockerham, C.C. Estimating F-statistics for the analysis of population structure. Evolution **1984**, 38, 1358–1370. **[Google Scholar]**

190. Bright, J.-A.; Taylor, D.; Curran, J.; Buckleton, J. Searching mixed DNA profiles directly against profile databases. Forensic Sci. Int. Genet. **2014**, 9, 102–110. **[Google Scholar] [CrossRef]**

191. Abarno, D.; Sobieraj, T.; Summers, C.; Taylor, D. The first Australian conviction resulting from a familial search. Aust. J. Forensic Sci. **2019**, 51, S56–S59. **[Google Scholar] [CrossRef]**

192. Taylor, D.; Abarno, D.; Rowe, E.; Rask-Nielsen, L. Observations of DNA transfer within an operational Forensic Biology Laboratory. Forensic Int. Genet. **2016**, 23, 33–49. **[Google Scholar] [CrossRef] [PubMed]**

193. Kruijver, M.; Meester, R.; Slooten, K. p-Values should not be used for evaluating the strength of DNA evidence. Forensic Sci. Int. Genet. **2015**, 16, 226–231. **[Google Scholar] [CrossRef] [PubMed]**

194. Budowle, B.; Onorato, A.J.; Callaghan, T.F.; Della Manna, A.; Gross, A.M.; Guerrieri, R.A.; Luttman, J.C.; McClure, D.L. Mixture Interpretation: Defining the Relevant Features for Guidelines for the Assessment of Mixed DNA Profiles in Forensic Casework. J. Forensic Sci. **2009**, 54, 810–821. **[Google Scholar] [CrossRef] [PubMed]**

195. Taylor, D.; Bright, J.-A.; Scandrett, L.; Abarno, D.; Lee, S.-I.; Wivell, R.; Kelly, H.; Buckleton, J. Validation of a top-down DNA profile analysis for database searching using a fully continuous probabilistic genotyping model. Forensic Sci. Int. Genet. **2021**, 52, 102479. **[Google Scholar] [CrossRef] [PubMed]**

196. Taylor, D.; Buckleton, J.; Bright, J.-A. Factors affecting peak height variability for short tandem repeat data. Forensic Sci. Int. Genet. **2015**, 21, 126–133. **[Google Scholar] [CrossRef] [PubMed]**

197. Bright, J.-A.; Curran, J.M. Investigation into stutter ratio variability between different laboratories. Forensic Sci. Int. Genet. **2014**, 13, 79–81. **[Google Scholar] [CrossRef]**

198. Kelly, H.; Bright, J.-A.; Kruijver, M.; Cooper, S.; Taylor, D.; Duke, K.; Strong, M.; Beamer, V.; Buettner, C.; Buckleton, J. A sensitivity analysis to determine the robustness of STRmix™ with respect to laboratory calibration. Forensic Sci. Int. Genet. **2018**, 35, 113–122. **[Google Scholar] [CrossRef]**

199. Kelly, H. Developmental validation of a software implementation of a flexible framework for the assignment of likeli-hood ratios for forensic investigations. Forensic Sci. Int. Rep. **2021**, 100231. **[Google Scholar] [CrossRef]**

200. Kruijver, M.; Bright, J.-A.; Kelly, H.; Buckleton, J. Exploring the probative value of mixed DNA profiles. Forensic Sci. Int. Genet. **2019**, 41, 1–10. **[Google Scholar] [CrossRef]**

201. Taylor, D.; Kruijver, M. Combining evidence across multiple mixed DNA profiles for improved resolution of a donor when a common contributor can be assumed. Forensic Sci. Int. Genet. **2020**, 49. **[Google Scholar] [CrossRef]**

202. Kruijver, M.; Taylor, D.; Bright, J.-A. Evaluating DNA evidence possibly involving multiple (mixed) samples, common donors and related contributors. Forensic Sci. Int. Genet. **2021**, 54, 102532. **[Google Scholar] [CrossRef]**

203. Allen, P.S.; Pugh, S.N.; Bright, J.-A.; Taylor, D.A.; Curran, J.M.; Kerr, Z.; Buckleton, J.S. Relaxing the assumption of unrelatedness in the numerator and denominator of likelihood ratios for DNA mixtures. Forensic Sci. Int. Genet. **2020**, 51, 102434. **[Google Scholar] [CrossRef] [PubMed]**

204. Regulator, F.S. The Forensic Science Regulator Guidance on DNA Mixture Interpretation FSR-G-222; The Forensic Science Regulator: Birmingham, UK, 2018; pp. 1–63. **[Google Scholar]**

205. Bright, J.-A.; Taylor, D.; McGovern, C.; Cooper, S.; Russell, L.; Abarno, D.; Buckleton, J. Developmental validation of STRmix™, expert software for the interpretation of forensic DNA profiles. Forensic Sci. Int. Genet. **2016**, 23, 226–239. **[Google Scholar] [CrossRef] [PubMed]**

206. Brookes, C.; Bright, J.-A.; Harbison, S.; Buckleton, J. Characterising stutter in forensic STR multiplexes. Forensic Sci. Int. Genet. **2012**, 6, 58–63. **[Google Scholar] [CrossRef]**

207. Kelly, H.; Bright, J.-A.; Buckleton, J.S.; Curran, J.M. Identifying and modelling the drivers of stutter in forensic DNA profiles. Aust. J. Forensic Sci. **2013**, 46, 194–203. **[Google Scholar] [CrossRef]**

208. Triggs, C.; Curran, J. The sensitivity of the Bayesian HPD method to the choice of prior. Sci. Justice **2006**, 46, 169–178. **[Google Scholar] [CrossRef]**

209. Bright, J.-A.; Stevenson, K.; Curran, J.M.; Buckleton, J.S. The variability in likelihood ratios due to different mechanisms. Forensic Sci. Int. Genet. **2015**, 14, 187–190. **[Google Scholar] [CrossRef]**

210. Taylor, D.; Buckleton, J.; Bright, J.-A. Does the use of probabilistic genotyping change the way we should view sub-threshold data? Aust. J. Forensic Sci. **2017**, 49, 78–92. **[Google Scholar] [CrossRef]**

211. Russell, L.; Cooper, S.; Wivell, R.; Kerr, Z.; Taylor, D.; Buckleton, J.; Bright, J. A guide to results and diagnostics within a STRmix™ report. Wiley Interdiscip. Rev. Forensic Sci. **2019**, 1, e1354. **[Google Scholar] [CrossRef]**

212. Moretti, T.; Just, R.S.; Kehl, S.C.; Willis, L.E.; Buckleton, J.S.; Bright, J.-A.; Taylor, D..; Onorato, A.J. Internal validation of STRmix for the interpetation of single source and mixed DNA profiles. Forensic Sci. Int. Genet. **2017**, 29, 126–144. **[Google Scholar] [CrossRef]**

213. Noël, S.; Noël, J.; Granger, D.; Lefebvre, J.-F.; Séguin, D. STRmix™ put to the test: 300,000 non-contributor profiles compared to four-contributor DNA mixtures and the impact of replicates. Forensic Sci. Int. Genet. **2019**, 41, 24–31. **[Google Scholar] [CrossRef]**

214. Duke, K.R.; Myers, S.P. Systematic evaluation of STRmix™ performance on degraded DNA profile data. Forensic Sci. Int. Genet. **2019**, 44, 102174. **[Google Scholar] [CrossRef] [Green Version]**

215. Lin, M.-H.; Bright, J.-A.; Pugh, S.N.; Buckleton, J.S. The interpretation of mixed DNA profiles from a mother, father, and child trio. Forensic Sci. Int. Genet. **2019**, 44, 102175. **[Google Scholar] [CrossRef] [PubMed] [Green Version]**

216. Buckleton, J.S.; Bright, J.-A.; Gittelson, S.; Moretti, T.R.; Onorato, A.J.; Bieber, F.R.; Budowle, B.; Taylor, D.A. The Probabilistic Genotyping SoftwareSTRmix: Utility and Evidence for its Validity. J. Forensic Sci. **2018**, 64, 393–405. **[Google Scholar] [CrossRef] [PubMed]**

217. Riman, S.; Iyer, H.; Vallone, P. Exploring DNA interpretation software using the PROVEDIt dataset. Forensic Sci. Int. Genet. Suppl. Ser. **2019**, 7, 724–726. **[Google Scholar] [CrossRef]**

218. Takano, M.H. R.4368—Justice in Forensic ALGORITHMS Act of 2019; 2019. **[Google Scholar]**

219. Access to STRmix™ Software by Defence Legal Teams (“Access Policy”); 2020. **[CrossRef]**

220. Adams, N.; Koppl, R.; Krane, D.; Thompson, W.; Zabell, S. Letter to the Editor-Appropriate Standards for Verification and Validation of Probabilistic Genotyping Systems. J. Forensic Sci. **2018**, 63, 339–340. **[Google Scholar] [CrossRef] [PubMed]**

221. Software and Systems Engineering Standards Committee of the IEEE Computer Society. IEEE Standard for System, Software, and Hardware Verification and Validation IEEE Std 1012™-2016; IEEE: New York, NY, USA, 2017. **[Google Scholar]**

222. The Queen v. Clinton James Tuite. S CR 2014 007, 23 October 2017.

04 AN ANALYTICAL FRAMEWORK FOR FORENSIC DNA INTERPRETATION

1. INTRODUCTION: AN OVERVIEW

This chapter explores a framework developed by forensic scientists, including forensic DNA scientists, to assist them in analyzing and communicating their findings in a fair, strong, rational, and transparent manner. This mode of reasoning was utilized as early as the late 19th century [1]. The formalization of this process was carried out by the Case Assessment and Interpretation team of the former Forensic Science Service of England and Wales in the 1990s [2]. The technique serves as a framework for logical thinking when dealing with unclear situations, regardless of the specific forensic field. However, in this context, our emphasis is on DNA analysis. The essential basis for reasoning in all forensic science disciplines, which we regard to be a paradigm, is extensively covered in various books [3,4,5,6,7,8] and interpretation guides [9,10,11,12].

2. INDETERMINACY IN THE CRIMINAL TRIAL

Within the framework of a criminal trial, there are only a limited number of elements that are definitively established as true: the court possesses an ambiguous understanding of crucial contested occurrences, yet it is imperative to render a conclusion. Disputed events may involve determining the paternity of a child, such as if "Mr. Smith is the biological father," or establishing the origin of blood found at a crime scene, such as whether "Ms. Jones is the source." In such instances, the court will enlist the assistance of DNA experts. Frequently, the court will hold high expectations and want unequivocal responses. Due to the CSI effect [13], individuals may have the misconception that DNA is distinct and hence capable of identifying the biological father of a child or determining the source of blood/DNA discovered at a crime scene. Nevertheless, the current approach lacks the capability to formally determine the identity of the child's father or the source of the trace. Only a limited number of forensic findings may be unequivocally presented as "facts" and allow for absolute certainty. Is this an issue of concern?

We contend that uncertainty is indeed present, and as elucidated by Dennis Lindley [14], instead of disregarding or attempting to quash it, the optimal strategy is to devise a rational method for handling it. This is achieved by utilizing the concept of probability, which offers a consistent and rational foundation for making decisions when faced with uncertainty.

3. THE FUNCTIONS OF A DNA SCIENTIST AND VARIOUS METHODS OF REPORTING (FACTUAL, INVESTIGATIVE, EVALUATIVE)

The information provided by DNA scientists might either be based on factual evidence or presented as subjective opinions. (In this context, we are discussing viewpoints that are formed using expertise and professional analysis, specifically, conclusions gained from forensic observations).

A factual report provides a detailed account of the actions taken and the observations made. The scientist refrains from drawing any conclusions or expressing any subjective interpretations regarding the significance of the findings. Objective reporting is suitable when conclusions are unambiguous. An illustrative instance would involve a report detailing the DNA profile of an individual, enabling its inclusion in a nationwide DNA repository. If the analysis of the observations requires specialized expertise, it would be deceptive to only display the information without providing an expert evaluation. For instance, suppose the scientist solely provided the account of the findings from a preliminary blood test. Merely asserting that the item underwent blood testing and yielded a positive outcome may lead to potential misinterpretation. It is important to note that a positive presumptive test for blood does not definitively prove that the substance is blood, especially during the investigative phase [15]. Likewise, if a report in a paternity case states that the child and the claimed father have one allele in common for all except one genetic marker, without providing an interpretation, it could be prone to misinterpretation.

Forensic scientists' perspectives can be categorized into two main types: "investigative" and "evaluative" [16]. It is important to clarify that forensic scientists do not engage in police investigations or work as investigators. The purpose of this differentiation is to emphasize that the inquiries faced during the inquiry and the legal processes typically take on a dissimilar structure. This results in a disparity in the inferential procedure [16,17] employed in formulating the opinion, which subsequently aids in addressing these inquiries. Table 1 illustrates many tasks that exemplify the distinct roles undertaken by DNA scientists. It is important to emphasize that there are instances where it can be challenging to clearly distinguish different functions.

Table 1. Differences between investigative and evaluative roles.

Investigative Role	Evaluative Role
Tends to be crime-focused.	Tends to be suspect-focused.
Tends to be at the beginning of the criminal justice process.	Tends to be at the culmination of the criminal justice process.
Helps the investigator make decisions.	Helps the court take decisions.
Type of questions: What happened? What is this? Who could be involved?	Type of questions: Is Mr Smith the source of the DNA or is it someone else? Did Mr Smith drive the car or was he a passenger?
Suggests explanations for the observations and gives guidance.	Evaluates the observations (i.e., results) given at least two mutually exclusive propositions.
Open-ended process.	More formal and structured.
Explanations need to encompass all realistic possibilities to avoid bias and avoid potentially misleading the inquiry.	Assigned probabilities should be calibrated; rates of misleading opinions should be low and documented.

An investigative opinion is formed when explanations are created to justify the observations. They are typically, but not solely, created when there is no person of interest (POI) involved. An expert analysis might be provided in a scenario where a potential rape victim lacks a distinct memory of the incident and no semen is detected. Possible reasons for the lack of sperm presence may include the use of a condom, absence of ejaculation, complete elimination of all traces of sperm, utilization of a vaginal douche, or the absence of sexual intercourse. The scientist's list of explanations may not be comprehensive, as there could be other potential explanations that have not been taken into account or have not been generated. These explanations are not necessarily mutually exclusive, meaning that multiple explanations could be true. For instance, it is possible that a condom was worn and the victim used a vaginal douche. Another instance of an investigative opinion could arise while conducting a DNA study on an athlete's urine to investigate potential doping. Consider a scenario where the DNA profile obtained from the urine sample does not match the DNA profile of the athlete, but there are multiple alleles that are common to both profiles. If no mistake has occurred, the athlete cannot be the originator of the urine in such a scenario. One plausible hypothesis for the results could be that a nearby family member is the origin of the urine. This could be proposed as a potential line of inquiry.

As previously stated, the delineation of responsibilities and the many forms of expertise offered by forensic scientists can be complex and ambiguous at times. Evaluating the significance of a DNA comparison for investigative purposes is quite justifiable. In situations where there is no suspect linked to the site, a database search is commonly conducted. The objective is to furnish investigation leads and information regarding the potential origin of the DNA. One key distinction is that during the early phases of a case, there may be an absence of a suspect or defendant. If the scientist intends to utilize the data in a legal setting, they must consider at least one option, such as the defense's interpretation of the facts. This can be derived from the defendant's statements, but it is not mandatory for the defense to provide information. It can also be based on case information obtained during the investigation, such as the defendant and the victim working at the same place. Additionally, it can be based on a plausible alternative that can be reasonably assessed for credibility by a judicial body. When there is a defendant involved in a case, scientists should provide an assessment of their findings, which should be based on a set of case-specific propositions (sometimes known as "allegations" or "hypotheses") and the surrounding circumstances. As per Willis et al. [9], evaluative reports for court use should be generated only if two specific conditions are fulfilled:

- The forensic practitioner has been asked by a mandating authority or party to examine and/or compare material (typically recovered trace material with reference material from known potential sources).
- The forensic practitioner seeks to evaluate the results with respect to particular competing propositions set by the specific case circumstances or as indicated by the mandating authority.

4. GUIDELINES AND PRINCIPLES FOR PRODUCING EVALUATIVE REPORTS

When choosing the approach for the evaluation of forensic findings, there is a need to first define what the desired properties of the interpretation framework are [**16,19**]. The desiderata of any approach to interpretation have been proposed as: balance, logic, transparency, and robustness. Not unsurprisingly, these have since been included in several guidelines on evaluative reporting [**9,10,12,20**]. This is not to say that investigative opinions do not have these properties. However, the principles of interpretation [**4,21,22**] apply mainly for forming evaluative opinions. This is because in the early stages of an investigation, there may be very little case information, little in the way of suggestions for what happened, and no suspect. In that case, it would not be possible to consider alternatives put forward by, for example, a defence team. Below, we consider only the principles for evaluative reporting as applied to issues relating to a POI when their case proceeds to court.

4.1. First Principle of Evaluative Reporting: Importance of Case Information

The first principle for forming evaluative opinions tells us that interpretation takes place in a framework of circumstances. Note that this is also true for our choice regarding the methods of analysis: we would need to know what the issue is. One can distinguish between aspects of the circumstances that are task-pertinent and task-irrelevant. The role of the forensic scientist can be divided in two parts: (1) understanding the uncertainties facing the fact finder and (2) helping the fact finder to resolve them. They will thus first need information to identify the issue(s) with which forensic science can help. Then, the scientist should devise and agree on an effective case strategy, including an assessment of the possible outcomes and their value, to help address the issue. Once the examinations have been completed and observations have been made, scientists will assign a probability to the specific observations, given propositions that are meaningful in the case and given the available information (task-pertinent case circumstances, but also expert knowledge). The probability they assign will be personal and conditional in the sense that it depends on what the individual knows, is told, and what is assumed. For a DNA scientist, case circumstances such as whether the persons of interest have legitimate access to the objects/persons/premises, what they say about the alleged incident in question, the activities that are alleged to have taken place, and the timelines, are all examples of task-pertinent information that will impact the value of the results. Examples of information that is not relevant for the DNA scientist and is potentially harmful because of bias could include (1) there is eyewitness evidence that points toward the POI, (2) there is a partial finger-mark that supports the proposition that a specified person touched the object, or (3) the POI had first confessed to the offence but later retracted that admission. As task-pertinent case information impacts the value of the findings, it is essential to give a signal that should the framework of circumstances change, it will be necessary to review the interpretation. We discuss examples of caveats in **Section 12**.

4.2. Second Principle of Evaluative Reporting: Two or More Competing Propositions Should Be Considered

To be balanced, when assessing the value of biological results, one must consider at least two propositions (i.e., statements that are either true or false, and that can be affirmed or denied). They will be formulated in pairs based on the case information (we discuss proposition formulation in **Section 7**) and should represent the views of the two parties as understood at the time of the writing of the report.

Propositions need to be mutually exclusive (if one is true, the other is not) and, if possible, exhaustive in the context of the case (i.e., one should not consider all propositions as default, but only those that are of interest to the court [**23**]). It is not feasible nor desirable to consider absolute exhaustiveness, and practice can proceed with an acceptable coverage, that is without the omission of a relevant proposition [**24**]. It is important to ensure that the propositions to be considered are based on case information. If, the case information changes and it is shown that the propositions considered are not meaningful anymore, a new evaluation will need to be performed and a new written statement issued.

4.3. Third Principle of Evaluative Reporting: Scientists Need to Assign Their Probability of the Findings, Not Their Probability of the (Alleged) Facts

To respect logic, forensic scientists shall assign the probability of their findings given the truth of propositions, not the probability of the propositions given the findings. It may seem obvious that scientists need to focus on the value of the findings. However, it is not a straightforward endeavour, and many scientists are tempted to give an opinion on propositions. An example could be the doping case discussed earlier: while the DNA scientist is in a position to assign the probability of the results given the urine is from the athlete's sister, it is not possible—based on the results only—to assign the probability that the urine is from the athlete's sister. To do so, one would need to consider all the information in the case (for example that the athlete has a sister).

4.4. Forth Principle of Evaluative Reporting: The Value of the Findings Is Expressed by the Ratio of the Probability of the Scientific Observations Given the Case Information and Given That Each, in Turn, of the Propositions Are True

To measure how the new evidence (e.g., DNA results) affects one's uncertainty about the proposition (e.g., the urine is from the sister) considering conditioning information, one can use a model which is known as Bayes' rule. It is a mathematical idealisation that the belief about a set of propositions is updated based on the (weight of the) evidence [25]. Note that Bayes' rule is seldom used in court (except maybe for paternity cases). Generally, the different pieces of evidence are combined intuitively by the fact finder without assigning any figure. This is done, for instance, when referring to "corroborating evidence". Notwithstanding, Bayes' rule provides a very useful framework for understanding how DNA results may be presented in a logical, transparent, and impartial way in legal proceedings.

Bayes' rule may be depicted in a format known as the odds form of Bayes' rule (Equation (1)). Odds are the ratio of the probability of the proposition being true divided by the probability of it being false.

$$\underbrace{\frac{\Pr(H_\mathrm{p}|I)}{\Pr(H_\mathrm{d}|I)}}_{\text{prior odds}} \times \underbrace{\frac{\Pr(E|H_\mathrm{p}, I)}{\Pr(E|H_\mathrm{d}, I)}}_{\text{likelihood ratio}} = \underbrace{\frac{\Pr(H_\mathrm{p}|E, I)}{\Pr(H_\mathrm{d}|E, I)}}_{\text{posterior odds}} \tag{1}$$

where "Pr" denotes probability, "H_p" the proposition summarising the prosecution's point of view, and "H_d" the proposition summarising the defence's point of view. The letter "I" stands for the information mentioned in the section on the first principle of interpretation, and "E" (for evidence) represents the scientific observations (i.e., results or findings). The vertical bar "|" is called the conditioning bar and can be read as "given" or "assuming that".

One of the most important lessons that can be learned from Bayes' rule, as depicted in this form, is the nature of the roles played by different actors in the judicial process. It can be seen there are three terms in the equation, and the important question is: who takes responsibility for each of these three?

The first term represents prior odds, where the probability of each proposition given the information is considered. Assessing the allegations or the facts in issue is, without doubt, the duty of the fact finders. The last term also represents odds, which again relate to the probability of the propositions, but this time considering in addition the DNA results (or other forensic observations). These are said to be posterior odds, as they represent one's updated belief after knowing the results (or the evidence) "E".

The second term is the likelihood ratio (LR for short), which is a measure of the value of the findings. It is defined in terms of the ratio of two conditional probabilities: (i) the probability of the findings given that one proposition is true and given the conditioning information; and (ii) the probability of the findings given that the other proposition is true and given the conditioning information. The two conditional probabilities forming the LR may be assigned either on the basis of (published) data and/or the general knowledge (base) of the forensic practitioner. It is a measure of the relative strength of support that particular findings give to one proposition against a stated alternative [**3,4,7,26,27**]. A LR is a ratio of probabilities; thus, by definition, it is a number (as probabilities are numbers between 0 and 1). If the LR is 1, results are uninformative, and they do not support one proposition over the other. If the LR is larger than one, results support the first proposition compared to the alternative. If the LR is smaller than 1 (e.g., 0.001), then results support the alternative proposition over the first proposition. (It is sometimes reported that LRs can be negative, that is smaller than 0. This is incorrect. LRs theoretically can range between 0 and infinity. Log(LR) can be negative, but not LRs).

The focus of the LR is always on the findings, never on the proposition. It should be seen as a reinforcing or weakening factor in the perception of the truth of propositions that existed without the technical findings. This factor measures the change produced by the findings on the odds of the fact in issue being true. (In the literature, this factor is also more generally called a Bayes Factor (BF). With simple propositions, a BF reduces to a LR, as discussed in [**28**]. However, when multiple propositions are used, the BF does not reduce to the LR: it is a ratio of weighted likelihoods). Because the focus of the LR is on the scientific result, it is clearly in the domain and remit of the scientists. It allows them to provide assistance through the use of their expertise to assign probabilities for their observations given the truth of the competing propositions.

In addition, without considering Bayes' rule, it appears quite sensible to say that scientists must give their opinion on the results and not on the disputed facts in issue. It is for the factfinder to render opinions on facts, and for DNA scientists to give the value of their results. When DNA scientists give their opinion on the alleged facts (or propositions) based only on the value of their results (i.e., LR), then they are said to transpose the conditional [**26,27**]. This is a very common error of logic and appears in many forms [**29**]. It has been called the "prosecutor's fallacy" [**30**], but it is just as frequently to be found on the lips of defenders, judges, and journalists. It is more properly known as the "fallacy of the transposed conditional" because it is a matter of confusion between two conditional probabilities: the probability of the findings given the propositions and the probability of the propositions given the findings. One can erroneously transpose the conditional when giving an opinion on a single probability or on a ratio of probabilities.

5. AVOIDING THE TRANSPOSED CONDITIONAL

Not transposing the conditional is difficult, and it would be satisfying if one could avoid it just by knowing about Bayes' rule and reporting a LR. It is so natural for the human mind to want an opinion on (alleged) facts, that it takes time and training to avoid this fallacy. There are several strategies that one can adopt to avoid this error of logic. Some of these were developed at the time when the Case Assessment Interpretation team from the former Forensic Science Service of England and Wales was training all their reporting officers; these are outlined in [**6**] and summarised below.

The first thing to investigate is whether the opinion pertains to the DNA results or to the proposition. The second aspect to check is that the sentence contains a word such as "if" or "given" and that these are associated with the propositions. If one has pen and paper, it is always a good idea to use notation, as spotting an error is then easier. Another coping strategy is to memorise correct and incorrect statements. When in doubt, one should re-phrase the statement of opinion along the lines of the correct format. Another strategy to ensure that there is no transposed conditional is to begin one's sentence with the term "The DNA results" and add the probabilistic statement and the conditioning.

A lot of practice is needed to avoid inadvertently transposing the conditional: we discuss examples of incorrect formulations in **Table 2**. One should remember to state both propositions, as a LR is relative.

Table 2. Statements with transposed conditionals and their associated correct statement.

Sr.	Incorrect or Ambiguous Statement (A)	Correct Statement (B)	Notation
1.	Given the DNA results, it is a billion times more likely that the DNA is from Ms Jones than from an unknown unrelated person.	The results are a billion times more probable if the DNA is from Ms Jones rather than if it is from an unknown unrelated person.	A: $Pr(H_p\|E,I)/Pr(H_d\|E,I)$ B: $Pr(E\|H_p,I)/Pr(E\|H_d,I)$ Note: In A, the use of the term "that"is always suspicious.
2.	The likelihood ratio calculated the probability that the DNA evidence observed in the profile originated from the applicant, rather than another person chosen at random from the Australian Caucasian population. (Sometimes, scientists will write "the probability that a randomly selected person would have this DNA profile is 1 in a billion.". However, the alternative source of the DNA is not "selected at random", but rather an unknown person, related or not to the persons of interest depending on the case).	The likelihood ratio represents the ratio of two probabilities: the probability of the result given that the DNA is from the applicant and the probability of the result given the DNA is from an unknown person from the Australian Caucasian population.	A: $Pr(H_p\|E,I)/Pr(H_d\|E,I)$ B: $Pr(E\|H_p,I)/Pr(E\|H_d,I)$ Note: a word such as « if » or « given » should always be present when using conditional probabilities.
3.	Participants of the proficiency test were asked whether their DNA results more probably originated due to the disputed activity or social interactions. (In the exercise, it read as "Participants were required to consider each DNA profile separately and assess whether they originated either due to primary or secondary transfer" however, it is best not to put the word transfer in the propositions as transfer/ persistence and recovery are factors that scientists will take into account in their evaluation.)	Participants of the proficiency test were asked whether their DNA results were more probable given the disputed activity than given social interactions.	A: $Pr(H_p\|E,I)/Pr(H_d\|E,I)$ B: $Pr(E\|H_p,I)/Pr(E\|H_d,I)$ Note: In A, the absence of the term "if [the proposition]"or "given [the proposition]"is a clue that the statement needs review.

Sr.	Incorrect or Ambiguous Statement (A)	Correct Statement (B)	Notation
4.	The probability that the DNA comes from a random unrelated person is one in a million.	The probability of the results if the DNA comes from a random unrelated person is one in a million.	A:$Pr(H_d\|I)$ B: $Pr(E\|H_d,I)$ Note: statement B is correct (not transposed) but not balanced since $Pr(E\|H_p,I)$ is missing.
5.	Considering the genetic characteristics of the trace, it is a million times more likely that Mr S is the source of the DNA rather than his uncle.	The genetic characteristics of the trace are a million times more likely if Mr S is the source of the DNA rather than his uncle.	A: $Pr(H_p\|E,I)/ Pr(H_d\|E,I)$ B: $Pr(E\|H_p,I)/Pr(E\|H_d,I)$ Note: in statement A, the phrase "considering the genetic characteristics of the trace" implies that the DNA characteristics represent the conditioning information (thus are present behind the conditional bar). However, the conditioning information should be the propositions and the information; the term "given" should be associated with the propositions and information, not with the results.
6.	As explained by this Court in Tuite [No 1] for each DNA sample where the suspect cannot be excluded as a contributor, a ratio was calculated which shows how much more likely it is that the suspect was the source of the DNA (or a contributor to it) than that some other person chosen at random from the population was the source (or a contributor).	As explained by this Court in Tuite [No 1] for each DNA sample where the suspect cannot be excluded as a contributor, a ratio was calculated which shows how much more likely the DNA results would be given the suspect were the source of the DNA (or a contributor to it) than given an unknown person from the population were the source (or a contributor).	A: LR defined incorrectly as $Pr(H_p\|E,I)/ Pr(H_d\|E,I)$ B: LR is defined as LR = $Pr(E\|H_p,I)/ Pr(E\|H_d,I)$

Sr.	Incorrect or Ambiguous Statement (A)	Correct Statement (B)	Notation
7.	The most favoured proposition is that S is the source of the DNA rather than an unknown unrelated person.	The DNA results strongly support the proposition that S, rather than an unknown unrelated person, is the source of the DNA.	Note: in A the use the term favour could be read as saying the first proposition is most likely. The term "support" is more appropriate.

All incorrect/ambiguous statements originate from statements, judgements [**31**], or scientific communications. The last statement "The most favoured proposition is that S is the source of the DNA" is ambiguous: it could lead the reader to think that the proposition which is the most favoured is the most probable. This is not the case, as depending on prior odds, the most probable proposition might not be the one that is the most supported by the results. An example is shown in **Table 3** using Bayes' rule. One can see that with a LR of 1 million and very low prior odds of 1 to 10 million, the posterior probability of the first proposition would be 9% (or 0.09); the most favoured or most likely proposition would be the alternative.

Table 3. Posterior probabilities with the same LR of a million, but different prior odds. In the first case, although results support the first proposition, the most favoured proposition is the alternative, with a probability of 91%. When prior odds are equal to the LR, the probability of the proposition is 50%. If prior odds are 1:1, then posterior odds are equal to the LR.

Prior Odds	LR	Posterior Odds	Posterior Probability of the First Proposition	Posterior Probability of the Alternative
1 to 10 million	1×10^6	1 to 10	9%	91%
1 to 1 million	1×10^6	1 to 1	50%	50%
1 to 10,000	1×10^6	100 to 1	99%	1%

One can note that, if the prior probability of the first proposition is zero, then whatever the LR, the posterior probability is zero as well. It would be rare to have this situation. According to [**14**], when assigning our probabilities, we should admit the possibility that we might be wrong. If we do, this rule denies probabilities of 1 or 0. (This rule is called Cromwell's rule, named after Oliver Cromwell, who said to the Church of Scotland, "I beseech you, in the bowels of Christ, think it possible you may be mistaken". Calling it Cromwell's rule is attributed to Dennis Lindley). The probability of an event given K is 1 if, and only if, K logically implies the truth of E (and of zero if K implies the falsity of E). To provide an illustration where there can be a prior probability of zero, we revisit the case where the issue was whether the urine was from the athlete or not. You will remember that the DNA was different from the athlete's DNA, but that the donor and the athlete shared many alleles. In that case, it was reported that the DNA profile comparison was of the order of a billion times more likely if the person's sister was the source of the urine, rather than if an unrelated person was. The DNA scientist reported that the probability that the urine originated from the sister was 99.9999999%. In those conditions, they conclude that it was practically proven that the urine was from the sister. This prompted the athlete's lawyer to write a letter to say that there was only a minor problem in that reasoning: the athlete did not have a sister (but she did have a half-sister). In this case, the probability of the proposition is zero. This also shows why it is best for scientists to give an opinion on the results, however large their LR. It is generally not considered the scientists' remit to give an opinion on facts (except, as mentioned earlier, in some countries for paternity cases), which is the case if they give posterior probabilities.

To calculate posterior probabilities using Bayes' rule in odds form (Equation (1)), one multiplies the prior odds by the LR. This gives us posterior odds. If the odds are a to b, to obtain the probability of the first proposition, one divides a by (a + b). If the odds are, for example, 1:1, the probability of the proposition is 1 divided by 2, thus 0.50 (or 50%, as probabilities can also be expressed as percentages).

It should be noted that, when being extra careful about not transposing the conditional, some think that it is incorrect to say "the results support the first proposition rather than the second". The use of the word "support" in this context was proposed in a manner analogous to H. Jeffreys [**32**]. It does not indicate that one proposition is more likely than the other, only that the results are more probable if the first proposition is true than if the alternative is. Because it is important to indicate what our results mean and do not mean, we recommend outlining this point in our statements.

6. HIERARCHY OF PROPOSITIONS

The concept of a hierarchy of propositions [**33**] applies to all forensic disciplines. It was developed initially for evaluative rather than investigative opinions, and one will note that the examples of propositions given in the early Case Assessment and Interpretation (CAI) publications were generally suspect-focused. Over time, the CAI development team found that the concept of a hierarchy of issues and propositions was equally applicable to investigative issues [**16**]. The classification of propositions into three main levels (source, activity, and offence) allows forensic scientists to contextualise the results, to consider the factors in their evaluation and to communicate to the client the purpose of the proposed examinations. The demarcation between the levels is not meant to be rigid, and it is recognised that sometimes levels will be difficult to distinguish. The levels simply provide a model framework that helps scientists to organise their thinking, actions, and decisions. The important point to stress to practitioners is: do not try to force all the issues you will encounter into one of the levels of the framework. Instead, just specify clearly in words the issue, and hence the propositions to consider. If the issue and propositions then fall neatly into one of the categories (i.e., one of the levels), so much the better, but do not worry if the issue/propositions do not seem to fit one of the categories. The important thing is that you have clearly specified the issue, with which the examinations can help, both for yourself and for the factfinders.

Table 4. Evaluative examples of pairs of mutually exclusive propositions at different levels in the hierarchy that DNA scientists could contribute to addressing provided they have knowledge that is needed but which otherwise would be unavailable to the court.

Level	Question/Issue	Results	Example of Pairs of Propositions
Source	Is the POI the source of the body fluid?	DNA profiling comparison.	Mr A is the source of the blood. An unknown unrelated person is the source of the blood.
Sub-source	Is the POI the source of the DNA?		Mr A is the source of the DNA. An unknown unrelated person is the source of the DNA.
Sub-sub-source	Is the POI the source of the part of the mixture?		Mr A is the major contributor of the DNA mixture. An unknown unrelated person is the major contributor of the DNA mixture.
Activity	Did the POI do the activity?	Presence/absence of DNA at different locations. Quantity/quality of the DNA. (DNA profiling comparison) *. Presumptive tests. Multiple traces from same activity.	Mr A and Ms B had penile-vaginal intercourse. Mr A and Ms B only had social activities as described in the case information. Mr Smith was the driver and Mr Jones the passenger at the relevant time. Mr Jones was the driver and Mr Smith the passenger at the relevant time.
Offence	Is the POI the offender?	Multiple traces possibly resulting from different activities compared to Mr A. Presence/absence of DNA. Quantity/quality of the DNA. (DNA profiling comparison) *. Presumptive tests.	Mr A is the burglar (in the sense of "Mr A did the specified activities that the burglar has allegedly done, as specified in the paragraph on case information"). Mr A has nothing to do with the burglary.
* In some cases, considering whether or not the DNA is from the POI can have an impact on the evaluation.			

6.1. Issue with Which the Forensic Scientist Can Help: Is Mr Smith's the Source of the DNA/Biological Material?

Initially, the proposal hierarchy indicated that it was only feasible to acquire a DNA profile from bodily fluids that were available in rather substantial amounts. Under those circumstances, it is reasonable to infer that the DNA profile originated from an identifiable bodily fluid, such as blood. This premise was called into doubt with the introduction of more refined procedures. This resulted in the emergence of additional levels in addressing the question of the source, namely the DNA level (or sub-source level) and the DNA contributor level (or sub-sub-source level [34]). These levels are relevant in cases where the question pertains to whether an individual is the source of a specific portion of the DNA mixture, such as a significant component. Below, we explore the circumstances in which it is appropriate to select source-level propositions or their corresponding sub-levels.

6.1.1. Source-Level Propositions

Source-level propositions are adequate given two conditions: first, the issue should be whether a given person is the source of the material. Second, there should be no risk for the court to misinterpret the findings in the context of the alleged activities. This would typically be the case when the material is found in such a quantity that there is (i) no need to consider its presence for reasons other than the alleged activity (i.e., it will be accepted by the fact finder that the material is relevant), and (ii) that the nature of the material can be safely assumed. The following example is adapted from [**9**], illustrating when considering the results of a DNA comparison given source-level propositions is not misleading:

"A large pool of fresh red bloodlike material is recovered at the point of entry at a burglary scene and the circumstances suggest it has originated from the offender(s), whomever they may be. A sample is delivered to the laboratory for DNA analysis. Combination of a positive presumptive test, large quantity and appearance allows the scientist to safely assume that it would be agreed that the stain is blood. The defendant, Mr D., says that he has never been in the premises and denies that the blood at the scene is from him. The set of propositions can be (1) the bloodstain came from the defendant and (2) the bloodstain came from an unknown individual." Assuming that the nature of the material will not be contested, the same term, "bloodstain", can be used in both propositions. It is sometimes believed that source-level propositions can be formulated when the nature of the material (e.g., blood, semen, saliva, cellular material) is disputed and that this accommodates consideration of the probability of presumptive tests. However, it does not as the probability of observing a positive (or a negative) result for the presumptive test would be equivalent whether the blood is from Mr D or from someone else. Therefore, if the nature of the material is disputed, it is, in general, more meaningful to consider activity-level propositions [**11**]: these will take into account the results of presumptive tests as well as the transfer, persistence, and the presence of the material as background (i.e., material from an unknown source present for unknown reasons).

6.1.2. Sub-Source-Level Propositions

The advent of highly sensitive methods has made it possible to produce DNA profiles from very small quantities of biological material [**35**]. With invisible or small stains, the nature of the material from which the DNA profile is produced is often unknown. In such cases, if the issue is who is the source of the DNA, one can assess the results of a DNA comparison given sub-source propositions (i.e., the source of the DNA, not of a given body fluid). These are especially useful for producing investigative leads. As mentioned in [**10**], one can use a LR in both the investigative and the evaluative phase. The main difference is that in the evaluation phase, there will generally be a suspect/defendant around whom the issues and propositions will be defined. In this situation, it will be necessary to take into account an alternative proposition, typically the defence's view of events, if that has been communicated to the scientist. This person may, for example, mention that they know the victim. Again, in such cases, assessing the results given activity-level propositions will generally be more meaningful. However, the DNA scientist operates in "investigative mode" where, for example, a database search is carried out because there is no suspect for the crime. Here, in the initial phase, what is of interest is to provide information about who could be the source of the DNA. An example of sub-source propositions would be: "The DNA is from candidate X" or "The DNA is from an unknown person". If the aim is to produce a useful lead, the person will not have been arrested yet, and de facto, the scientist will have been provided with no alternative proposition or information. The person making the investigative decision (here, for example, to arrest the candidate or not) will not be the court but, in some jurisdictions, an investigating magistrate, or in others, a police investigator. When there is very little case information, the value of the comparison needs to be much higher for the person making the decision (e.g., to arrest the candidate or not). In addition, for cost effectiveness, one may also want to avoid investigating many false leads. This explains why larger LRs will often be needed for investigative purposes.

6.1.3. Sub-Sub-Source-Level Propositions

If the issue is whether a POI is the major (or minor) contributor of a DNA mixture, then one can consider sub-sub-source propositions [**34**]. An example of sub-sub-source propositions would be: "Mr A is the major contributor to the DNA mixture" or "An unknown person is the major contributor to the DNA mixture". If it is important that the POI is compatible with the major component, then this generally is an indication that the issue lies in the activities and that scientists can add value by considering activity-level propositions. If the relative quantity is not an important factor, then sub-source propositions are generally preferred to sub-sub-source, as the former allow accounting for all the results (and not only part of the mixture).

6.2. Issue with Which the Forensic Scientist Can Help: Did Mr Smith Perform the Activities Alleged by the Prosecution or Those Alleged by the Defence?

The next level in the hierarchy of propositions is the activity level. The evaluation of given activity-level propositions generally involves assessment of the extrinsic characteristics (e.g., quality of the DNA profile, relative quantity of DNA, where the DNA was sampled from) and should be considered when transfer, persistence, or background have a significant impact on the understanding of the value of the findings in the context of relevant case circumstances and the alleged activities [**9**,**11**,**36**]. Depending on the case and the information content of the profile, the source of the DNA might be contested or agreed. When the source of the DNA is not contested, but the activities leading to the deposition of the DNA are, one does not necessarily need to consider the source of the DNA anymore For investigative purposes, the DNA profile of the trace and of the person still need to be compared. To determine the value of this comparison, one will assign a LR given sub-source-level propositions. However, if there is no dispute and thus only one proposition (i.e., the DNA is from the POI), this LR value is not relevant. It is the LR given activity-level propositions that is meaningful. It is sometimes believed that to consider activity-level propositions, one needs to agree on the source of the DNA. This is not true: in this type of evaluation, one can consider both possibilities (i.e., that the DNA is from the POI or not). If so, one has associated sub-source propositions. However, depending on the rarity of the DNA profile, this consideration will have little impact on the value of the findings given activity-level propositions. Indeed, as indicated by the England and Wales Court of Appeal [**37**]: "It makes the task of the jury so much easier if they do not have to plough through and listen to evidence that is simply not in dispute." Let us look at an example where the issue is one of activity. Assume a stolen car crashed into a group of pedestrians, killing one and injuring others. Two people escaped from inside the car and ran away.

Acting on information, the police quickly arrested two men, Mr Smith and Mr Jones. Both admitted to being in the car at the time of the collision, but both denied being the driver, instead accusing the other of being the driver. The issue would be: "Did Mr Smith or Mr Jones drive the car at the relevant time?". The activity-level propositions would be: "Mr Smith drove the car at the relevant time and Mr Jones was the passenger." The alternative would be the reverse: "Mr Jones was the driver and Mr Smith the passenger".

As both the driver's and the passenger's airbags were activated at the time of the collision, an examination of the airbags for biological material could help to address the issue. Another typical case where sub-source-level propositions might not be meaningful, would be when a person has legitimate access to the object or person on which examinations have been performed (e.g., a gun found in the POI's car). In such cases, the source of the DNA (i.e., the person) may well not be contested (which does not mean that the DNA does not need to be analysed, only that, depending on the results, these may not need to be assessed). It is worth noting that activity-level propositions allow for the assessment of the absence of evidence [**33**,**38**]. The saying "The absence of (matching) evidence is not evidence of absence" is not always true. To know when it is, formal evaluation is needed. (As much as possible we try and avoid the term match for two reasons: first, laypersons believe that saying there is a match means that the DNA is from the person; second, scientists can at best state they were unable to see any difference they judge relevant. This does not mean that the two profiles are identical: indeed, two separate identities cannot be identical because, given sufficient resolution, all distinct entities are distinguishable from each other, even when two items come from the same source). Activity-level propositions also facilitate the combination of DNA results from different items that were touched because of the same activity (e.g., the two airbags, and possibly the steering wheel, in the example above). Finally, one should note that sometimes it may be difficult to distinguish offence from activity. As an example, a proposition such as "Mr A stabbed Mr B." or "Ms A shot Mr B." may be considered either as an offence and/or an activity-level proposition. Remember, as indicated previously, the lines of demarcation in the hierarchy should not be seen as rigid: it is meant to organise thinking, actions, and decisions.

6.3. Issue with Which the Forensic Scientist Can Help: Is Mr Smith the Offender or Does He Have Nothing to Do with the Offence?

The issue for the court is always the offence, which is at the top level of the hierarchy. An example of a pair of competing offence-level propositions could be: "Mr Smith committed the burglary" and "Mr Smith had nothing to do with the burglary". It should be remembered that propositions and case information are closely entwined so that in the case information, more detail would be given indicating, for example, that Mr Smith visited the jewellery store 3 days prior to the burglary. It is sometimes cautioned that offence-level propositions are not the domain of the scientist but of the court. Although this is true, this statement applies to all levels of propositions, as scientists offer their opinion on the results and not on propositions (or else, they would transpose the conditional). This is valid whatever the level, and offence level is not special in that sense. However, the evaluation of findings given offence-level propositions is special in the sense that it is rare that forensic scientists add value by considering propositions at the offence level, compared to a level lower in the hierarchy. Indeed, in many cases, the difference between activities and offence lies in the intent or consent, and in that case, obviously, biological results cannot help discriminating between these two levels. A typical case where DNA scientists cannot add value would be if they considered "rape" instead of "vaginal/penile penetration or consensual sex" [**39**]. Biological results do not give any information on the issue of consent, pre-meditation, nor intent, thus DNA scientists cannot help the court address those issues. In these situations, DNA scientists should not rise in the hierarchy, as they would not use any specialised knowledge, nor add value, when considering the offence rather than the activities.

However, the consideration of offence-level propositions allows adding value when there are multiple forensic findings that need to be combined by a forensic scientist. Such a case could be a burglary implying multiple activities: for example, breaking glass, jumping out of window, opening a safe. In this situation, offence-level propositions would enable combining the different results (e.g., shoe-marks, fibres, and DNA profile comparisons). The list of the activities would be very similar to what constitutes an offence in that case. Offence-level propositions have also been proposed to explore the impact of other factors such as relevance [**40,41**].

7. FORMULATION OF PROPOSITIONS

Within a forensic case, people (e.g., the police, the defence, or witnesses) will make various claims or statements. These are either true or false and can be affirmed or refuted. It is once they are formalised by the scientist that these claims will be referred to as propositions. (Some people use the term hypothesis to designate propositions used for the evaluation of findings. We prefer to keep this term for situations where scientific experiments are performed to "test" a hypothesis. As discussed in [**3**], this enables distinguishing between both concepts, and it is only when a proposition is formulated for empirical testing that we will call it a hypothesis). As described in [**33**], propositions need to be mutually exclusive (if one is true, the other is false) and formulated in pairs (e.g., views put forward by the parties to the cases) against a background of information and assumptions. They should also be amenable to a reasoned assignment of credibility by a judicial body [**9**]. There may be more than two propositions, but in the context of a criminal trial there will be two views. For the formalisation of propositions, the basic criterion is that they should be formulated in such a way that it is reasonable for the scientist to address a question of the form: "What is the probability of the observations given this proposition and given the framework of circumstances?" [**12**].

There are other important criteria to keep in mind when formulating propositions. For example, propositions are about causes and as such will be assessed by the decision maker (e.g., factfinder). If propositions contain factors that are to be considered in the evaluation, these factors cannot be assessed by the scientists anymore: being part of the proposition, they will be assessed by the decision maker. Formulation of propositions needs to adhere to specific criteria and appropriate phrasing. As it is a difficult task that requires expertise, the DNA scientist is in the best position to formalise the propositions, and one cannot expect that prosecution or defence formally define the so-called "Prosecution or Defence propositions" themselves. (The defence proposition may be compound. For example, if the alternative is that the DNA is from an unknown person, this unknown person may be unrelated or a sibling or a cousin). These terms are used to indicate that the propositions represent the views of these two parties as understood from the case information available (i.e., that the propositions were formulated against the background of information available from the parties). However, should one of these not accept the propositions considered by the scientist, a new evaluation will be needed. Ideally the formulation of propositions should be discussed between the parties and the DNA scientist before doing the work.

There have been many publications on the formulation of propositions [**10,11, 18,23,33,42,43,44,45,46**]. In **Table 5**, we give the criteria to which they should adhere and examples of poorly worded propositions, and their corresponding, more meaningful formulations are discussed in **Table 6**. It is important to emphasise that case information and propositions are entwined and will both appear in a statement. What goes in the information and the proposition will depend on the case. However, because we repeat propositions in our statements and in court, it is preferable to keep them short and snappy.

Table 5. Criteria that help spotting whether propositions are formulated in a meaningful way.

Criteria for Propositions	Basis of the Criteria
They come in pairs, so there are at least two propositions.	To ensure a balanced view representing both parties.
They are based on the views of the parties and contextual information.	So that the evaluation is relevant to the case.
They are formal and relate to inductive inference.	To allow scientists logically to assess their findings
They are mutually exclusive.	If not, a LR cannot be used.
They represent the positions that prosecution and defence respectively would be expected to take at court.	So that there is one value of the findings and not several values (one LR, not several).
Propositions are about "causes", not results.	To enable the scientists to add value and expertise that is needed for the understanding the case.

Table 6. Examples of propositions that should be avoided and how to formulate them in a more meaningful way.

Sr.	Examples to Avoid	More Meaningful Examples	Comments
1.	Mr Smith was not the passenger.	Mr Smith was the driver.	If propositions are vague, it is difficult to assign a probability, unless this is specified in the paragraph summarising task-pertinent information.
2.	The DNA is from someone other than Mr Smith.	The DNA is from an unknown person.	
3.	Mr Smith was in recent contact with the victim.	Mr Smith visited the victim's house as described in the case information.	
4.	The matching profile comes from Mr Smith.	The DNA is from Mr Smith.	"Matching profile" is a result: it should not be included in the proposition.
5.	The male DNA is from Mr Smith or someone of his paternal lineage.	The male DNA is from Mr Smith.	Here, it is Mr Smith who would be on trial, not his paternal lineage. If one needs to consider a person from the paternal lineage, this should be done in the alternative. It is the methods that depend on the issue and not the reverse (i.e., propositions do not depend on methods).
6.	Mr A's DNA was transferred on the drug package via Officer B.	Officer B arrested Mr A before seizing the drug package.	As written, the statement says that "DNA was transferred". This is essentially an explanation for the observations. The probability of the findings given this explanation is approaching 1. The probability of DNA being transferred needs to be taken into account by the scientist when evaluating results given activity-level propositions and the case information. That transfer has occurred cannot be included in the proposition for evaluation.

In the evaluative stage, propositions should not be findings-led, and thus, ideally, the formulation of propositions should be made without knowing the results. This is an essential, early component of the recommended process of Case Assessment and Interpretation. In DNA casework—especially for investigative purposes—when considering sub-source propositions, the alternative source is generally by default an unknown person. If the propositions are standard and if knowing the findings does not impact the value of the comparison, then it is acceptable. However, if there is an impact, it is more problematic. An example, of a findings-led proposition could be "Mr A is the minor contributor of the DNA mixture", because Mr A happens to be compatible with the minor contributor. Another could be to change the number of contributors because there is one exclusion at a locus if the mixture is considered as a two-person mixture, but not if it is assigned as a three-person mixture. Regarding the number of contributors to a mixture, one should note that there is no need to consider a specific number. It is sensible in some cases to consider a variable number of contributors [**44**,**47**]. A last example of findings-led propositions would be the situation where there are two candidates for the same mixture. If one chooses a different set of propositions based on whether they explain the mixture together or not, then the propositions could be findings-led. In such cases, a suggested solution is again to consider multiple propositions [**48**].

8. FORMULATION OF THE ALTERNATIVE IN THE ABSENCE OF INFORMATION FROM THE PERSON(S) OF INTEREST

A POI is under no obligation to provide information and may give a no-comment interview. In such a case, scientists will formulate an alternative that appears the most reasonable based on what they know [**9**,**12**]. The investigation might provide information, for example that the victim and defendant visit the same gym, suggesting that activity-level propositions might be appropriate. One can also suggest the negation of the first proposition (e.g., Mr Smith is not the source of the DNA), provided we are explicit on what is meant by "not" [**46**]. This ought to be explained in the paragraph describing the case information. The implication of adopting such a negation should be set out clearly for the receivers and users of the opinion—it tends to maximise the value of the observations in support of the main proposition over the alternative. Some scientists do point this out in their reports. The important considerations regarding, for example, from whom the DNA comes (e.g., if not from Mr Smith) will be clearly disclosed. A caveat should indicate that should these assumptions not be relevant to the case, a new interpretation and perhaps further analysis will be necessary based on the new case information and new alternative.

9. DISTINCTION BETWEEN EXPLANATIONS AND PROPOSITIONS

It is particularly important to distinguish propositions from explanations when the issue is activity, as these explanations are more and more commonly offered by the parties. In the context of the Case Assessment and Interpretation model [**2**,**18**], explanations have been recognised as intermediate considerations when exploring less formal alternatives. Explanations can be very useful in the investigative stage: they provide new leads and outline what information is needed. Explanations will be generated based on the observations and generally do not qualify as formal propositions for the evaluative stage. If the explanation is prescriptive, the probability of the observations given this explanation will be one. Examples of prescriptive explanations could be "The trace has been contaminated with the suspect's DNA", "The persons were in contact recently and transferred DNA directly," or if we want to state the obvious, "The stain came from someone with the same DNA profile". Explanations may be speculative or fanciful. Contrary to propositions, they do not depend on case information and are not necessarily mutually exclusive. Examples of various types of explanations are given in **Table 7.**

Table 7. Examples of explanations that can be given as investigative opinions, but not evaluative.

Observations	Explanations
DNA profile of Mr Smith is compatible with the DNA profile of the trace.	The DNA was planted by the police.
	The real offender has the same DNA profile
	His DNA was transported from his beer can to the door by the wind.
	The government synthesised a DNA profile with the same allelic designations as him.
	The DNA is from his lost twin.
	There was contamination.
	The DNA was secondarily transferred.
	The person was recently in contact with the object.
No semen.	There was no ejaculation.
	A condom was used.
	There was no intercourse.
	There was intercourse but all trace of semen was lost following a vaginal douche.
	The swab taken did not recover the material that was present because of bad procedures.

In the context of DNA, especially when the issue is how the DNA was deposited, one should avoid, or at least outline the limitations of, considering explanations in court: in this process the scientist cannot assign the value of the results which then could easily be misunderstood. As indicated in [**49**], "'bare' explanations are likely to be of limited assistance to fact-finders, and might even be regarded as potentially misleading and, sometimes, pernicious." We will revisit this aspect in the section on communication and reporting.

10. A NOTE ON MULTIPLE PROPOSITIONS

While it is not feasible to achieve absolute exhaustiveness, it is important that all the relevant case information is considered when formulating the propositions. This can imply having two main propositions, but several sub-propositions. Indeed, if the scientist omits a proposition that is relevant, it is possible to have results that support a proposition that would not be supported if all pertinent information had been considered. In the context of mixtures, one may have to consider different numbers of contributors [**44,47**], different persons of interest [**48**], or different degrees of relatedness between the POI and the alternative source and/or different populations [**50,51**]. It has also been shown that for close relatives, considering multiple propositions (but two views) achieves better sensitivity and specificity [**52**]. An example of multiple propositions (two main propositions and associate sub-propositions) with two persons of interest—Mr A and Mr B—could be for the evaluation of the comparison of Mr A's DNA profile with a two-person DNA mixture:

- Mr A is a contributor
- Mr A and Mr B are the source of the DNA mixture.
- Mr A and an unknown are the source of the DNA mixture.
- Mr A is NOT a contributor
- Mr B and an unknown are the source of the DNA mixture.
- Two unknown persons are the source of the DNA mixture.

11. PRE-ASSESSMENT

The division of forensic science and the utilization of DNA databases in investigations highlight the significance of case information in formulating an acceptable case strategy and providing meaningful responses. An significant result of the Case Assessment and Interpretation initiative was the formalization of a process known as case pre-assessment [49,53,54]. The majority of the processes outlined include the process of analyzing and discussing the problem before conducting investigations and allocating resources. It might be argued that this approach simply represents effective forensic methodology.

11.1. Revisiting Good Forensic Practices for Evaluative Reporting

In order to provide optimal service, the initial step will involve identifying the requirements of the situation and examining how one may assist in resolving the issue. After explicitly identifying and discussing the questions with the mandating authority, a comprehensive examination approach may be formulated and mutually agreed upon with the client. Subsequently, the work can be executed, and the results together with their subsequent interpretation can be provided. While this procedure may seem uncomplicated, its practical application might prove challenging. Initially, due to the lack of comprehensive training provided to the police, they may not fully comprehend the significance of case facts in determining the most effective examination approach, thus resulting in their unawareness of some limits. Furthermore, in numerous instances, the task will first be executed to furnish an exploratory clue. After the production of the lead, it is possible that the criminal justice system may not always be cognizant of the fact that the case information provided by the person of interest (POI) can significantly alter the significance of the outcomes.

Effective case management necessitates task-relevant information, including the disputed allegations, statements from persons of interest (if obtainable), and details regarding the recovery location and method of items (e.g., found inside the car of the person of interest). The case circumstances assist scientists in comprehending the issues at hand and determining the appropriate types of opinions to provide, whether investigative or evaluative. The selection of the examination strategy will be guided by administrative details, such as the deadline and the budget. Prior contemplation of the case and one's expectations prior to undertaking the actual work offers numerous benefits, such as guaranteeing (i) the meaningfulness and cost-effectiveness of the work performed, and (ii) prompting the scientist to consider and record the anticipated outcomes based on the truth of each proposition, thereby reducing the likelihood of post-hoc rationalization or bias. Even the most rational scientists, when faced with the results, tend to justify their expectations, making them seem more probable upon observation. Considering the various potential outcomes guarantees the coherence of the assigned probabilities. Prior evaluation is especially beneficial when DNA scientists need to contemplate phenomena such as transfer and persistence.

11.2. An Example of Post-HocRationalisation That Can Be Avoided Using Pre-Assessment

Suppose we have a scenario in which the prosecution claims that Mr. S engaged in digital penetration of Ms. J's vagina. According to Mr. S, he spent the night solely attending to Ms. J due to her excessive alcohol consumption. Mr. S's nails are swabbed for DNA 3 hours after the events. Suppose we did not conduct any preliminary evaluation of the case, meaning we did not outline all the possible results of the examination and their respective probabilities. Given the information that a complete female DNA profile was obtained from the swab taken from the right hand, it can be inferred that this outcome was anticipated or likely to occur if the prosecution's claim were valid, falling within the realm of our predicted possibilities. Nevertheless, if a fragmented female profile had been acquired, it would be reasonable to acknowledge the potentiality that Mr. S has cleansed his hands. Assuming the statement is accurate, it would imply that we would have anticipated obtaining a fragmented profile. Regardless of the result, there is a tendency to justify it. If we were unaware of the result, we would not be influenced by it. Similarly, the POI may feel inclined to rationalize the findings when presented with the results. To ensure optimal conditions, it is advisable to: (i) allocate probabilities to potential outcomes without any prior knowledge of the actual results (this can be accomplished by an independent scientist or by employing a pre-existing Bayesian Network [55]), (ii) gather accounts from the involved parties regarding their perspectives on the events, without disclosing the outcomes. In theory, this should not pose any issues, as the purported facts should not rely on the outcomes.

12. COMMUNICATION, REPORTING, AND TESTIMONY

To exchange information, the messenger (e.g., the DNA scientist) needs to convey the value of the findings clearly, and the recipient of information (e.g., judiciary, police investigator) needs to understand the message in the intended manner. This implies that DNA scientists explain their reasoning and the meaning of the results in an accessible way to a large audience, who will have different education, backgrounds, languages, and expectations. As discussed in [**56**], more research is needed to address the effective presentation of forensic findings. In this section, we briefly explore the topic, but are of the opinion that, to tackle this challenge, DNA scientists should master the key concepts of interpretation. This will be easier if they have received formal education in forensic interpretation.

For efficient communication, it is also important to adapt to the audience. As alluded to earlier, the recipient of forensic information does not come without preconceived ideas: in one case, they may have the impression that DNA is unique; science is exact, precise, and gives answers that are independent of human judgement. In another case, they may think that DNA is too complex and cannot be helpful. There can easily be a disconnection between prior (mis) knowledge and the reality of forensic DNA interpretation. Another point is that, if communication takes place in the context of a given case, then according to [**57**], "the audience's pre-existing beliefs or attitudes towards the communicator, topic or object of uncertainty might influence or change the effects of uncertainty communication". Thus, not only will the communicator have a bearing on how the value of the evidence is perceived, but so will the other case information available to the recipient of information. For these reasons, formal education outside the courtroom is certainly the best means to ensure that the nature of forensic opinions is well communicated and understood. Having forensic interpretation courses in the curriculum of law degrees, as is the case in some universities (e.g., Lausanne, Switzerland), helps ensure that the future judiciary and advocates understand key concepts such as uncertainty, probability, and likelihood ratios.

The establishment of a shared language enhances communication by facilitating the clear articulation of both intended and unintended meanings, with the aid of a dictionary. Furthermore, it is important to recognize that certain terms (such as guess, subjective, match, assumption) carry significant connotations and are susceptible to misinterpretation. Therefore, it is advisable to avoid using these words wherever feasible or provide a clear explanation when they are used.

12.1. Reporting: General Desiderata

The desiderata, as well as the principles of interpretation, that have been proposed for evaluation of the results apply to reporting (orally or in writing). In addition, it has been proposed that the goals of communication should be truthfulness, candour, and comprehensibility [**23**]. The pursuit of one goal often requires the sacrifice of the others. The tension between these three goals can be illustrated by a triangle where each goal represents an angle (see **Figure 1**, Buckleton, personal communication). Candour implies that experts adhere to a code of conduct and only report in their area of expertise.

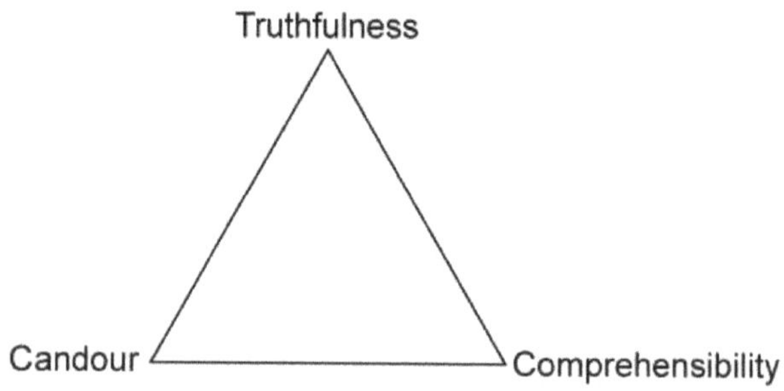

Figure 1. Triangle representing the tensions between the goals of communication.

12.2. Statement Writing

The specific criteria for composing a statement will vary depending on the jurisdiction, however, it is advisable to adhere to established recommendations for optimal performance [9,21]. These ideas offer guidance on the content of the statement and advise the reader to avoid certain terms and phrases that are still commonly used today, such as "consistent with," "association," "link," "contact," "support," or "refute." Refute, being a categorical assertion, is not seen as the converse of support. Support can vary in intensity, but refutation does not have varying degrees. Instead of using the phrase "whether the results support or refute," one may use the phrase "whether the results support one proposition in comparison to the alternative or neither proposition." Due to their ambiguous nature, these phrases typically fail to effectively communicate the significance of the findings.

To get accurate results, it is important for DNA scientists to possess scientific expertise and consider the relevant conditions of the case. Therefore, statements should have a detailed paragraph that describes the available information and the assumptions made. The problem must be accurately recognized, proposals must be prepared, and scientists should express their readiness to assist in addressing any alternative proposals in the event that the circumstances change or if there has been a misunderstanding. Given that the case information is not a compilation of "facts," it is crucial to note that if there are any changes in the case information, it will be essential to reassess the interpretation. The subsequent section will provide a detailed account of the items, focusing on methodological features commonly known as "Technical issues." These aspects encompass many elements like as the methodologies employed for analysis and interpretation, as well as considerations surrounding the transfer, persistence, and recovery of DNA. The findings of the analysis will be presented and assessed. When dealing with intricate scenarios, such as determining the value of findings based on activity-level propositions, it is helpful to include a paragraph that discusses the probability of the results given the case information and each proposition. This will enable the reader to comprehend the rationale behind the reasoning and the origin of the data. Providing a definition of an LR and clarifying its limitations can assist illustrate the distinction between the likelihood of the findings based on the supplied propositions and information, and the likelihood of the propositions based on the finds and information. It is important to explicitly disclose the constraints of the interpretation and the problems being examined. Table 8 presents a selection of practical precautions that we recommend.

Table 8. Examples of useful caveats in written statements.

Reason for the Caveat	Example
Underline the importance of case information and propositions.	The evaluation presented in this report is crucially dependent on the information provided to the examiner and on the propositions addressed. Any change in the framework of circumstances or in either of the propositions should be seen as sufficient reason for a new evaluation. If some information were found to be incorrect, or if new information were made available, I would need to re-evaluate the value of the findings. Re-evaluation will be more effective if performed in advance of a trial.
Explain what a LR is and is not.	A likelihood ratio indicates if and to what extent the DNA analysis results support one proposition over another. It is not possible, on this basis alone, to determine which is the most probable proposition. To assign the probability of a proposition, the DNA analysis results should be combined with other information in the case. This is generally not considered to be the remit of the DNA scientist.

Reason for the Caveat	Example
Alert on the difference between source and activity issues.	This report does not provide any information on the mechanisms or actions that led to the deposition of the recovered biological material. It only provides information regarding its origin (e.g., who is the source of the DNA). Should there be any issue regarding the transfer mechanisms that led to the detection of this material, the results should be evaluated given the alleged activities.
Delineate the meaning of a verbal scale.	The likelihood ratio is a numerical value. Words can be assigned to brackets of numerical values and used as a descriptor of the results' support for a proposition. Several verbal equivalence tables have been published, and it is above all a convention.

12.3. The Use of Verbal Equivalents

In order to convey the significance of the LR, various verbal equivalents (also known as verbal scales) have been proposed [4, 58, 59]. When a quantitative likelihood ratio (LR) is provided, the LR value should be stated first [9] and may be supplemented by a verbal equivalent [56, 59, 60]. For instance, a likelihood ratio of around 1000 has been attributed, indicating that the DNA findings are 1000 times more likely if Mr. Smith is the DNA source compared to his absent sibling. Hence, the DNA evidence corroborates the claim that Mr. Smith is the originator of the DNA, as opposed to his inaccessible sibling. The level of support can be characterized as robust. Verbal equivalents are unnecessary if one comprehends the meaning of an LR. In order to demonstrate the theoretical updating of views based on DNA results, it would be more effective to incorporate a table including a few instances of previous odds and the impact of the results (i.e., the obtained likelihood ratio) on posterior odds. (For individuals who lack familiarity with odds, it is also feasible to convert odds into probabilities.) Additionally, this approach offers the benefit of illustrating the distinction between likelihood ratios (LRs), prior odds, and posterior odds.

There is a belief that distinct verbal scales are required for DNA, namely autosomal DNA, due to the significantly bigger likelihood ratios (LRs) compared to other disciplines like mtDNA or fibres. Contrary to the above statement, DNA scientists argue that a DNA comparison with a likelihood ratio (LR) of 1000 lacks informative value due to their focus on investigative work in the present era. In such a scenario, it is often necessary to employ greater likelihood ratios (LRs) in order to prevent an excessive number of candidates from the national DNA database (and a surplus of misleading leads). Moreover, in cases when there is little supplementary evidence, the authorities may require more discerning outcomes to determine whether an individual should be apprehended or not. Another possible explanation, which is not necessarily contradictory, is that DNA experts are accustomed to dealing with extremely high likelihood ratios (LRs) and hence consider a value of 1000 as insignificant, similar to how billionaires could view it as "pocket money". According to many publications [4,9,61], it is recommended to use the same linguistic equivalents regardless of the field of study and the type of results (autosomal DNA, Y-STR, or mtDNA comparisons). Therefore, it is necessary to utilize the same verbal scale when reporting findings for activity- or sub-source-level propositions, regardless of whether the results are intended for missing persons, paternity, or sibling instances. Verbal scales [21,58,59,60,62,63] have been the subject of extensive discussion.

There are three specific points where a general agreement appears to exist: (1) If the likelihood ratio (LR) value is equal to "one", then the results should be regarded as uninformative. It is the results themselves, rather than the LR, that lack informative value. Likewise, it is the outcomes and not the LR that offer validation for one proposition in comparison to the other. The LR quantifies the level of support provided by the results for either of the propositions. Hence, the observations offer no support in answering the given propositions. If the likelihood ratios (LRs) are greater than one, it indicates support for the first proposition. (3) If the likelihood ratios (LRs) are less than one, the findings provide evidence in favor of the alternative hypothesis. Standardization of verbal scales is challenging due to the reliance on conventions, resulting in the proposal of several scales with differing resolutions and nomenclature. While verbal counterparts are inadequate, focusing solely on the LR value does not appear to be very promising either, as research has demonstrated that individuals struggle to comprehend the notion of LRs when considered independently. Although an optimal approach for conveying the significance of scientific discoveries has not been determined, this does not imply that we should alter the evaluation process (just as we would not modify DNA analysis procedures due to public comprehension limitations). Nevertheless, unless there is a broader comprehension of the principles of LR and probability, it is OK for the DNA scientist to include a verbal explanation, as long as the LR value is presented prior to it.

12.4. Testimony

In court, there is an increasing focus on the manner in which the DNA was deposited. Nevertheless, only a limited number of DNA experts are willing to produce a report on this subject, and a few may be inclined to postpone their responses and address the questions directly in a courtroom setting. The current situation [12,64] is suboptimal due to the challenging nature of evaluating biological outcomes. Therefore, it must adhere to the identical standards as any other assessment, which include being accompanied by a peer-reviewed written statement that is accessible to the defense.

During legal proceedings, DNA experts may be required to provide the statistical significance of the results based on sub-source propositions. They may also be requested to respond to hypothetical queries, which often involve providing explanations rather than making assertions. For instance, consider the following scenario: "If the accused had shaken hands with the actual perpetrator, would it not be feasible to obtain DNA evidence from my client in such a situation?" It is conceivable that one could argue in favor of this possibility. Nevertheless, as mentioned in reference [65], the question arises as to how the fact-finder can interpret the DNA evidence and its implications when presented with a substantial likelihood ratio (LR) for the sub-source propositions and a range of potential explanations for the transfer resulting from specific activities.

Inquiries regarding the potential for DNA transfer necessitate a nuanced response. Typically, when a case is brought to court, DNA scientists can provide more valuable assistance to the fact-finders by evaluating the significance of the DNA findings within the specific circumstances of the case. It is important to note that when responding to inquiries about the possibility of secondary transfer, one would be expressing an opinion about the claimed behaviors involving secondary transfer. Moreover, when discussing the DNA's origin and stating that "The vagina is the most probable source of the DNA" [37], it becomes ambiguous if it is a transposed conditional or a posterior probability if the assignment of prior odds is not specified. If the fluid's inherent properties indicate an active state (such as in the case of vaginal cells), this poses a dilemma, as the characteristics of the substance immediately pertain to the matter under the jurisdiction of the court.

If the questions regarding how DNA was transferred appear reasonable to the court, it is recommended to ask for a recess [**12,25**] and perform a proper evaluation of the results given what is alleged.

If DNA scientists are unable to evaluate the significance of the observations due to time constraints, insufficient case information, or lack of expertise, they should explicitly state that, in the absence of additional information, the findings should be deemed uninterpretable (and therefore uninformative) and likely inadmissible due to the potential for bias.

13. AN EXAMINATION OF LIKELIHOOD RATIOS

Now that you are familiar with the main concepts of interpretation, we would like to discuss aspects relating to what LRs are, if they can be estimated, how precise they should be, and whether it is problematic to transpose the conditional when LRs are very large.

13.10. The concepts of likelihood ratio and probability

Scientists should know how to explain what a likelihood ratio is. As described earlier, a LR is a ratio of two conditional probabilities given competing propositions and conditioning information. However, what is a probability? A probability is a number between zero and one that represents our uncertainty with regard to the truth of some aspect of the universe in the past, present, or future. All probabilities are conditional: they depend on what you know, what you are told, and what you assume. In some simple situations, such as coin-tossing, there might be little disagreement between people about the truth of a statement such as "the coin will land showing a head". In general, though, the central component of knowledge means that different people will have different probabilities for the same thing. We say that probability is personal. In relation to any uncertain event there is no "correct" probability, so we say that probabilities are "assigned" rather than "estimated".

Because a likelihood ratio is the ratio of two probabilities, it necessarily follows that a LR is personal also. Thus, in relation to any particular pair of propositions in a DNA case, there is no "correct" LR: different scientists will bring different levels of knowledge (and understanding) to bear. What we require is that the scientist to whom we pay attention is well calibrated: that is, we expect that the scientist can be relied upon to assign large values to the LR in cases where the prosecution proposition is actually true and to assign small values to the LR in cases where the defence proposition is actually true. This concept of calibration is critical to software systems that are created to assist scientists in assigning LRs and to the publications supporting advanced DNA probabilistic genotyping calculations, include extensive studies of ground truth cases. A ground truth case is one that has been artificially created; in its simplest form, it will consist of two sets of data and the truth with regard to whether the two are from the same original source (H_p true) or not (H_d true) is known without doubt. The distribution of LRs from H_p-true ground truth cases should peak at high values (greater than one); the distribution from H_d-true ground truth cases should peak at small values (less than one). If considering, for example, the source of a DNA mixture recovered on a scene, because people can share part of their DNA, it is expected that some non-donors will share alleles adventitiously and have a LR larger than one fortuitously. This is even more true when comparing mixed/partial DNA profile with individuals who are closely related to contributors or due to co-ancestry effects **[52]**. There are sophisticated measures for assessing calibration experiments quantitatively, but one simple one is known as "Turing's rule". This follows from a theorem, attributed by IJ Good to Alan Turing **[66,67]**, that shows that the "expected value of a LR in favour of a wrong proposition is one". This implies that the average value of the LR in a large H_d-true calibration experiment should be approximately one: in practice, this means a highly skewed distribution, with most LRs close to zero and the odd one or two substantially greater than one. For example, suppose that a LR of a million is computed given sub-source propositions. It follows that if we simulated profiles of millions of non-donors, we would expect roughly 1 in every million non-donor DNA profiles to yield a LR of 1 million when compared to the DNA profile of the trace. We would also expect 999,999 out of every million non-donor profiles to yield a LR of 0 when compared to the DNA profile of the trace. The average LR of these ground truth comparisons is then 1.

Good (ibid) also showed how he and Turing regarded the logarithm of the LR as a measure of evidential weight, and this view appears highly relevant to the forensic field. This notion contributes to the idea of expressing verbal conventions in rough correspondence to orders of magnitude of the LR [**58**]. It also suggests the notion that precise values of the LR are not needed for effective communication of evidential weight to jurors. Hence, our suggestion is to report LRs to one significant figure. If a LR of 10,256.32 were computed, we would conclude that the findings are of the order of 10,000 more probable if... than if...This allows us to convey that it is the order of magnitude that is important.

For LRs smaller than one (i.e., when results support the alternative), it has been suggested to reverse the propositions and adopt the same rounding rules. Indeed, numbers smaller than one are difficult to understand: for example, if our LR is 0.01, shall we say results are 0.01 times less (or more?) likely if the first proposition were true rather than if the alternative were true? It is easier to report that results are 100 times more likely if the alternative proposition were true rather than if the first proposition were true.

Current population genetic models condone the multiplying together of genotype probabilities across many loci, and this in turn leads to extremely large LRs—billions, trillions, quadrillions, and still further. When this issue first arose in the UK, Foreman and Evett [**68**] argued that the extent of investigations into the independence assumptions implicit in this process was insufficient to justify the robustness of LRs in excess of one billion. So, when the Forensic Science Service introduced the ten locus STR system into casework, the largest magnitude of LR quoted was one billion. This was expected to be a temporary expedient, but to this day, there still seems to be little in the way of large-scale between-locus dependence effects. This seems to cause little embarrassment, and it is common to see LRs of the order 10^{20} reported in DNA cases (It should be noted that with very small numbers, there are some analogies that are misleading. An example is the "several planets earth" or the "galaxy" argument used, for example, in the Jama Case [**69**]. "The range, it was said, within which the calculation was made was between 1 in 45 billion and 1 in 14 trillion. [...] In other words, it would appear to be necessary to search well beyond this planet and conceivably this galaxy to find a match". This argument leads the layperson to think that DNA is sufficient for individualisation, when it is not [**70**]). In some countries, for example, the UK [**71**], it is still current practice to report all LRs that are computed as greater than 10^9 to be "of the order of one billion", even though the number of loci in routine use is much greater than the original 10 at the time of the Foreman and Evett study. This seems to cause no problem, but it is a peculiar state of affairs. In addition, it has been advocated that one should consider the possibility of an error, [**72**] as DNA analysis is not error free [**73**]. When we do, the value of the results will be largely dominated by this probability [**3**,**7**,**74**].

13.2. *Does transposing the conditional really matter when using high likelihood ratios (LRs)?*

Some might advocate that we should not split hairs and that if the LR is very high, then the effect of prior odds is washed away and it is not a real issue if the scientist transposes the conditional. Reporting and testimony represent the end-product of the scientist's job. Whether or not it would be acceptable in some cases to let the court believe that the results allow the scientist to assign a posterior probability, is a matter of ethics and code of conduct. The scientist's remit is scientific results and their value in the context of the alleged facts, not the facts themselves. It is the duty of factfinders to consider both the results and the alleged facts.

14. AT A GLANCE

Comprehending and expressing doubt is a challenging undertaking. Given that it is impossible to eliminate uncertainty, we must confront it and incorporate it into our actions [14]. For DNA scientists, this entails implementing methods to guarantee that results are accurately evaluated and effectively conveyed. The initial phase is identifying the problem that can be addressed by forensic science and utilizing the framework we have provided. This enables scientists to systematically evaluate and communicate the significance of their findings in a clear and transparent manner. This ensures that the logical rules associated to specific sub-source-level propositions are not transferred to activity-level propositions [75]. It is crucial to recognize that DNA, while highly valuable, is not a panacea. There will be instances where relying just on DNA comparisons would not yield useful results. If the individual in question possesses authorized authorization to the entity or individual, and it can be reasonably assumed that the DNA originates from said individual, then it is not very logical to contemplate the likelihood of the outcomes supposing the DNA is derived from an unidentified individual, as this is not the claim being made. Another scenario could arise where the focus is not on the individual providing the DNA, but rather on the actions that resulted in the deposition of the material. If both parties claim to have engaged in very similar behaviors, the DNA analysis will not be able to differentiate between their claims. The trier of facts must be informed of these points.

In order to enhance communication, achieve harmonization, and elevate the standards of interpretation, various steps could be implemented: (1) Allocate resources to enhance the formal education of the individuals who play crucial roles in communication, namely the messenger and the recipient of the information. (2) Equip the forensic community with suitable tools and expertise to effectively carry out their tasks. (3) Include the act of interpreting information as an integral component of the accreditation process. Implementing technical assessors and comprehensive competence examinations would enable the supervision of the assessment of DNA results, considering both sub-source and activity-level propositions. This would guarantee that DNA scientists strictly follow the principles of interpretation as recommended in the codes of practice and conduct for evaluative views by the Forensic Science Regulator of England and Wales [12]. It is worth mentioning that certain nations, including the Netherlands, have taken steps to ensure and enhance the quality of court experts' involvement in the legal proceedings through initiatives led by The Netherlands Register of Court Experts [76,77]. Other countries should consider this approach to ensure that experts are adequately qualified and certified for both types of reporting.

15. SUMMARY

In recent decades, the forensic community has made significant efforts to establish a systematic framework for forensic interpretation. This framework is crucial for ensuring the fair and secure administration of justice. We critically examine the existing findings and guidelines and offer practical illustrations of their implementation in casework. Following a discourse on the ambiguity prevalent in criminal trials and the various responsibilities that DNA scientists may assume, we hereby provide the fundamental principles of interpretation for evaluative reporting. We demonstrate the utility of their application in mitigating a prevalent logical error and propose effective techniques for DNA scientists to prevent the misplacement of the conditional statement. Next, we examine the hierarchy of propositions and elucidate its significance as a fundamental concept in evaluating biological findings. We also explore the distinctions in evaluating outcomes based on propositions at the source level vs the activity level. We demonstrate the significance of doing pre-assessment, particularly when the inquiries pertain to the purported activities, and when the scientists must take into account transfer and persistence in order to provide guidance to the court. Lastly, we will engage in a discourse regarding the composition of statements and the delivery of testimony. This document offers instructions on how DNA scientists can effectively communicate their findings in a fair, clear, and rational manner.

REFERENCES

1. Taroni, F.; Champod, C.; Margot, P. Forerunners of Bayesianism in early forensic science. J. Forensic Identif. **1999**, 49, 285–310. **[Google Scholar]**

2. Jackson, G. The Development of Case Assessment and Interpretation (CAI) in Forensic Science. Ph.D. Thesis, University of Abertay, Dundee, UK, 2011. **[Google Scholar]**

3. Aitken, C.; Taroni, F.; Bozza, S. Statistics and the Evaluation of Evidence for Forensic Scientists, 3rd ed.; John Wiley & Sons: Chichester, UK, 2021. **[Google Scholar]**

4. Evett, I.W.; Weir, B.S. Interpreting DNA Evidence—Statistical Genetics for Forensic Scientists; Sinauer Associates, Inc.: Sunderland, MA, USA, 1998. **[Google Scholar]**

5. Kaye, D.H. The Double Helix and the Law of Evidence; Harvard University Press: Cambridge, MA, USA, 2010. **[Google Scholar]**

6. Buckleton, J.S.; Bright, J.-A.; Taylor, D. Forensic DNA Evidence Interpretation, 2nd ed.; CRC Press: Boca Raton, FL, USA, 2016. **[Google Scholar]**

7. Robertson, B.; Vignaux, G.A.; Berger, C.E.H. Interpreting Evidence, 2nd ed.; Wiley & Sons: Chichester, UK, 2016. **[Google Scholar]**

8. Aitken, C.G.G.; Stoney, D.A. The Use of Statistics in Forensic Science, 1st ed.; Ellis Horwood Series in Forensic Science; CRC Press: Boca Raton, FL, USA, 1991. **[Google Scholar]**

9. Willis, S.M.; McKenna, L.; McDermott, S.D.; O'Donnell, G.; Barrett, A.; Rasmusson, B.; Höglund, T.; Berger, C.E.H.; Sierps, M.J.; Lucena-Molina, J.J.; et al. ENFSI Guideline for Evaluative Reporting in Forensic Science: Strengthening the Evaluation of Forensic Results Across Europe (STEOFRAE). 2015. Available online: **http://enfsi.eu/wp-content/uploads/2016/09/m1_guideline.pdf** (accessed on 14 May 2022).

10. Gill, P.; Hicks, T.; Butler, J.M.; Connolly, E.; Gusmao, L.; Kokshoorn, B.; Morling, N.; van Oorschot, R.A.H.; Parson, W.; Prinz, M.; et al. DNA commission of the International society for forensic genetics: Assessing the value of forensic biological evidence—Guidelines highlighting the importance of propositions: Part I: Evaluation of DNA profiling comparisons given (sub-) source propositions. Forensic Sci. Int. Genet. **2018**, 36, 189–202. **[Google Scholar] [CrossRef] [PubMed] [Green Version]**

11. Gill, P.; Hicks, T.; Butler, J.M.; Connolly, E.; Gusmão, L.; Kokshoorn, B.; Morling, N.; van Oorschot, R.A.H.; Parson, W.; Prinz, M.; et al. DNA commission of the International society for forensic genetics: Assessing the value of forensic biological evidence—Guidelines highlighting the importance of propositions. Part II: Evaluation of biological traces considering activity level propositions. Forensic Sci. Int. Genet. **2020**, 44, 102186. **[Google Scholar] [CrossRef] [PubMed] [Green Version]**

12. Forensic Science Regulator. Development of Evaluative Opinion. FSR-C-118; 2021. Available online: **https://assets.publishing.service.gov.uk/government/uploads/system/uploads/attachment_data/file/960051/FSR-C-118_Interpretation_Appendix_Issue_1__002_.pdf** (accessed on 14 May 2022).
13. Edmond, G.; Cole, S.A. Legal aspects of forensic science. In Encyclopedia of Forensic Sciences, Second ed.; Siegel, J.A., Saukko, P.J., Houck, M.M., Eds.; Academic Press: Waltham, MA, USA, 2013; pp. 466–470. **[Google Scholar]**
14. Lindley, D.V. Understanding Uncertainty; John Wiley & Sons, Ltd.: Hoboken, NJ, USA, 2006. **[Google Scholar]**
15. Samie, L.; Champod, C.; Delemont, S.; Basset, P.; Hicks, T.; Castella, V. Use of Bayesian Networks for the investigation of the nature of biological material in casework. Forensic Sci. Int. **2022**, 331, 111174. **[Google Scholar] [CrossRef] [PubMed]**
16. Jackson, G.; Jones, S.; Booth, G.; Champod, C.; Evett, I.W. The nature of forensic science opinion—A possible framework to guide thinking and practice in investigations and in court proceedings. Sci. Justice **2006**, 46, 33–44. **[Google Scholar] [CrossRef]**
17. Nordby, J.J. Dead Reckoning: The Art of Forensic Detection; CRC Press LLC.: Boca Raton, FL, USA, 2000. **[Google Scholar]**
18. Evett, I.W.; Jackson, G.; Lambert, J.A. More on the hierarchy of propositions: Exploring the distinction between explanations and propositions. Sci. Justice **2000**, 40, 3–10. **[Google Scholar] [CrossRef]**
19. Jackson, G. The scientist and the scales of justice. Sci. Justice **2000**, 40, 81–85. **[Google Scholar] [CrossRef]**
20. Association of Forensic Science Providers. Standards for the formulation of evaluative forensic science expert opinion. Sci. Justice **2009**, 49, 161–164. **[Google Scholar] [CrossRef]**
21. Evett, I.W.; Jackson, G.; Lambert, J.A.; McCrossan, S. The impact of the principles of evidence interpretation on the structure and content of statements. Sci. Justice **2000**, 40, 233–239. **[Google Scholar] [CrossRef]**
22. Berger, C.E.H.; Buckleton, J.; Champod, C.; Evett, I.W.; Jackson, G. Evidence evaluation: A response to the court of appeal judgment in R v T. Sci. Justice **2011**, 51, 43–49. **[Google Scholar] [CrossRef]**

23. Gittelson, S.; Kalafut, T.; Myers, S.; Taylor, D.; Hicks, T.; Taroni, F.; Evett, I.W.; Bright, J.A.; Buckleton, J. A practical guide for the formulation of propositions in the Bayesian approach to DNA evidence interpretation in an adversarial environment. J. Forensic Sci. **2016**, 61, 186–195. **[Google Scholar] [CrossRef] [PubMed]**

24. Biedermann, A.; Hicks, T.; Taroni, F.; Champod, C.; Aitken, C. On the use of the likelihood ratio for forensic evaluation: Response to Fenton et al. Sci. Justice **2014**, 54, 316–318. **[Google Scholar] [CrossRef] [PubMed]**

25. OSAC. Best Practice Recommendation for Evaluative Forensic DNA Testimony OPEN COMMENT VERSION (2022-S-0024). Draft OSAC Proposed Standard; 2022. Available online: **www.nist.gov/system/files/documents/2022/01/04/OSAC%202022-S-0024%20BPR%20for%20Evaluative%20Forensic%20DNA%20Testimony.OPEN%20COMMENT%20VERSION.pdf** (accessed on 14 May 2022).

26. Evett, I.W. Avoiding the transposed conditional. Sci. Justice **1995**, 35, 127–131. **[Google Scholar] [CrossRef]**

27. Aitken, C.G.G.; Roberts, P.; Jackson, G. Fundamentals of Probability and Statistical Evidence in Criminal Proceedings; Working Group on Statistics the Law of the Royal Statistical Society: 2011; Volume Practitioner Guide No.1. Available online: **https://www.maths.ed.ac.uk/~cgga/Guide-1-WEB.pdf** (accessed on 14 May 2022).

28. Taroni, F.; Marquis, R.; Schmittbuhl, M.; Biedermann, A.; Thiéry, A.; Bozza, S. Bayes factor for investigative assessment of selected handwriting features. Forensic Sci. Int. **2014**, 242, 266–273. **[Google Scholar] [CrossRef]**

29. Koehler, J.J. Forensic fallacies and a famous judge. Jurimetrics **2014**, 54, 211–219. **[Google Scholar]**

30. Thompson, W.C.; Schumann, E.L. Interpretation of statistical evidence in criminal trials: The prosecutor's fallacy and the defence attorney's fallacy. Law Hum. Behav. **1987**, 11, 167–187. **[Google Scholar] [CrossRef]**

31. Supreme Court of Victoria (Australia)—Court of Appeal. Tuite v The Queen 49 VR 196, 200 2015 Maxwell ACJ, Redlich and Weinberg JJA. Available online: **https://jade.io/article/397203** (accessed on 19 May 2022).

32. Jeffreys, H. Theory of Probability, 3rd ed.; Clarendon Press: Oxford, UK, 1983. **[Google Scholar]**

33. Cook, R.; Evett, I.W.; Jackson, G.; Jones, P.J.; Lambert, J.A. A hierarchy of propositions: Deciding which level to address in casework. Sci. Justice **1998**, 38, 231–240. **[Google Scholar] [CrossRef]**

34. Taylor, D.; Bright, J.A.; Buckleton, J. The 'factor of two' issue in mixed DNA profiles. J. Theor. Biol. **2014**, 363, 300–306. **[Google Scholar] [CrossRef]**

35. Evett, I.W.; Gill, P.D.; Jackson, G.; Whitaker, J.; Champod, C. Interpreting small quantities of DNA: The hierarchy of propositions and the use of Bayesian networks. J. Forensic Sci. **2002**, 47, 520–530. **[Google Scholar] [CrossRef]**

36. Taroni, F.; Biedermann, A.; Vuille, J.; Morling, N. Whose DNA is this? How relevant a question? (A note for forensic scientists). Forensic Sci. Int. Genet. **2013**, 7, 467–470. **[Google Scholar] [CrossRef] [Green Version]**

37. England and Wales Court of Appeal (Criminal Division) Decisions, Weller, R. v [2010] EWCA Crim 1085 (04 March 2010). Available online: **http://www.bailii.org/ew/cases/EWCA/Crim/2010/1085.html** (accessed on 19 May 2022).

38. Taroni, F.; Bozza, S.; Hicks, T.; Garbolino, P. More on the question 'When does absence of evidence constitute evidence of absence?' How Bayesian confirmation theory can logically support the answer. Forensic Sci. Int. **2019**, 301, e59–e63. **[Google Scholar] [CrossRef] [PubMed]**

39. Taylor, D.; Kokshoorn, B.; Biedermann, A. Evaluation of forensic genetics findings given activity level propositions: A review. Forensic Sci. Int. Genet. **2018**, 36, 34–49. **[Google Scholar] [CrossRef] [PubMed] [Green Version]**

40. Evett, I.W. Establishing the evidential value of a small quantity of material found at a crime scene. J. Forensic Sci. Soc. **1993**, 33, 83–86. **[Google Scholar] [CrossRef]**

41. Stoney, D.A. Transfer Evidence. In The Use of Statistics in Forensic Science, 1st ed.; Ellis Horwood Series in Forensic Science; Aitken, C.G.G., Stoney, D.A., Eds.; CRC Press: Boca Raton, FL, USA, 1991; pp. 107–138. **[Google Scholar]**

42. Biedermann, A.; Hicks, T. The importance of critically examining the level of propositions when evaluating forensic DNA results. Front. Genet. **2016**, 7, 8. **[Google Scholar] [CrossRef] [Green Version]**

43. Buckleton, J.; Bright, J.-A.; Taylor, D.; Evett, I.; Hicks, T.; Jackson, G.; Curran, J.M. Helping formulate propositions in forensic DNA analysis. Sci. Justice **2014**, 54, 258–261. **[Google Scholar] [CrossRef]**

44. Buckleton, J.; Taylor, D.; Bright, J.A.; Hicks, T.; Curran, J. When evaluating DNA evidence within a likelihood ratio framework, should the propositions be exhaustive? Forensic Sci. Int. Genet. **2021**, 50, 102406. **[Google Scholar] [CrossRef]**

45. Hicks, T.; Biedermann, A.; de Koeijer, J.A.; Taroni, F.; Champod, C.; Evett, I.W. The importance of distinguishing information from evidence/observations when formulating propositions. Sci. Justice **2015**, 55, 520–525. **[Google Scholar] [CrossRef]**

46. Taylor, D.; Kokshoorn, B.; Hicks, T. Structuring cases into propositions, assumptions, and undisputed case information. Forensic Sci. Int. Genet. **2020**, 44, 102199. **[Google Scholar] [CrossRef] [Green Version]**

47. Taylor, D.; Bright, J.A.; Buckleton, J. Interpreting forensic DNA profiling evidence without specifying the number of contributors. Forensic Sci. Int. Genet. **2014**, 13, 269–280. **[Google Scholar] [CrossRef]**

48. Hicks, T.; Kerr, Z.; Pugh, S.; Bright, J.A.; Curran, J.; Taylor, D.; Buckleton, J. Comparing multiple POI to DNA mixtures. Forensic Sci. Int. Genet. **2021**, 52, 102481. **[Google Scholar] [CrossRef]**

49. Jackson, G.; Roberts, P.; Aitken, C. Guidance for Judges, Lawyers, Forensic Scientists and Expert Witnesses. 4. Case Assessment and Interpretation of Expert Evidence. 2015. Available online: **https://rss.org.uk/RSS/media/File-library/Publications/rss-case-assessment-interpretation-expert-evidence.pdf** (accessed on 14 May 2022).

50. Buckleton, J.S.; Walsh, K.A.J.; Evett, I.W. Who is "Random Man"? J. Forensic Sci. Soc. **1991**, 31, 463–468. **[Google Scholar] [CrossRef]**

51. Balding, D.J. Weight-of-Evidence for Forensic DNA Profiles; Wiley: Chichester, UK, 2005. **[Google Scholar]**

52. Kalafut, T.; Pugh, S.; Gill, P.; Abbas, S.; Semaan, M.; Mansour, I.; Curran, J.; Bright, J.A.; Hicks, T.; Wivell, R.; et al. A mixed DNA profile controversy revisited. J. Forensic Sci. **2021**, 67, 128–135. **[Google Scholar] [CrossRef] [PubMed]**

53. Cook, R.; Evett, I.W.; Jackson, G.; Jones, P.J.; Lambert, J.A. A model for case assessment and interpretation. Sci. Justice **1998**, 38, 151–156. **[Google Scholar] [CrossRef]**

54. Jackson, G.; Jones, P. Case Assessment and Interpretation. In Encyclopedia of Forensic Science; Jamieson, A., Moenssens, A., Eds.; John Wiley & Sons, Ltd.: Chichester, UK, 2009; pp. 483–497. **[Google Scholar]**

55. Taroni, F.; Aitken, C.; Bozza, S.; Garbolino, P.; Biedermann, A. Bayesian Networks and Probabilistic Inference in Forensic Science, 2nd ed.; John Wiley & Sons, Ltd.: Chichester, UK, 2014. **[Google Scholar]**

56. Neumann, C.; Kaye, D.; Jackson, G.; Reyna, V.; Ranadive, A. Presenting Quantitative and Qualitative Information on Forensic Science Evidence in the Courtroom. Chance **2016**, 29, 37–43. **[Google Scholar] [CrossRef]**

57. van der Bles, A.M.; van der Linden, S.; Freeman, A.L.J.; Mitchell, J.; Galvao, A.B.; Zaval, L.; Spiegelhalter, D.J. Communicating uncertainty about facts, numbers and science. R. Soc. Open Sci. **2019**, 6, 181870. **[Google Scholar] [CrossRef] [Green Version]**

58. Aitken, C.G.G.; Taroni, F. A verbal scale for the interpretation of evidence. Sci. Justice **1998**, 38, 279–281. **[Google Scholar] [CrossRef]**

59. Marquis, R.; Biedermann, A.; Cadola, L.; Champod, C.; Gueissaz, L.; Massonnet, G.; Mazzella, W.D.; Taroni, F.; Hicks, T. Discussion on how to implement a verbal scale in a forensic laboratory: Benefits, pitfalls and suggestions to avoid misunderstandings. Sci. Justice **2016**, 56, 364–370. **[Google Scholar] [CrossRef] [Green Version]**

60. Martire, K.A.; Watkins, I. Perception problems of the verbal scale: A reanalysis and application of a membership function approach. Sci. Justice **2015**, 55, 264–273. **[Google Scholar] [CrossRef]**

61. Nordgaard, A.; Ansell, R.; Drotz, W.; Jaeger, L. Scale of conclusions for the value of evidence. Law Probab. Risk **2011**, 11, 1–24. **[Google Scholar] [CrossRef] [Green Version]**

62. Eldridge, H. Juror comprehension of forensic expert testimony: A literature review and gap analysis. Forensic Sci. Int. Synerg. **2019**, 1, 24–34. **[Google Scholar] [CrossRef]**

63. Sjerps, M.; Biesheuvel, D.B. The interpretation of conventional and 'Bayesian' verbal scales for expressing expert opinion: A small experiment among jurists. Forensic Linguist. **1999**, 6, 214–227. **[Google Scholar] [CrossRef]**

64. Hicks, T.; Biedermann, A.; Taroni, F.; Champod, C. Problematic reporting in DNA cases: The need for accredited formats and certified reporting competence. Forensic Sci. Int. Genet. Suppl. Ser. **2019**, 7, 205–207. **[Google Scholar] [CrossRef]**

65. Jackson, G.; Biedermann, A. "Source" or "activity". What is the level of issue in a criminal trial? Significance **2019**, 16, 36–39. **[Google Scholar] [CrossRef]**

66. Good, I.J. Probability and the Weighing of Evidence; Charles Griffin & Company Limited: London, UK, 1950. **[Google Scholar]**

67. Taylor, D.; Buckleton, J.; Evett, I. Testing likelihood ratios produced from complex DNA profiles. Forensic Sci. Int. Genet. **2015**, 16, 165–171. **[Google Scholar] [CrossRef] [PubMed]**

68. Foreman, L.A.; Evett, I.W. Statistical Analysis to Support Forensic Interpretation of a New Ten-Locus STR Profiling System. Int. J. Leg. Med. **2001**, 114, 147–155. **[Google Scholar] [CrossRef]**

69. Vincent, F.H.R. Report: Inquiry into the Circumstances That Led to the Conviction of Mr Farah Abdulkadir Jama. 2010. Available online: **https://www.parliament.vic.gov.au/papers/govpub/VPARL2006-10No301.pdf** (accessed on 14 May 2022).

70. Biedermann, A.; Vuille, J. Understanding the logic of forensic identification decisions (without numbers). Sui Generis **2018**, 83, 397–413. **[Google Scholar] [CrossRef]**

71. Hopwood, A.J.; Puch-Solis, R.; Tucker, V.C.; Curran, J.M.; Skerrett, J.; Pope, S.; Tully, G. Consideration of the probative value of single donor 15-plex STR profiles in UK populations and its presentation in UK courts. Sci. Justice **2012**, 52, 185–190. **[Google Scholar] [CrossRef]**

72. Koehler, J.J.; Chia, A.; Lindsey, S. The random match probability in DNA evidence: Irrelevant and prejudicial? Jurimetr. J. **1995**, 35, 201–219. **[Google Scholar]**

73. Kloosterman, A.; Sjerps, M.; Quak, A. Error rates in forensic DNA analysis: Definition, numbers, impact and communication. Forensic. Sci. Int. Genet. **2014**, 12, 77–85. **[Google Scholar] [CrossRef]**

74. Coquoz, R.; Comte, J.; Hall, D.; Hicks, T.; Taroni, F. Preuve Par l'ADN-la Génétique au Service de la Justice, 3rd ed.; Presses Polytechniques et UniversitairesRomandes: Lausanne, Switzerland, 2013. **[Google Scholar]**

75. Biedermann, A.; Champod, C.; Jackson, G.; Gill, P.; Taylor, D.; Butler, J.; Morling, N.; Hicks, T.; Vuille, J.; Taroni, F. Evaluation of forensic DNA traces when propositions of interest relate to activities: Analysis and discussion of recurrent concerns. Front. Genet. **2016**, 7, 215. **[Google Scholar] [CrossRef] [Green Version]**

76. Doyle, S. Quality Management in Forensic Science, 1st ed.; Academic Press: London, UK, 2018. **[Google Scholar]**

77. van Oorschot, R.A.H.; Meakin, G.E.; Kokshoorn, B.; Goray, M.; Szkuta, B. DNA transfer in forensic science: Recent progress towards meeting challenges. Genes **2021**, 12, 1766. **[Google Scholar] [CrossRef] [PubMed]**

05 OPEN-SOURCE AND COMMERCIAL SOFTWARE OPTIONS FOR THE ANALYSIS OF FORENSIC SEQUENCING DATA: AN OVERVIEW

1. INTRODUCTION: AN OVERVIEW

In the past decade, the discipline of genetics has been significantly impacted by the advancements in Next-generation sequencing (NGS) technologies. Massively parallel sequencing (MPS), also known as high-throughput genomics, is a method developed on multiple platforms that offers genome-scale insights for various fields including medical diagnostics, epidemiology, population genetics, and forensic genetics. The proliferation of vast datasets poses novel issues in the areas of data storage and security, analysis, interpretation, and comparable reporting, all of which must adhere to established forensic genetics standards.

The field of forensic genetics often requires its scientists to have widespread knowledge in related fields such as general genetics, chemistry, physics, physiology, and pathology; however, bioinformatics was rarely among the skills in demand previously. With the introduction of MPS to the field came the generation of a greater amount of data. Due to the lack of readily available user-friendly software, such scarce skills became not just desirable but necessary for early adopters. In the beginning, software to interpret the sequencing data was only developed by research laboratories, naturally with none of the usual emphasis on an attractive graphical user interface (GUI) but focused on functionality and required the users to comfortably navigate the command line. Most analysts working in the forensic DNA laboratories are familiar with running software on the Windows operating system; even those using their Macintosh with the Unix-based operating system rarely would open their terminals and engage in command line operations. Suddenly, the need for data analysis required skills in navigating a whole new world of software running on Unix- and Linux-based computers, and while purchasing such computers was simple enough, gaining the skills to use the software may seem more challenging [**8**]. Such limitations were recognized and, with time, more software options were developed from research laboratories for the needs of the forensic community, some even offering versions run on Windows or more accessible web-based software. To date, several commercial options also entered the arena, offering to close the gap by providing visual, easy to use and ready-to-export solutions, which would satisfy those in need of quick answers and no particular desire to look 'under the hood'.

Some forensic laboratories already established analysis of the mitochondrial DNA (mtDNA) using Sanger sequencing, and for those laboratories the introduction of MPS brings benefits mostly from the upscaling of the sequencing processes, lowering costs and manual workload, speeding up and automating the analyses. Furthermore, MPS of mtDNA may allow insight into more nuanced phenomena, such as low-level heteroplasmy, length heteroplasmy, and better detection of low-level mixtures. Short tandem repeat (STR) typing, however, had never used sequencing as a standard for forensic analysis, therefore the analysis of this new type of data introduces challenges. DNA analysts are familiar with interpreting STR data from capillary electrophoresis (CE) electropherograms from the last two decades, and many of the CE features are transferable to sequencing, e.g., the length-based allele names, the electrophoretic peaks, and the stutter artifacts. The application of sequencing offers an extra dimension of information for the markers, which drives the ongoing efforts to standardize the nomenclature of the sequence-level data, with the requirement to be back-compatible with the length-based allele names. Software solutions developed individual reporting formats that are sometimes difficult to reliably compare; however, most of these also provide a visual representation of the data, comparable to the already familiar electropherograms, and detailed counts of coverage read depth, similar to CE relative fluorescence unit (RFU) values. Despite the variable formats, these efforts aim to provide a human-readable sequence structure, as well as a sequence string format for universal comparison of the detected sequence variants. One area of non-consensus is the degree or range of reporting of the flanking regions surrounding the markers. While this is mostly influenced by the chemistry used, interpretation of these regions may be optional, dependent on settings, or may even be omitted; therefore becoming a potential source of discrepancy between analysis methods. Similar to reporting from CE data, the analysts will be required to report which kit they used, supplemented with the genomic range of reporting to avoid such discrepancies. While adjustments to reporting will become straightforward with nomenclature standardization and the available software options are increasingly user-friendly, the most critical adaptation for the analysis of STR sequencing data is reaching a comfort level with this data type, developing some basic bioinformatic skills to process data and interpret sequence variants routinely or in challenging cases.

Below is a concise collection of the different software and algorithm choices now accessible for analyzing sequencing data, with a specific emphasis on their application in forensic investigations. Our objective is to offer a comprehensive manual for forensic experts who are beginning to incorporate these innovative sequencing techniques into their regular forensic DNA analysis procedures.

2. JUSTIFICATION FOR THE UTILIZATION OF HIGH-THROUGHPUT SEQUENCING DATA ANALYSIS TECHNIQUES FOR SHORT TANDEM REPEATS (STRS)

True to the proverbial concept of bioinformatics, that 'there is more than one way to solve a problem', individual algorithms indeed differ, but regardless of which programming language they use, on which operating systems they run or which sequencing data type, or platform they can process, the general approach is broadly similar and summarized on the schematic graph in **Figure 1**.

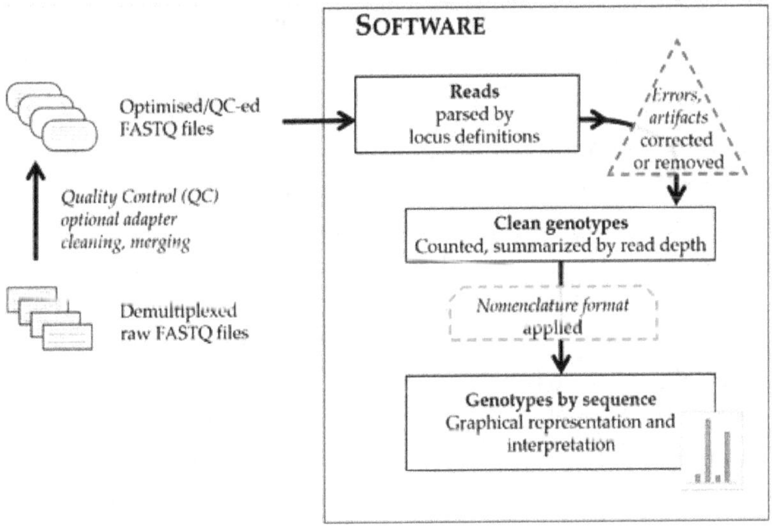

Figure 1. Schematic representation of general forensic MPS data processing steps.

The input files are text files containing sequence data in different formats generated by the sequencing platforms: files of sequence data with or without quality values for each base call in each read (FASTQ or FASTA), or sequence alignment files and their indices (BAM and BAI). The sequencing reads from the input files are parsed by using a defined set of attributes with characteristics of the targeted markers by which to filter. The terminology of the software describing these attributes significantly differ, therefore **Table 1** compares not just the software themselves, but the verbiage for the files providing locus definitions and names for the landmarks of the targeted loci. These files provide configurations for the analyses in respect to the range and specificity of sequence targeted, by allowing strict or flexible matching to the short sequences landmarking the targeted loci and their immediate flanking regions. These landmark sequences anchor the reads to the selected loci, and often coincide with known or presumed primer regions of the amplicons. The targeted markers are also described by their repeat motifs and/or structure, which increases the locus-specificity and allows for the precise recognition of allele variants. Approaches differ as to whether software only recognizes a predefined set of allele variants aligning reads to these references, or could recognize and call undefined, novel variants, and furthermore, capable of creating various possible combinations of expected alleles just from the provided repeat blocks of the array. Regardless of the approach, the reads of each marker are tallied and summarized in the form of a read depth value (or coverage) for each allele. The recognition of a group of reads as alleles are also facilitated by adjustable analytical thresholds separating signal from noise.

The relationship between observed sequences is often used to categorize calls as true alleles or their derivatives (stutter or reads with errors). Some software offers options to flag, remove, and/or correct potential artifacts and errors from sequencing. At the end of the process, allele calls are designated based on adequate coverage surpassing thresholds for interpretation and being excluded as artifacts.

The common denominator of any software approach is the generation of sequence strings as the ultimate comparable form of sequence alleles, a requirement [**9**,**10**] for publishing population study sequence variants that allow for concordance checking between methods; with the caveat of different analysis ranges may still generate discrepancies between different methods. While such sequence strings are easily comparable by computer programs, this is not true for human analysts, therefore the software also reports a human-friendly format of the sequence alleles in their preferred nomenclature. These usually are presented in a 'bracketed' form with the counts of the repeat blocks summarized using brackets (e.g., [GATA]8); furthermore, these formats could address the marker, genomic location analyzed, the length equivalent of the allele and may also include any flanking region variation observed when compared to the human reference genome (usually the most recent version, GRCh38). Most software, apart from the standard outputs of the sequence strings, read depths and a form of bracketed nomenclature, also provide a visual output: a graphical representation of the detected alleles in a familiar histogram format, which being similar to the electropherogram peaks aids the transition of analysts from STR typing by CE to sequencing.

Table 1. Summary of characteristics of software for the interpretation of MPS data of forensic markers.

Software	Versions	Author/Vendor	Year	Accessibility	Runs on	Locus Definition	Landmarks for Loci
STRait Razor	v1.0	Warshauer et al. [**11**]	2013	free	Unix/Linux	config file	'anchor'
	v2.0	Warshauer et al. [**12**]	2015	free	Unix/Linux		
	v2s	King et al. [**13**]	2017	free	Unix/Linux		
	v3.0	Woerner et al. [**14**]	2017	free	all platforms		
	Online	King et al. [**15**]	2021	free	online/ all platforms		
FDSTools	TSSV	Anvar et al. [**16**]	2014	free	Unix/Linux	library file	'flank'
	v1.0	van der Gaag et al. [**17**]	2016	free	Unix/Linux		
	v1.1.1	Hoogenboom et al. [**18**]	2017	free	Unix/Linux		
	v2.0	Hoogenboom et al. [**19**]	2021	free	all platforms	STRNaming	
STRinNGS	v1.0	Friis et al. [**20**]	2016	on request	Unix/Linux	configuration file	'flanking sequences'
	v2.0	Jonck et al. [**21**]	2020	free	Unix/Linux		
MyFLq	v1.1	Van Neste et al. [**22,23**]	2014	free	online/Unix/ Linux	panels	'recognition elements'
toaSTR	v1.0	Ganschow et al. [**24**]	2018	free	online	allele database	'primer'
Altius	Cloud	Bailey et al. [**25**]	2017	on request	online	lookup table	'target regions'
ExactID	v2.0	Battelle [**26**]	2015	commercial	Windows	config file	default

Software	Versions	Author/Vendor	Year	Accessibility	Runs on	Locus Definition	Landmarks for Loci
GeneMarker HTS	v1.0	SoftGenetics [**27**]	2017	commercial	Windows	default	default
MixtureAce	v1.0	NicheVision [**28**]	2018	commercial	Windows	default	default
CLC Genomics Workbench	AQME	Sturk-Andreaggi et al. [**29**]	2017	commercial	all platforms	non STR	non STR
Universal Analysis Software	v2.3	Verogen [**30**]	2021	commercial	Windows	default	default
Converge Forensic Analysis Software	v2.2	Thermo Fisher [**31**]	2019	commercial	Windows	BED files	default

A new phenomenon introduced by using bioinformatic software for forensic DNA analysis is the occasional appearance of bioinformatic null alleles. These are the bioinformatic equivalents of null alleles in CE where sequence variation underneath the primer binding sites could impair or prevent amplification of the actual alleles. In the case of bioinformatic nulls, the amplification is not compromised and the sequencing reads are present in the raw data files, but there is an unexpected sequence variation underneath the landmark regions of a locus that a software uses to recognize locus-specific reads. While most software allows for 'wobble' or approximate matching in these landmark regions, this sequence variation can be significant enough for the software to fail to recognize and analyze the true reads in the filtering process, thus resulting in a null allele. The best prevention of bioinformatic nulls being reported in profiles is the use of a secondary data analysis method, which can be particularly useful in forensic validations or population studies. Using a sequencing platform-specific software in combination with another commercial, free or open-source software can largely eliminate the chance of bioinformatic nulls remaining unrecognized. In the case of the custom loci set developed in-house, where only open-source software can be used, it is good practice to use multiple software to call alleles, or at least use the same software with different settings in their locus definition files specifying different landmark regions, to avoid the occasional bioinformatic nulls.

Analysis of sequencing data requires access to adequate storage and safeguarding of the generated data. Local protocols need to be developed for the long-term maintenance and expansion of these resources, considering the size of the data files is not comparable to those originating from CE, often measured in gigabytes per run. Most of the following tools can be run on a standard laptop or desktop, but high-performance computing resources can be beneficial when processing a lot of samples.

3. FREELY AVAILABLE SOFTWARE

In the early stages of the application of massively parallel sequencing to the forensic field, most solutions were developed in academic settings as a necessary research tool to be able to characterize and analyze data generated by sequencing platforms [**11,16,20,22**]. These approaches often focused on STR markers, occasionally offering options to analyze mtDNA data as well [**18**]. These software are freely available but assume the users have a basic level of bioinformatics skills allowing them to navigate and operate through the command line. Such basic skills can be obtained either through professional training [**32**] or self-taught courses via one of the several available online tutorials on 'how to Linux' [**33**]. Once the basic command-line skills are comfortably obtained, the following software can be run just as confidently through a terminal window as clicking an icon in a GUI.

While there are a few software options available through web-based interfaces [**23,24,25**], some developers offer [**21,34**] or transition to [**35**] providing a version of their software that can be downloaded as a 'Docker image'. This is a 'ready to use' packet of the program and all its dependencies required to run the application successfully, regardless of the underlying resources available locally [**36**]. A program, the Docker engine, facilitates the use of such packets on both Linux and Windows-based applications. While similar to virtual machines, this solution is more flexible and portable, as the isolated environment does not require a part of the hardware to be closed off, but rather creates such containers on a software level. This form of software availability improves not only data security, satisfying those who cannot allow data file exchange outside of their local laboratory but can also make these applications more accessible for those who are just beginning their journey with software operated through the command line.

3.1. STRait Razor

This software, designed to analyze reads from sequenced amplicons targeting STRs, was first published in 2013. Its evolution went through iterations from STRait Razor [**11**], v2.0 [**12**], v2s [**13**], v3.0 [**14**], and STRait Razor Online (SRO) [**15**] improving its processing speeds and output files, extending its analysis to the flanking regions and providing secondary analysis tools, such as additional workbooks for visual interpretation of the data using histograms and reporting sequence alleles following the International Society for Forensic Genetics (ISFG) early considerations [**37**].

The software uses FASTQ files as an input and versions prior to SRO required command line navigation. Detailed help files and guides are available, instructing users how to run an analysis by entering a command with the desired options. The file that sets the locus definitions is referred to as the 'config file' and the landmarks on each side of the loci are called the 'anchors'. These modifiable config files are included for the currently available main sequencing kits, or custom files can be generated by the user. The output are simple text files, which can be processed further either by the provided Excel workbooks, the online platform, or custom scripts for the advanced users. These additional processes can summarize the results in a tabular and a visual format and facilitate additional insights such as allele nomenclature, stutter analysis, or sequencing error profiles. While previous versions could be run on the command line (using a Mac or a Linux computer), the v3.0 of this software can also run using the Command Prompt in Windows. The latest version (SRO) introduces the main functionality of the software in an online tool format, suitable for quick analysis of individual files, without the use of a Unix or Linux environment. The online format significantly decreases the need for bioinformatics skills; however, for batch processing a large number of files or for the use of custom settings running the downloaded command-line version of SRO is more practical. The software includes config files for the commercially available sequencing kits and a default set of predefined alleles to call theses from the sequencing reads it analyzes, therefore any undefined sequence allele by default would require the user to establish an appropriate nomenclature. In such cases, the software may label the unrecognized variant as 'novel' by default, however, the variant may have been reported in more up-to-date literature or increasingly available databases [**38,39,40**].

The software is a general starting point for those interested in exploring their data further, specifically to be able to provide an unrestricted reporting of the flanking region variants [**41**]. It has proven useful in providing a secondary analysis to commercial software outputs as a means for eliminating bioinformatic null alleles [**42**].

3.2. FDSTools

This software is also designed to analyze reads from amplified STRs, with later versions offering the capability to analyze mtDNA results [**43**] from sequencing data. The evolution of the software through its iterations starts with the standalone TSSV tool [**16**] recognizing repetitive motifs in the reads, which was integrated into the FDSTools bundles v1.0, later v1.1.1 [**17,18**]. The latest version (v2.0) was expanded by an integrated nomenclature package STRNaming [**19**]. The software is a bundle of several tools to be used in the analyses of sequencing data from raw FASTQ files. Analyzed loci and their analysis attributes are defined by a 'library file', including their landmark regions referred to as 'flanks'. Results include coverage values with options for different outputs including bracketed and string formats. The package includes several additional tools for stutter analysis and correction, databasing, and visualizations as well. The addition of the STRNaming module eliminates the need for user input on the locus definition files. Instead, the program now automatically recognizes repetitive sequences in the reference sequence using these as the preset preferences for bracketing interpretation of the sequence reads and, as such, automates nomenclature classification of the called alleles. The addition of this module facilitates the ongoing efforts to reach a unified nomenclature for the standard human forensic STR markers [**37,44,45**].

The software is a good starting point as a secondary analysis option with additional flexibility for those interested in building custom solutions for their more specific needs beyond standard reports [**17,46,47**]. The offered modular tools and customization are ideal for stutter analysis or the visualization of stutter restoration to the respective parent allele [**48**]. Those who appreciate graphics generated in a report-ready format will find the graphical HTML outputs useful [**17**]. Beyond the standard or custom niche sets of STR markers of human forensics, the software is an ideal tool for those developing wildlife forensic markers with the need for flexible software adaptable to species identification from novel STR multiplexes [**49**].

3.3. STRinNGS

The software STRinNGS v1.0 [**20**] was one of the early approaches available on request developed by researchers. This tool required command-line skills to analyze the data and use the output files in further scripts to summarize stutter and error profiles observed. The recently released v2.0. [**21**] is openly available to download for local use and has been updated to provide a more refined set of criteria for improved reliability in allele calling including error filtering, identifying stutter reads, and flagging unusual sequences for manual review. STRinNGS accepts FASTQ files as input and runs the settings via its locus definition file which is referred to as the 'configuration file' where it defines the marker landmarks as 'flanking sequences'. To accommodate the need for quality control (QC), the software offers an output format that can be used directly for submission to STRidER [**9**]. This site (**https://strider.online/**) is dedicated to the QC of autosomal STR population data sets, providing unique identification numbers as proof of data passing their checks.

The software is a good alternative as a secondary analysis to eliminate bioinformatic nulls in the analysis and is now an improved tool that helps the analyst with the manual review by providing several optional flags and settings. The software reports a format in line with guidance from the forensic community [**9,10,37**] as well as its own developed format for allele nomenclature which is easily comparable with other free software outputs for concordance. It provides clear indications of the genomic locations, the length-based alleles, the sequence structures, and the flanking variations [**50**] and, for the convenience of the user, includes the sequence strings analyzed.

3.4. MyFLq

One of the earliest software solutions for forensic STR data analysis from MPS was developed [**22**] in a form of a web-based user-friendly application using FASTA or FASTQ files for input. In the past, this was also available as an integrated online tool on BaseSpace [**23**], for use with Illumina sequencing data output. For the practicality of analyzing sensitive data locally, a desktop version of the software is also available to download [**22**] or provided as a Docker-container file [**34**] to be downloaded as a functional package and run locally. To help recognize non-predefined true alleles, MyFLq can estimate whether an unrecognized allele is truly a novel allele or a result of errors. The landmarks defining the loci analyzed are referred to as 'primers', however, this does not necessarily mean that they completely overlap with the primers in the amplification reaction. The approach uses a dynamic calculation of the flanking regions and the region of interest (ROI), rather than a static definition of repeat region and flanking regions. The ROI, the variable part of the sequence, is compared to the reference alleles and allows an easy interpretation of SNPs as well as STR length polymorphisms within the analyzed region. The output is a report of the sequences with their sequence and the derived length alleles as well, including visualization of the results.The use of this software can be interesting for those who want an alternative analysis when comparing methods and those who are interested in viewing their data in a simple, non-bracketed nomenclature format. MyFLq has the potential to work with SNP and mtDNA data as well. This approach could also be useful for working with new STRs or non-human STRs, capitalizing on the flexible approach of locus analysis which can adjust to a dynamically growing reference allele database.

3.5. ToaSTR

This software offers a user-friendly graphical web-based solution for the analysis of STR data from sequencing. It does not require bioinformatics expertise from the users as it provides an intuitive GUI to analyze data from FASTQ or FASTA files. Web-based software options often face questions about data security and laboratories may be restricted from uploading sensitive data to the web, therefore the developers currently provide access to this secure web-based tool upon request [**24**]. Those who require further assurance will welcome the recent update that will move the web-based application at the end of 2021 to a Docker-based format [**35**], allowing the software to be downloaded as a functional unit operating securely locally.ToaSTR defines the analyzed loci together as a 'panel' and refers to the landmark sequences as 'recognition elements'. The panels to be analyzed are customizable and therefore independent of the sequencing platforms and kits [**51**]. The software includes predictive stutter modeling allowing an automatic classification of the observed sequences and the differentiation of artifacts. The reporting nomenclature format of ToaSTR is aligned to the ISFG considerations [**37**] and includes graphical visualization of the results.Prior to the implementation of the updated software format, the web-based version remains valuable for assessing training data and trials, as well as for mobile demonstrations that necessitate prompt and visually captivating results.

3.6. Altius

Altius is an autonomous and secure software that operates in the Cloud. It is specifically designed to efficiently analyze large amounts of data from FASTQ files. Users can access this user-friendly graphical user interface (GUI) through a web browser without needing any specialized knowledge in bioinformatics. The software has the ability to analyze MPS data from a specific group of STRs (autosomal, X- and Y-STRs) [52,53] produced by several platforms, including the MinION. The analysis is highly reliable and capable of handling batch data processing [25]. The locus identification characteristics utilized in this study are derived from STRaitRazor v2.0 [12]. A lookup table is created to compile the definitions of the loci, which enables the software to accurately identify the specific loci of interest. The findings are stored in a MySQL database and can be exported as reports. These reports include the complete sequence strings, a visual representation of the results, and a nomenclature format that complies with the guidelines of ISFG [37]. The software ensures data security through the utilization of Amazon Web Services capabilities, enabling users to customize access-control methods according to their specific needs. Altius grants access to its secure cloud system upon request and subsequent authentication.

4. COMMERCIAL SOFTWARE

In addition to the readily accessible academic software, there are various alternatives provided by commercial enterprises. These solutions can be used either as an additional option to the vendors' own sequencing chemical and platform, or as independent tools for examining the raw data output from different sequencers. Typically, these programs are designed to be easy for users to navigate, with visually pleasing graphical interfaces. They offer a restricted range of options for customizing procedures, aiming to deliver a smooth and trouble-free analytical experience. The programs also generate graphical output that is familiar and presentable, along with results that are ready for presenting. Several of them provide choices for mtDNA analysis as well as STR data analysis, both produced on the sequencing platforms. Commercial software aims to facilitate the adoption of MPS by new users, enhancing their proficiency in working with sequence data. Nevertheless, it offers limited control over the algorithms and occasional problem-solving may necessitate the support of the software providers. The properties of these systems are appealing to high-throughput regular laboratories, and the dependable convenience they provide could rationalize the expense.

4.1. GeneMarker HTS (SoftGenetics, State Collage, PA)

GeneMarker HTS [27] offers an integrated solution for analyzing sequencing data from mtDNA, STRs, and SNPs generated on either Illumina or Ion Torrent platforms. The software is validated for mtDNA data analysis [**54,55**]. It can be used to analyze the mtDNA control region or the whole mtDNA genome, as required [**56**]. The STR analysis utilizes an in-built panel for the Promega PowerSeq 46GY kit (Promega, Madison, WI, USA), using FASTQ files generated from an Illumina MiSeq (Illumina, San Diego, CA, USA), alternatively, a panel for custom chemistries can be used for analyzing data from other kits. MtDNA and STR analysis (including flanking region variations) can be performed individually or simultaneously. GeneMarker HTS reports the length-equivalent of the sequence alleles, provides sequence strings and a visual interpretation of the results using histograms. An audit trail of changes and analysis settings are logged, and user access rights are controlled by its database. Demo and trial versions, training materials, and product support are available. GeneMarker HTS operates under Windows.

4.2. ExactID (Battelle, Colombus, OH)

Battelle's ExactID [**26**] offers another fully integrated agnostic software solution designed for professional use in government agencies and crime laboratories. The sequencing platform-independent software analyzes data from FASTQ files generated from various chemistries targeting forensic markers, such as autosomal, X- and Y-STRs [**57,58**], SNPs, microhaplotypes, and mtDNA. The analysis settings are defined in 'config files' for the various marker panels. The user-friendly GUI offers a familiar display of the observed alleles in a histogram format along with the length-equivalent alleles and the bracketed sequence alleles in line with the ISFG considerations [**37**] for STRs. The software can recognize previously undefined alleles and to report flanking region variation. The results can be exported in multiple formats: .pdf file with tabular and graphical summaries, .csv files for further external analysis, and an additional .sef file format for evidence preservation. Furthermore, ExactID offers additional intelligence leads by interpreting data relating to phenotypic markers and biogeographical ancestry using the Battelle Avatar plugin. Audit trail and user access control are provided by the software. ExactID operates under Windows.

4.3. MixtureAce (NicheVision, Akron, OH)

MixtureAce [**28**] the plugin tool for the ArmedXpert software offers a user-friendly option to analyze MPS data from FASTQ files for STR (autosomal, X- and Y-STR) markers [**59,60**] with the benefit of the integrated hash-based Sequence Identifier (SID) nomenclature [**61**], a unique abbreviated format of sequence-based alleles designed to identify the relationships between sequences. MixtureAce uses the SIDs to recognize reads of stutter or other predefined artifacts using customizable thresholds and thus facilitates the recognition of reads not filtered out as true alleles. Undefined artifacts still need to be manually curated [**60**]. The software reports within the ranges of sequences encompassing the STRs following the UAS flanking region report [**44**]. This ready-to-use solution can report from a single source or interpret mixed samples using another ArmedXpert plugin: Mixture Interpretation. MixtureAce operates under Windows.

4.4. CLC Genomics Workbench (QIAGEN, Hilden, Germany)

CLC Genomics Workbench [**62**] is a genomic bioinformatic tool collection developed by and offered from Qiagen for comprehensive sequencing data analysis in general. This tool allows customization of its collection with plugins, such as the AQME [**29**], the toolbox specifically developed in collaboration with AFDIL to accommodate forensic-specific mtDNA sequence analysis for data generated from any MPS platform. AQME also includes haplogroup estimation and phylogenetically consistent nomenclature to facilitate reporting of the results. This specific plugin can be applied within the CLC Workbench framework.

4.5. Universal Analysis Software (Verogen, San Diego, CA)

Universal Analysis Software (UAS) [**30**] is the custom software of the MiSeqFGx sequencing platform that can analyze sequencing data from forensic markers using specific modules for the ForenSeq line of kits. Currently available chemistries target STRs (autosomal, X- and Y-STRs), SNPs, and mtDNA. Raw data is directly processed from the sequencer to generate demultiplexed raw sequence output FASTQ files. This is then further analyzed within the software using alignment to the human reference sequence and variant calling from the sequences at the range reported by the software. To extend the reported range outside of the repeat region an additional flanking region report is also available in the form of an excel file. To further analyze variation outside of expected flanking region variations, the raw FASTQ files can also be exported and processed by external software for independent analysis and concordance. The software is validated together with the platform and chemistry as the MiSeq Forensic Genomics System [**63,64**] supported by training and direct product support from the vendor.

The GUI is designed to be intuitive and user-friendly and with default and additional modules for different forensic genomic applications for the FGx platform, such as the STR analysis module or the data analysis for mtDNA sequencing chemistries. A supplementary analysis generates investigative leads, such as the estimation of phenotypic markers (hair and eye color) and biogeographical ancestry estimation of the samples [**65,66**]. Furthermore, genomic applications can analyze data generated from dedicated SNP panels for SNP-based identification of degraded remains; or can pre-format the generated data for downstream use in databases specific to the application of forensic genetic genealogy (FGG). FGG is an investigative tool for identifying distant kinship of a sample using databases built from ‘direct-to-consumer’ (DTC) genealogy DNA test results, data volunteered by citizen scientists. The generated data is formatted to be comparable with the markers in the database allowing to facilitate the investigation of serious crimes or to identify unidentified human remains [**67**].

4.6. Converge Forensic Analysis Software (Thermo Fisher, Waltham, MA)

Converge Forensic Analysis Software [**31**] is the comprehensive validated software customized to the HID Ion S5 sequencing platforms of Thermo Fisher. Converge is designed for this specific sequencing platform and visualizes the analyzed results obtained from the Torrent Server via the HID Genotyper plugin. It has modules specific to workflows of the offered chemistries targeting specific forensic markers: STRs including multiple markers for sex-determination [**68**], mtDNA control region, or the full mitochondrial genome [**69**]. Additional modules beyond STR analysis include those interpreting data from kits targeting selected SNP sets, which can establish identity from degraded samples [**70**,**71**] or can provide investigative leads and estimate biogeographic ancestry [**72**]. Data organization in Converge is optimized and streamlined around case management. The software and chemistries are validated for mtDNA analysis [**73**] and the users are supported by training and documentation from the vendor.

Via the HID Genotyper plugin, the generated sequencing reads are demultiplexed and aligned to the default reference sequence in regions specified by the BED file. The BED files are specific to the chemistries targeting different marker sets. Both the chosen reference and the BED files can be customized. The generated data can be downloaded as alignment files (BAM and BAI) or alternatively can also be generated as FASTQ files to download for independent analysis and concordance analysis.

The GUI is designed to be intuitive for the sequence-based data and follows the familiar look of the vendor's CE-based software (GeneMapper ID-X, Thermo fisher, Waltham, MA, USA) and it can integrate and compare the two data types for casework, paternity, and kinship calculations. For markers that are not currently supported by the offered kits and the software (for example chemistry targeting multiple Y chromosomal markers), sequencing can be performed using a custom set of amplicons [**74**,**75**]. The generated raw data then can be downloaded and analyzed with the available independent software options.

5. OTHER SOFTWARE OPTIONS FOR WHOLE GENOME SEQUENCING (WGS) DATA

Without exhausting the list there are other software options available [**76**,**77**], and many were designed to identify and analyze STR markers from genome-wide sequencing data without a forensic focus. STRs, in general, may be medically relevant or used as markers for population genetics, and specific software has also been designed to identify other relevant tandem repeats to facilitate medical diagnosis or genotype of these markers [**78**,**79**,**80**,**81**,**82**,**83**]. Recent reviews [**84**,**85**] also provided an overview of several alternative software that can generate STR profiles from whole-genome sequencing data [**86**,**87**,**88**,**89**,**90**,**91**,**92**,**93**,**94**].

While these may not be the immediate focus of forensic analysts mainly interested in reporting the sequencing data from the targeted amplification of markers specifically curated for forensic purposes, WGS data analysis methods could prove useful in exploring alternative approaches with already available data sources or in research projects.

6. TIPS, TRICKS, AND MORE TOOLS

Despite the evolution of software solutions for forensic MPS data, occasionally data analysis can come to a halt if suspicious results are observed. This could be an unexpected null or supernumerary allele, unreasonably low coverage, or confusing sequence structure. In case of concern, there are always a few options to investigate the reason for discrepancies. For example, one can investigate the observed coverage values in relation to the expected inter-locus balance, which can indicate failure to detect an allele in heterozygotes interpreted falsely as homozygotes (bioinformatic null alleles). Any software can potentially generate bioinformatic null calls, i.e., the inability to recognize and report a specific variant. The best approach to confirm any unexpected instances is to use multiple software (or at least multiple settings) for the analysis and perform a concordance check-in between analysis methods.In-built software of the sequencing platforms (UAS and Converge) can offer investigative leads using SNP data from some of their chemistries. Additionally, the user can harvest the relevant SNP data and independently verify certain phenotypic traits: eye and hair color using the constantly updated and freely available tools (**https://hirisplex.erasmusmc.nl/**) hosted at the Erasmus MC University. The website offers options for a manual or automated upload of the SNP genotype data to verify the prediction of these phenotypic traits using the established results from relevant studies (IrisPlex [**95**], HIrisPlex [**96**], HIRISPlex-S [**97,98,99**]).

Visualizing genetic variations frequently aids in comprehending the manner in which certain alterations in nucleotides give rise to atypical sequence configurations. The Integrative Genomics Viewer (IGV) [100] is a valuable tool for visualizing alignment and variant calling files, allowing for manual comparison with the reference sequence. If the consensus sequence of the reads is not readily apparent through manual review, an alternative tool called VisCoSe may be useful. VisCoSe has the capability to compute and compare consensus sequences from several datasets [101]. Performing independent Quality Control of the raw data before analysis is a recommended practice. This involves monitoring the primary features of the dataset both before and after any extra clean-up operations. One way to accomplish this is by utilizing the FastQC tool [102]. Utilizing supplementary tools such as Trimmomatic, Cutadapt, and seqtk for meticulous adapter trimming, or employing FLASH, BBMerge, or CASPER for combining paired-end reads, can potentially enhance the subsequent analysis. There are situations where employing supplementary data cleansing technologies can enhance the analysis of raw data.

Eliminating inaccurate readings and low-quality segments of readings that are specific to the chemistry and platform can result in clear and certain identification of alleles. Additionally, this process can enhance the coverage values obtained from the dataset. Open datasets that are now accessible provide a valuable resource for individuals who are not yet involved in massively parallel sequencing but are interested in gaining more knowledge about data analysis before developing a local workflow. An example of such a source is the Forensic DNA Open Dataset, which is made available by the NIST Applied Genetics Group [109] and can be accessed at https://doi.org/10.18434/M32157. Open datasets containing whole-genome sequencing (WGS) data can be accessed through various sources. One such source is the data portal of the 1000 Genomes Project, which provides access to WGS data. Another source is the International Genome Sample Resource (IGSR), which also offers open datasets for WGS data. These projects provide variants that can be viewed using the 1000 Genome Browsers hosted at the National Center for Biotechnology Information (NCBI).

7. AT A GLANCE

The objective of this evaluation was to present a concise and easily understandable summary of the software choices now available. It recognizes the difficulties faced by forensic specialists who are not experts in bioinformatics in this particular subject. This review would be advantageous for DNA analysts who are currently knowledgeable in CE-based analysis and tools but lack experience in high-throughput sequencing, or for those who intend to produce sequencing data in the future.

All the software solutions offered exhibit satisfactory performance, and the choice of selecting one (or, as recommended here, multiple) over others may depend on personal preference, financial constraints, or compatibility with existing equipment. By actively investigating these different possibilities, routine forensic casework laboratories will enhance their comprehension of the sequence-level diversity of forensic markers and the benefits of integrating sequence data analysis into their workflows. Gaining proficiency in fundamental bioinformatics is crucial in order to effectively harness the new opportunities presented by MPS in the discipline.

8. SUMMARY

The primary obstacles to incorporating novel techniques for forensic DNA analysis in standard laboratories frequently involve the financial investment and the specialized knowledge necessary to locally apply and authenticate these technologies. Over the past decade, a number of commercially accessible choices expressly designed for forensic purposes have emerged in the field of next-generation sequencing. These options provide dependable and verified solutions. However, the current perception is that the readily accessible knowledge and skills to evaluate, interpret, and comprehend such data are still falling behind. This review provides a basic introduction for novice forensic scientists who are starting to use next-generation sequencing in their local laboratories. Given that many professionals in this field lack a background in bioinformatics, they may encounter challenges in understanding the new terminology and analysis choices that are now available. This document provides a concise overview of the open-source and commercial software currently available for analyzing forensic sequencing data. It aims to serve as a helpful resource for individuals who are new to the forensic application of massively parallel sequencing.

REFERENCES

1. Chen, M.; Zhao, H. Next-generation sequencing in liquid biopsy: Cancer screening and early detection. Hum. Genom. **2019**, 13, 34. **[Google Scholar] [CrossRef] [Green Version]**
2. John, G.; Sahajpal, N.S.; Mondal, A.K.; Ananth, S.; Williams, C.; Chaubey, A.; Rojiani, A.M.; Kolhe, R. Next-Generation Sequencing (NGS) in COVID-19: A Tool for SARS-CoV-2 Diagnosis, Monitoring New Strains and Phylodynamic Modeling in Molecular Epidemiology. Curr. Issues Mol. Biol. **2021**, 43, 845–867. **[Google Scholar] [CrossRef]**
3. Gonzalez-Quezada, B.A.; Creary, L.E.; Munguia-Saldana, A.J.; Flores-Aguilar, H.; Fernandez-Vina, M.A.; Gorodezky, C. Exploring the ancestry and admixture of Mexican Oaxaca Mestizos from Southeast Mexico using next-generation sequencing of 11 HLA loci. Hum. Immunol. **2019**, 80, 157–162. **[Google Scholar] [CrossRef]**
4. Borsting, C.; Morling, N. Next generation sequencing and its applications in forensic genetics. Forensic Sci. Int. Genet. **2015**, 18, 78–89. **[Google Scholar] [CrossRef] [PubMed]**
5. Bruijns, B.; Tiggelaar, R.; Gardeniers, H. Massively parallel sequencing techniques for forensics: A review. Electrophoresis **2018**, 39, 2642–2654. **[Google Scholar] [CrossRef] [PubMed] [Green Version]**
6. Alonso, A.; Barrio, P.A.; Muller, P.; Kocher, S.; Berger, B.; Martin, P.; Bodner, M.; Willuweit, S.; Parson, W.; Roewer, L.; et al. Current state-of-art of STR sequencing in forensic genetics. Electrophoresis **2018**, 39, 2655–2668. **[Google Scholar] [CrossRef]**
7. Ballard, D.; Winkler-Galicki, J.; Wesoly, J. Massive parallel sequencing in forensics: Advantages, issues, technicalities, and prospects. Int. J. Legal Med. **2020**, 134, 1291–1303. **[Google Scholar] [CrossRef]**

8. Alonso, A.; Muller, P.; Roewer, L.; Willuweit, S.; Budowle, B.; Parson, W. European survey on forensic applications of massively parallel sequencing. Forensic Sci. Int. Genet. **2017**, 29, e23–e25. **[Google Scholar] [CrossRef] [PubMed]**
9. Bodner, M.; Bastisch, I.; Butler, J.M.; Fimmers, R.; Gill, P.; Gusmao, L.; Morling, N.; Phillips, C.; Prinz, M.; Schneider, P.M.; et al. Recommendations of the DNA Commission of the International Society for Forensic Genetics (ISFG) on quality control of autosomal Short Tandem Repeat allele frequency databasing (STRidER). Forensic Sci. Int. Genet. **2016**, 24, 97–102. **[Google Scholar] [CrossRef]**
10. Gusmao, L.; Butler, J.M.; Linacre, A.; Parson, W.; Roewer, L.; Schneider, P.M.; Carracedo, A. Revised guidelines for the publication of genetic population data. Forensic Sci. Int. Genet. **2017**, 30, 160–163. **[Google Scholar] [CrossRef]**
11. Warshauer, D.H.; Lin, D.; Hari, K.; Jain, R.; Davis, C.; Larue, B.; King, J.L.; Budowle, B. STRait Razor: A length-based forensic STR allele-calling tool for use with second generation sequencing data. Forensic Sci. Int. Genet. **2013**, 7, 409–417. **[Google Scholar] [CrossRef]**
12. Warshauer, D.H.; King, J.L.; Budowle, B. STRait Razor v2.0: The improved STR Allele Identification Tool--Razor. Forensic Sci. Int. Genet. **2015**, 14, 182–186. **[Google Scholar] [CrossRef] [PubMed]**
13. King, J.L.; Wendt, F.R.; Sun, J.; Budowle, B. STRait Razor v2s: Advancing sequence-based STR allele reporting and beyond to other marker systems. Forensic Sci. Int. Genet. **2017**, 29, 21–28. **[Google Scholar] [CrossRef]**
14. Woerner, A.E.; King, J.L.; Budowle, B. Fast STR allele identification with STRait Razor 3.0. Forensic Sci. Int. Genet. **2017**, 30, 18–23. **[Google Scholar] [CrossRef] [PubMed]**
15. King, J.L.; Woerner, A.E.; Mandape, S.N.; Kapema, K.B.; Moura-Neto, R.S.; Silva, R.; Budowle, B. STRait Razor Online: An enhanced user interface to facilitate interpretation of MPS data. Forensic Sci. Int. Genet. **2021**, 52, 102463. **[Google Scholar] [CrossRef] [PubMed]**
16. Anvar, S.Y.; van der Gaag, K.J.; van der Heijden, J.W.; Veltrop, M.H.; Vossen, R.H.; de Leeuw, R.H.; Breukel, C.; Buermans, H.P.; Verbeek, J.S.; de Knijff, P.; et al. TSSV: A tool for characterization of complex allelic variants in pure and mixed genomes. Bioinformatics **2014**, 30, 1651–1659. **[Google Scholar] [CrossRef] [Green Version]**
17. van der Gaag, K.J.; de Leeuw, R.H.; Hoogenboom, J.; Patel, J.; Storts, D.R.; Laros, J.F.J.; de Knijff, P. Massively parallel sequencing of short tandem repeats-Population data and mixture analysis results for the PowerSeq system. Forensic Sci. Int. Genet. **2016**, 24, 86–96. **[Google Scholar] [CrossRef] [Green Version]**

18. Hoogenboom, J.; van der Gaag, K.J.; de Leeuw, R.H.; Sijen, T.; de Knijff, P.; Laros, J.F. FDSTools: A software package for analysis of massively parallel sequencing data with the ability to recognise and correct STR stutter and other PCR or sequencing noise. Forensic Sci. Int. Genet. **2017**, 27, 27–40. **[Google Scholar] [CrossRef] [Green Version]**

19. Hoogenboom, J.; Sijen, T.; van der Gaag, K.J. STRNaming: Generating simple, informative names for sequenced STR alleles in a standardised and automated manner. Forensic Sci. Int. Genet. **2021**, 52, 102473. **[Google Scholar] [CrossRef] [PubMed]**

20. Friis, S.L.; Buchard, A.; Rockenbauer, E.; Borsting, C.; Morling, N. Introduction of the Python script STRinNGS for analysis of STR regions in FASTQ or BAM files and expansion of the Danish STR sequence database to 11 STRs. Forensic Sci. Int. Genet. **2016**, 21, 68–75. **[Google Scholar] [CrossRef] [PubMed]**

21. Jonck, C.G.; Qian, X.; Simayijiang, H.; Borsting, C. STRinNGS v2.0: Improved tool for analysis and reporting of STR sequencing data. Forensic Sci. Int. Genet. **2020**, 48, 102331. **[Google Scholar] [CrossRef]**

22. Van Neste, C.; Vandewoestyne, M.; Van Criekinge, W.; Deforce, D.; Van Nieuwerburgh, F. My-Forensic-Loci-queries (MyFLq) framework for analysis of forensic STR data generated by massive parallel sequencing. Forensic Sci. Int. Genet. **2014**, 9, 1–8. **[Google Scholar] [CrossRef] [PubMed] [Green Version]**

23. Van Neste, C.; Gansemans, Y.; De Coninck, D.; Van Hoofstat, D.; Van Criekinge, W.; Deforce, D.; Van Nieuwerburgh, F. Forensic massively parallel sequencing data analysis tool: Implementation of MyFLq as a standalone web- and Illumina BaseSpace((R))-application. Forensic Sci. Int. Genet. **2015**, 15, 2–7. **[Google Scholar] [CrossRef] [PubMed]**

24. Ganschow, S.; Silvery, J.; Kalinowski, J.; Tiemann, C. toaSTR: A web application for forensic STR genotyping by massively parallel sequencing. Forensic Sci. Int. Genet. **2018**, 37, 21–28. **[Google Scholar] [CrossRef]**

25. Bailey, S.F.; Scheible, M.K.; Williams, C.; Silva, D.; Hoggan, M.; Eichman, C.; Faith, S.A. Secure and robust cloud computing for high-throughput forensic microsatellite sequence analysis and databasing. Forensic Sci. Int. Genet. **2017**, 31, 40–47. **[Google Scholar] [CrossRef]**

26. Battelle. ExactID®. Available online: **https://www.battelle.org/government-offerings/homeland-security-public-safety/security-law-enforcement/forensic-genomics/exactid** (accessed on 1 October 2021).

27. SoftGenetics. GeneMarker®HTS. Available online: **https://softgenetics.com/GeneMarkerHTS.php** (accessed on 1 October 2021).

28. NicheVision. ArmedXpert™ MixtureAce™. Available online: **https://nichevision.com/mixtureace/** (accessed on 1 October 2021).

29. Sturk-Andreaggi, K.; Peck, M.A.; Boysen, C.; Dekker, P.; McMahon, T.P.; Marshall, C.K. AQME: A forensic mitochondrial DNA analysis tool for next-generation sequencing data. Forensic Sci. Int. Genet. **2017**, 31, 189–197. **[Google Scholar] [CrossRef]**

30. Verogen. Universal Analysis Software v2.0 Reference Guide (VD2019002). Available online: **https://verogen.com/wp-content/uploads/2021/05/universal-analysis-software-v2-0-reference-guide-vd2019002-d.pdf** (accessed on 1 October 2021).

31. ThermoFisher. User Guide: Converge Software v2.2—Setup and Reference (100039539E). Available online: **https://assets.thermofisher.com/TFS-Assets/LSG/manuals/100039539_ConvergeSftwre_UG.pdf** (accessed on 1 October 2021).

32. EBI. EMBL-EBI Training Courses. Available online: **https://www.ebi.ac.uk/training/** (accessed on 1 October 2021).

33. The Linux Foundation. Introduction to Linux (Free Course). Available online: **https://training.linuxfoundation.org/training/introduction-to-linux/** (accessed on 1 October 2021).

34. Van Neste, C. MyFLq Site on GitHub—Docker Container. Available online: **https://github.com/beukueb/myflq** (accessed on 1 October 2015).

35. LABCON-OWL. toaSTR—Announcement: Transition to a Docker-Based Application. Available online: **https://www.toastr.de/** (accessed on 1 October 2021).

36. Docker. Docker Containers. Available online: **https://www.docker.com/resources/what-container** (accessed on 1 October 2021).

37. Parson, W.; Ballard, D.; Budowle, B.; Butler, J.M.; Gettings, K.B.; Gill, P.; Gusmao, L.; Hares, D.R.; Irwin, J.A.; King, J.L.; et al. Massively parallel sequencing of forensic STRs: Considerations of the DNA commission of the International Society for Forensic Genetics (ISFG) on minimal nomenclature requirements. Forensic Sci. Int. Genet. **2016**, 22, 54–63. **[Google Scholar] [CrossRef] [PubMed] [Green Version]**

38. Gettings, K.B.; Borsuk, L.A.; Ballard, D.; Bodner, M.; Budowle, B.; Devesse, L.; King, J.; Parson, W.; Phillips, C.; Vallone, P.M. STRSeq: A catalog of sequence diversity at human identification Short Tandem Repeat loci. Forensic Sci. Int. Genet. **2017**, 31, 111–117. **[Google Scholar] [CrossRef] [Green Version]**

39. Van Neste, C.; Van Criekinge, W.; Deforce, D.; Van Nieuwerburgh, F. Forensic Loci Allele Database (FLAD): Automatically generated, permanent identifiers for sequenced forensic alleles. Forensic Sci. Int. Genet. **2016**, 20, e1–e3. **[Google Scholar] [CrossRef]**

40. Willuweit, S. Challenges and Paradigm Shifts by the Adoption of MPS in Forensic Casework—Lessons Learned from the Collaborative DNASeqEx Project So Far; HIDS: Vienna, Austria, 2017. **[Google Scholar]**

41. Wendt, F.R.; King, J.L.; Novroski, N.M.M.; Churchill, J.D.; Ng, J.; Oldt, R.F.; McCulloh, K.L.; Weise, J.A.; Smith, D.G.; Kanthaswamy, S.; et al. Flanking region variation of ForenSeq DNA Signature Prep Kit STR and SNP loci in Yavapai Native Americans. Forensic Sci. Int. Genet. **2017**, 28, 146–154. **[Google Scholar] [CrossRef]**

42. Gettings, K.B.; Borsuk, L.A.; Steffen, C.R.; Kiesler, K.M.; Vallone, P.M. Sequence-based U.S. population data for 27 autosomal STR loci. Forensic Sci. Int. Genet. **2018**, 37, 106–115. **[Google Scholar] [CrossRef] [PubMed] [Green Version]**

43. van der Gaag, K.J.; Desmyter, S.; Smit, S.; Prieto, L.; Sijen, T. Reducing the Number of Mismatches between Hairs and Buccal References When AnalysingmtDNAHeteroplasmic Variation by Massively Parallel Sequencing. Genes **2020**, 11, 1355. **[Google Scholar] [CrossRef]**

44. Gettings, K.B.; Ballard, D.; Bodner, M.; Borsuk, L.A.; King, J.L.; Parson, W.; Phillips, C. Report from the STRAND Working Group on the 2019 STR sequence nomenclature meeting. Forensic Sci. Int. Genet. **2019**, 43, 102165. **[Google Scholar] [CrossRef] [Green Version]**

45. Phillips, C.; Gettings, K.B.; King, J.L.; Ballard, D.; Bodner, M.; Borsuk, L.; Parson, W. "The devil's in the detail": Release of an expanded, enhanced and dynamically revised forensic STR Sequence Guide. Forensic Sci. Int. Genet. **2018**, 34, 162–169. **[Google Scholar] [CrossRef] [PubMed] [Green Version]**

46. Huszar, T.I.; Jobling, M.A.; Wetton, J.H. A phylogenetic framework facilitates Y-STR variant discovery and classification via massively parallel sequencing. Forensic Sci. Int. Genet. **2018**, 35, 97–106. **[Google Scholar] [CrossRef] [Green Version]**

47. Claerhout, S.; Verstraete, P.; Warnez, L.; Vanpaemel, S.; Larmuseau, M.; Decorte, R. CSYseq: The first Y-chromosome sequencing tool typing a large number of Y-SNPs and Y-STRs to unravel worldwide human population genetics. PLoS Genet. **2021**, 17, e1009758. **[Google Scholar] [CrossRef]**

48. de Leeuw, R.H.; Garnier, D.; Kroon, R.; Horlings, C.G.C.; de Meijer, E.; Buermans, H.; van Engelen, B.G.M.; de Knijff, P.; Raz, V. Diagnostics of short tandem repeat expansion variants using massively parallel sequencing and componential tools. Eur. J. Hum. Genet. **2019**, 27, 400–407. **[Google Scholar] [CrossRef] [Green Version]**

49. Beasley, J.; Shorrock, G.; Neumann, R.; May, C.A.; Wetton, J.H. Massively parallel sequencing and capillary electrophoresis of a novel panel of falcon STRs: Concordance with minisatellite DNA profiles from historical wildlife crime. Forensic Sci. Int. Genet. **2021**, 54, 102550. **[Google Scholar] [CrossRef] [PubMed]**

50. Hussing, C.; Huber, C.; Bytyci, R.; Mogensen, H.S.; Morling, N.; Borsting, C. Sequencing of 231 forensic genetic markers using the MiSeqFGx forensic genomics system—an evaluation of the assay and software. Forensic Sci. Res. **2018**, 3, 111–123. **[Google Scholar] [CrossRef]**

51. Silvery, J.; Ganschow, S.; Wiegand, P.; Tiemann, C. Developmental validation of the monSTR identity panel, a forensic STR multiplex assay for massively parallel sequencing. Forensic Sci. Int. Genet. **2020**, 46, 102236. **[Google Scholar] [CrossRef]**

52. Silva, D.; Sawitzki, F.R.; Scheible, M.K.R.; Bailey, S.F.; Alho, C.S.; Faith, S.A. Genetic analysis of Southern Brazil subjects using the PowerSeq AUTO/Y system for short tandem repeat sequencing. Forensic Sci. Int. Genet. **2018**, 33, 129–135. **[Google Scholar] [CrossRef] [PubMed]**

53. Silva, D.; Scheible, M.K.; Bailey, S.F.; Williams, C.L.; Allwood, J.S.; Just, R.S.; Schuetter, J.; Skomrock, N.; Minard-Smith, A.; Barker-Scoggins, N.; et al. Sequence-based autosomal STR characterization in four US populations using PowerSeq Auto/Y system. Forensic Sci. Int. Genet. **2020**, 48, 102311. **[Google Scholar] [CrossRef]**

54. Holland, M.M.; Pack, E.D.; McElhoe, J.A. Evaluation of GeneMarker® HTS for improved alignment of mtDNA MPS data, haplotype determination, and heteroplasmy assessment. Forensic Sci. Int. Genet. **2017**, 28, 90–98. **[Google Scholar] [CrossRef] [PubMed]**

55. Brandhagen, M.D.; Just, R.S.; Irwin, J.A. Validation of NGS for mitochondrial DNA casework at the FBI Laboratory. Forensic Sci. Int. Genet. **2020**, 44, 102151. **[Google Scholar] [CrossRef] [PubMed] [Green Version]**

56. Wisner, M.; Erlich, H.; Shih, S.; Calloway, C. Resolution of mitochondrial DNA mixtures using a probe capture next generation sequencing system and phylogenetic-based software. Forensic Sci. Int. Genet. **2021**, 53, 102531. **[Google Scholar] [CrossRef] [PubMed]**

57. Gettings, K.B.; Kiesler, K.M.; Faith, S.A.; Montano, E.; Baker, C.H.; Young, B.A.; Guerrieri, R.A.; Vallone, P.M. Sequence variation of 22 autosomal STR loci detected by next generation sequencing. Forensic Sci. Int. Genet. **2016**, 21, 15–21. **[Google Scholar] [CrossRef] [PubMed] [Green Version]**

58. Montano, E.A.; Bush, J.M.; Garver, A.M.; Larijani, M.M.; Wiechman, S.M.; Baker, C.H.; Wilson, M.R.; Guerrieri, R.A.; Benzinger, E.A.; Gehres, D.N.; et al. Optimization of the Promega PowerSeq Auto/Y system for efficient integration within a forensic DNA laboratory. Forensic Sci. Int. Genet. **2018**, 32, 26–32. **[Google Scholar] [CrossRef] [PubMed]**

59. Young, B.A.; Gettings, K.B.; McCord, B.; Vallone, P.M. Estimating number of contributors in massively parallel sequencing data of STR loci. Forensic Sci. Int. Genet. **2019**, 38, 15–22. **[Google Scholar] [CrossRef]**

60. Sharma, V.; Young, B.; Armogida, L.; Khan, A.; Wurmbach, E. Evaluation of ArmedXpert software tools, MixtureAce and Mixture Interpretation, to analyze MPS-STR data. Forensic Sci. Int. Genet. **2021**, 56, 102603. **[Google Scholar] [CrossRef]**

61. Young, B.; Faris, T.; Armogida, L. A nomenclature for sequence-based forensic DNA analysis. Forensic Sci. Int. Genet. **2019**, 42, 14–20. **[Google Scholar] [CrossRef]**

62. QIAGEN. CLC Genomics Workbench. Available online: **https://digitalinsights.qiagen.com/products-overview/discovery-insights-portfolio/analysis-and-visualization/qiagen-clc-genomics-workbench/** (accessed on 1 October 2021).

63. Jager, A.C.; Alvarez, M.L.; Davis, C.P.; Guzman, E.; Han, Y.; Way, L.; Walichiewicz, P.; Silva, D.; Pham, N.; Caves, G.; et al. Developmental validation of the MiSeqFGx Forensic Genomics System for Targeted Next Generation Sequencing in Forensic DNA Casework and Database Laboratories. Forensic Sci. Int. Genet. **2017**, 28, 52–70. **[Google Scholar] [CrossRef] [Green Version]**

64. Hollard, C.; Ausset, L.; Chantrel, Y.; Jullien, S.; Clot, M.; Faivre, M.; Suzanne, E.; Pene, L.; Laurent, F.X. Automation and developmental validation of the ForenSeq() DNA Signature Preparation kit for high-throughput analysis in forensic laboratories. Forensic Sci. Int. Genet. **2019**, 40, 37–45. **[Google Scholar] [CrossRef]**

65. Sharma, V.; Jani, K.; Khosla, P.; Butler, E.; Siegel, D.; Wurmbach, E. Evaluation of ForenSeq Signature Prep Kit B on predicting eye and hair coloration as well as biogeographical ancestry by using Universal Analysis Software (UAS) and available web-tools. Electrophoresis **2019**, 40, 1353–1364. **[Google Scholar] [CrossRef]**

66. Fregeau, C.J. Validation of the VerogenForenSeq DNA Signature Prep kit/ Primer Mix B for phenotypic and biogeographical ancestry predictions using the Micro MiSeq(R) Flow Cells. Forensic Sci. Int. Genet. **2021**, 53, 102533. **[Google Scholar] [CrossRef]**

67. Kling, D.; Phillips, C.; Kennett, D.; Tillmar, A. Investigative genetic genealogy: Current methods, knowledge and practice. Forensic Sci. Int. Genet. **2021**, 52, 102474. **[Google Scholar] [CrossRef]**

68. Barrio, P.A.; Martin, P.; Alonso, A.; Muller, P.; Bodner, M.; Berger, B.; Parson, W.; Budowle, B.; Consortium, D. Massively parallel sequence data of 31 autosomal STR loci from 496 Spanish individuals revealed concordance with CE-STR technology and enhanced discrimination power. Forensic Sci. Int. Genet. **2019**, 42, 49–55. **[Google Scholar] [CrossRef] [PubMed]**

69. Strobl, C.; Eduardoff, M.; Bus, M.M.; Allen, M.; Parson, W. Evaluation of the precision ID whole MtDNA genome panel for forensic analyses. Forensic Sci. Int. Genet. **2018**, 35, 21–25. **[Google Scholar] [CrossRef]**

70. Avila, E.; Felkl, A.B.; Graebin, P.; Nunes, C.P.; Alho, C.S. Forensic characterization of Brazilian regional populations through massive parallel sequencing of 124 SNPs included in HID ion Ampliseq Identity Panel. Forensic Sci. Int. Genet. **2019**, 40, 74–84. **[Google Scholar] [CrossRef] [PubMed]**

71. Turchi, C.; Previdere, C.; Bini, C.; Carnevali, E.; Grignani, P.; Manfredi, A.; Melchionda, F.; Onofri, V.; Pelotti, S.; Robino, C.; et al. Assessment of the Precision ID Identity Panel kit on challenging forensic samples. Forensic Sci. Int. Genet. **2020**, 49, 102400. **[Google Scholar] [CrossRef]**

72. Pereira, V.; Mogensen, H.S.; Borsting, C.; Morling, N. Evaluation of the Precision ID Ancestry Panel for crime case work: A SNP typing assay developed for typing of 165 ancestral informative markers. Forensic Sci. Int. Genet. **2017**, 28, 138–145. **[Google Scholar] [CrossRef] [PubMed]**

73. Cihlar, J.C.; Amory, C.; Lagace, R.; Roth, C.; Parson, W.; Budowle, B. Developmental Validation of a MPS Workflow with a PCR-Based Short Amplicon Whole Mitochondrial Genome Panel. Genes **2020**, 11, 1345. **[Google Scholar] [CrossRef] [PubMed]**

74. Ralf, A.; van Oven, M.; Montiel Gonzalez, D.; de Knijff, P.; van der Beek, K.; Wootton, S.; Lagace, R.; Kayser, M. Forensic Y-SNP analysis beyond SNaPshot: High-resolution Y-chromosomal haplogrouping from low quality and quantity DNA using Ion AmpliSeq and targeted massively parallel sequencing. Forensic Sci. Int. Genet. **2019**, 41, 93–106. **[Google Scholar] [CrossRef]**

75. de la Puente, M.; Phillips, C.; Xavier, C.; Amigo, J.; Carracedo, A.; Parson, W.; Lareu, M.V. Building a custom large-scale panel of novel microhaplotypes for forensic identification using MiSeq and Ion S5 massively parallel sequencing systems. Forensic Sci. Int. Genet. **2020**, 45, 102213. **[Google Scholar] [CrossRef] [Green Version]**

76. Wang, D.; Tao, R.; Li, Z.; Pan, D.; Wang, Z.; Li, C.; Shi, Y. STRsearch: A new pipeline for targeted profiling of short tandem repeats in massively parallel sequencing data. Hereditas **2020**, 157, 8. **[Google Scholar] [CrossRef]**

77. Lee, J.C.; Tseng, B.; Chang, L.K.; Linacre, A. SEQ Mapper: A DNA sequence searching tool for massively parallel sequencing data. Forensic Sci. Int. Genet. **2017**, 26, 66–69. **[Google Scholar] [CrossRef]**

78. Budis, J.; Kucharik, M.; Duris, F.; Gazdarica, J.; Zrubcova, M.; Ficek, A.; Szemes, T.; Brejova, B.; Radvanszky, J. Dante: Genotyping of known complex and expanded short tandem repeats. Bioinformatics **2019**, 35, 1310–1317. **[Google Scholar] [CrossRef]**

79. Costa, I.P.D.; Almeida, B.C.; Sequeiros, J.; Amorim, A.; Martins, S. A Pipeline to Assess Disease-Associated Haplotypes in Repeat Expansion Disorders: The Example of MJD/SCA3 Locus. Front. Genet. **2019**, 10, 38. **[Google Scholar] [CrossRef] [PubMed]**

80. Holtgrewe, M.; Stolpe, O.; Nieminen, M.; Mundlos, S.; Knaus, A.; Kornak, U.; Seelow, D.; Segebrecht, L.; Spielmann, M.; Fischer-Zirnsak, B.; et al. VarFish: Comprehensive DNA variant analysis for diagnostics and research. Nucleic Acids Res. **2020**, 48, W162–W169. **[Google Scholar] [CrossRef] [PubMed]**

81. Liu, Q.; Tong, Y.; Wang, K. Genome-wide detection of short tandem repeat expansions by long-read sequencing. BMC Bioinform. **2020**, 21 (Suppl. 21), 542. **[Google Scholar] [CrossRef]**

82. Tang, H.; Kirkness, E.F.; Lippert, C.; Biggs, W.H.; Fabani, M.; Guzman, E.; Ramakrishnan, S.; Lavrenko, V.; Kakaradov, B.; Hou, C.; et al. Profiling of Short-Tandem-Repeat Disease Alleles in 12,632 Human Whole Genomes. Am. J. Hum. Genet. **2017**, 101, 700–715. **[Google Scholar] [CrossRef] [PubMed]**

83. Dashnow, H.; Lek, M.; Phipson, B.; Halman, A.; Sadedin, S.; Lonsdale, A.; Davis, M.; Lamont, P.; Clayton, J.S.; Laing, N.G.; et al. STRetch: Detecting and discovering pathogenic short tandem repeat expansions. Genome Biol. **2018**, 19, 121. **[Google Scholar] [CrossRef] [Green Version]**

84. Liu, Y.Y.; Harbison, S. A review of bioinformatic methods for forensic DNA analyses. Forensic Sci. Int. Genet. **2018**, 33, 117–128. **[Google Scholar] [CrossRef]**

85. Halman, A.; Oshlack, A. Accuracy of short tandem repeats genotyping tools in whole exome sequencing data. F1000Research **2020**, 9, 200. **[Google Scholar] [CrossRef] [Green Version]**

86. Gymrek, M.; Golan, D.; Rosset, S.; Erlich, Y. lobSTR: A short tandem repeat profiler for personal genomes. Genome Res. **2012**, 22, 1154–1162. **[Google Scholar] [CrossRef] [PubMed] [Green Version]**

87. Highnam, G.; Franck, C.; Martin, A.; Stephens, C.; Puthige, A.; Mittelman, D. Accurate human microsatellite genotypes from high-throughput resequencing data using informed error profiles. Nucleic Acids Res. **2013**, 41, e32. **[Google Scholar] [CrossRef] [PubMed] [Green Version]**

88. Fungtammasan, A.; Ananda, G.; Hile, S.E.; Su, M.S.; Sun, C.; Harris, R.; Medvedev, P.; Eckert, K.; Makova, K.D. Accurate typing of short tandem repeats from genome-wide sequencing data and its applications. Genome Res. **2015**, 25, 736–749. **[Google Scholar] [CrossRef] [Green Version]**

89. Willems, T.; Zielinski, D.; Yuan, J.; Gordon, A.; Gymrek, M.; Erlich, Y. Genome-wide profiling of heritable and de novo STR variations. Nat. Methods **2017**, 14, 590–592. **[Google Scholar] [CrossRef] [PubMed] [Green Version]**

90. Tang, H.; Nzabarushimana, E. STRScan: Targeted profiling of short tandem repeats in whole-genome sequencing data. BMC Bioinform. **2017**, 18 (Suppl. 11), 398. **[Google Scholar] [CrossRef] [Green Version]**

91. Mousavi, N.; Margoliash, J.; Pusarla, N.; Saini, S.; Yanicky, R.; Gymrek, M. TRTools: A toolkit for genome-wide analysis of tandem repeats. Bioinformatics **2020**, 37, 731–733. **[Google Scholar] [CrossRef] [PubMed]**

92. Kojima, K.; Kawai, Y.; Misawa, K.; Mimori, T.; Nagasaki, M. STR-realigner: A realignment method for short tandem repeat regions. BMC Genom. **2016**, 17, 991. **[Google Scholar] [CrossRef] [Green Version]**

93. Kristmundsdottir, S.; Sigurpalsdottir, B.D.; Kehr, B.; Halldorsson, B.V. popSTR: Population-scale detection of STR variants. Bioinformatics **2017**, 33, 4041–4048. **[Google Scholar] [CrossRef]**

94. Bolognini, D.; Magi, A.; Benes, V.; Korbel, J.O.; Rausch, T. TRiCoLOR: Tandem repeat profiling using whole-genome long-read sequencing data. Gigascience **2020**, 9, giaa101. **[Google Scholar] [CrossRef]**

95. Walsh, S.; Liu, F.; Ballantyne, K.N.; van Oven, M.; Lao, O.; Kayser, M. IrisPlex: A sensitive DNA tool for accurate prediction of blue and brown eye colour in the absence of ancestry information. Forensic Sci. Int. Genet. **2011**, 5, 170–180. **[Google Scholar] [CrossRef]**

96. Walsh, S.; Liu, F.; Wollstein, A.; Kovatsi, L.; Ralf, A.; Kosiniak-Kamysz, A.; Branicki, W.; Kayser, M. The HIrisPlex system for simultaneous prediction of hair and eye colour from DNA. Forensic Sci. Int. Genet. **2013**, 7, 98–115. **[Google Scholar] [CrossRef] [PubMed] [Green Version]**

97. Walsh, S.; Chaitanya, L.; Clarisse, L.; Wirken, L.; Draus-Barini, J.; Kovatsi, L.; Maeda, H.; Ishikawa, T.; Sijen, T.; de Knijff, P.; et al. Developmental validation of the HIrisPlex system: DNA-based eye and hair colour prediction for forensic and anthropological usage. Forensic Sci. Int. Genet. **2014**, 9, 150–161. **[Google Scholar] [CrossRef]**

98. Walsh, S.; Chaitanya, L.; Breslin, K.; Muralidharan, C.; Bronikowska, A.; Pospiech, E.; Koller, J.; Kovatsi, L.; Wollstein, A.; Branicki, W.; et al. Global skin colour prediction from DNA. Hum. Genet. **2017**, 136, 847–863. **[Google Scholar] [CrossRef] [Green Version]**

99. Chaitanya, L.; Breslin, K.; Zuniga, S.; Wirken, L.; Pospiech, E.; Kukla-Bartoszek, M.; Sijen, T.; Knijff, P.; Liu, F.; Branicki, W.; et al. The HIrisPlex-S system for eye, hair and skin colour prediction from DNA: Introduction and forensic developmental validation. Forensic Sci. Int. Genet. **2018**, 35, 123–135. **[Google Scholar] [CrossRef] [Green Version]**

100. Robinson, J.T.; Thorvaldsdottir, H.; Winckler, W.; Guttman, M.; Lander, E.S.; Getz, G.; Mesirov, J.P. Integrative genomics viewer. Nat. Biotechnol. **2011**, 29, 24–26. **[Google Scholar] [CrossRef] [PubMed] [Green Version]**

101. Spitzer, M.; Fuellen, G.; Cullen, P.; Lorkowski, S. VisCoSe: Visualization and comparison of consensus sequences. Bioinformatics **2004**, 20, 433–435. **[Google Scholar] [CrossRef] [Green Version]**

102. BabrahamBioinformatics. FastQC: A Quality Control Tool for High Throughput Sequence Data. Available online: **http://www.bioinformatics.babraham.ac.uk/projects/fastqc/** (accessed on 1 October 2010).

103. Bolger, A.M.; Lohse, M.; Usadel, B. Trimmomatic: A flexible trimmer for Illumina sequence data. Bioinformatics **2014**, 30, 2114–2120. **[Google Scholar] [CrossRef] [PubMed] [Green Version]**

104. Martin, M. Cutadapt removes adapter sequences from high-throughput sequencing reads. EMBnet. J. **2011**, 17, 10–12. **[Google Scholar] [CrossRef]**

105. Li, H. Seqtk: A Fast and Lightweight Tool for Processing FASTA or FASTQ Sequences. Available online: **https://github.com/lh3/seqtk** (accessed on 1 October 2013).

106. Magoc, T.; Salzberg, S.L. FLASH: Fast length adjustment of short reads to improve genome assemblies. Bioinformatics **2011**, 27, 2957–2963. **[Google Scholar] [CrossRef] [PubMed]**

107. Bushnell, B.; Rood, J.; Singer, E. BBMerge—Accurate paired shotgun read merging via overlap. PLoS ONE **2017**, 12, e0185056. **[Google Scholar] [CrossRef]**

108. Kwon, S.; Lee, B.; Yoon, S. CASPER: Context-aware scheme for paired-end reads from high-throughput amplicon sequencing. BMC Bioinform. **2014**, 15 (Suppl. 9), S10. **[Google Scholar] [CrossRef] [PubMed] [Green Version]**

109. NIST Applied Genetics Group. Forensic DNA Open Dataset. Available online: **https://data.nist.gov/od/id/mds2-2157** (accessed on 1 October 2019). **[CrossRef]**

110. 1000 Genomes Project. The International Genome Sample Resource (IGSR) Data Portal. Available online: **https://www.internationalgenome.org/data-portal/data-collection** (accessed on 1 October 2017).

111. Clarke, L.; Fairley, S.; Zheng-Bradley, X.; Streeter, I.; Perry, E.; Lowy, E.; Tasse, A.M.; Flicek, P. The international Genome sample resource (IGSR): A worldwide collection of genome variation incorporating the 1000 Genomes Project data. Nucleic Acids Res. **2017**, 45, D854–D859. **[Google Scholar] [CrossRef] [Green Version]**

112. Fairley, S.; Lowy-Gallego, E.; Perry, E.; Flicek, P. The International Genome Sample Resource (IGSR) collection of open human genomic variation resources. Nucleic Acids Res. **2020**, 48, D941–D947. **[Google Scholar] [CrossRef] [PubMed]**

113. NCBI. 1000 Genomes Browser. Available online: **https://www.ncbi.nlm.nih.gov/variation/tools/1000genomes/** (accessed on 1 October 2019).

06 ANIMAL FORENSIC GENETICS

1. INTRODUCTION: AN OVERVIEW

The predicament of endangered emblematic species, such as tigers, rhinoceroses, and elephants, receives significant media coverage. Moreover, the strong emotional connections that humans form with domesticated animals, specifically dogs and cats, are so significant that the mistreatment of pets holds a prominent place in the human consciousness. It may appear paradoxical that the forensic investigation and prosecution of suspected incidents involving non-human animals has consistently been given lesser priority than human identification. As an additional illustration pertaining to research in this field, the ISFG congress often dedicates only a small portion of its program to discussions on DNA in wildlife crime and non-human DNA profiling, while allocating numerous days to the topic of human identification. The low priority assigned to this matter is multifaceted, with a primary factor being the historical perception that investigations involving non-human material necessitated lower criteria compared to those applied in human identification cases. Previously, a significant portion of DNA typing for non-human organisms was conducted in unaccredited laboratories, mostly found in academic institutions. However, there is currently a shift occurring, as several facilities are obtaining complete ISO17025 accreditation. The inclusion of a review as part of a Special Issue serves as another proof of the ongoing recognition of non-human DNA typing as a valuable tool in forensic investigations. This review is divided into two primary sections. The first section examines the similarities between identifying individual dogs and cats using methods similar to human DNA profiling. The second section discusses traditional wildlife forensic testing, which focuses on determining the species present and utilizes mitochondrial DNA sequence analyses.

2. FORENSIC LABORATORIES SPECIALIZING IN WILDLIFE ANALYSIS

Genetic testing to enforce national legislation is rarely performed by the same operational laboratories that undertake human identification. This is primarily attributable to time and cost constraints, and the fact that most operational laboratories are accredited to undertake standard operating procedures relevant to human identification only. Most wildlife forensic investigations are undertaken by universities on an ad hoc basis and performed by university academics who may not routinely undertake work for the criminal justice system. Good laboratory practice has been encouraged, and guidelines have been suggested for Quality Control and Quality Assurance within an academic-based wildlife forensic laboratory [**1**]. There are notable exceptions. These include the US Fish & Wildlife Laboratory in Ashland, Oregon (**https://www.fws.gov/lab/** (accessed on 12 March 2021)), the Scotland-based Wildlife DNA Forensics Laboratory (**http://www.sasa.gov.uk/** (accessed on 12 March 2021)) and the Australian Museum in Sydney (**http://www.Australianmuseum.com** (accessed on 12 March 2021)); these laboratories have attained ISO17025 accreditation.

3. ANALYSIS OF SHORT TANDEM REPEATS (STRS) IN ANIMAL FORENSIC SCIENCE

Dogs and cats are two pet species that are commonly in close contact with humans. According to the North American Pet Insurance Association (NAPHIA), 65% of households in the USA, or 85 million homes, have a dog (**https://www.iii.org/fact-statistic/facts-statistics-pet-statistics** (accessed on 12 March 2021)). Equally over 9 million dogs and 8 million cats are owned in the UK (according to statista.com), this is about 25% of all homes. It is not surprising therefore that hairs from either dogs or cats are found associated with forensic evidence such as clothing, car seats, and household soft furnishing, an example is shown in **Figure 1**.

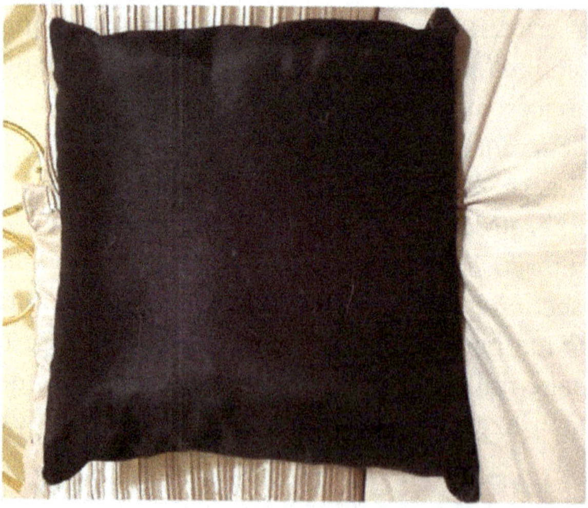

Figure 1. Showing how easy it is for cat hairs to transfer onto soft furnishing, in this case a cushion. These cat hairs can be valuable associative forensic evidence. Note also that these hairs can be transferred to another substrate by secondary transfer.

Such items onto which cat or dog hairs can be transferred, may themselves be associative evidence or be a substrate for secondary transfer to further items that may be of forensic relevance in an investigation. Therefore, it was with the first case of cat hairs to identify a person of interest and lead to a conviction.

3.1. Feline STR Typing

Snowball the cat became famous in arena of forensic DNA profiling for aiding in the resolution of an alleged homicide [2]. The work was initiated by the Royal Canadian Mounted Police (RCMP) after a 32-year-old woman from Prince Edward Island, Canada, was reported missing on 3 October 1994. This occurred in a remote wooded area. A man's jacket was found close to the abandoned car of the missing person, along with other items. White hairs clinging to the lining of the jacket were identified by the RCMP's laboratory to be from a cat. The only suspect in the case happened to own a white cat called Snowball.

Ten dinucleotide STR loci were used in a comparison of the DNA profiles from the hairs taken from the jacket to a hair samples that had been taken from Snowball; these ten loci were found to match. Now the issue was to determine the probability of this match and therefore a population genetic database was generated from cats in Prince Edward Island. In addition, a second database was generated from outbred cats from the Eastern United States [3]. The resulting match probabilities were 2.2×10^{-8} and 6.9×10^{-7} for the Prince Edward Island and the U.S. population databases, respectively [3].

The cat DNA evidence was accepted by the court, and in combination with additional human DNA evidence, was presented to the jury at the Supreme Court of Prince Edward Island. On 19 July 1996, the jury convicted the defendant of second-degree murder [2].

This first case was ground-breaking and showed the real potential of such evidence. The case required a number of steps: developing microsatellite markers, ensuring that the loci were variable, developing primer sets, ensuring the loci were not linked, testing to confirm that they could be co-amplified, developing an allelic database that was representative to allow for the use of robust statistics to support any matching DNA types. These steps are all part of the characterisation of hypervariable STR loci used in human identification, although the use of commercially available products circumvents this massive undertaking.

The first uses of STR loci used dinucleotide repeat markers, but these suffer from a number of stochastic effects, particularly increase in stutter peaks. Feline STR testing was developed further by a group in Germany who characterised 14 hypervariable STR markers, predominantly tetranucleotide repeats, and developed and allelic ladder [4]. These work adhered to the recommendations of the

International Society for Forensic Genetics [**1**]. To allow initial use of these 14 STRs in casework, the authors surveyed 122 unrelated cats in the local area and created an allelic database. Another key point to this work is that, with careful primer design, all 14 STR loci produced amplicons smaller than 260 bases; an important point when working on DNA from hairs and therefore likely to be degraded. An important aspect of this work is that the authors isolated and sequenced each locus to report on the underlying repeat structure. This type of work not only shows a model for the future, but also allowed interlaboratory testing to be performed.

Since this first case, there has been extensive research into increasing the number of hypervariable loci for both cats and dogs.

3.2. Canine STR Typing

A group based in Portugal characterised nine STR loci, all of which were tetranucleotide repeats, which were combined into one multiplex PCR [**5**]. The primer design ensured that the largest allele was still smaller than 350 bases. The authors had also isolated and characterised each of the nine loci so that the repeat sequence could be reported accurately. The authors had access to 113 dog samples to test the multiplex for all the standard conditions as expected in human identification. In combination, and based on the 113 sample set, the authors reported a very high discriminating power (matching probability = $1.63/10^{10}$). This type of work was the foundation for further canine studies.

This assay was extended by two more loci and used in the identification of wolves (Canis lupus) [**6**]. Dogs (Canis lupus familiaris) are a subspecies of the grey wolf and therefore the authors surmised rightly that the same primers would work effectively on wolf as on dogs. Wolves in European come into conflict with humans and are frequently blamed for killing livestock or attacking humans. A case study looked at one such case where a male had received many injuries to the body and claimed to been attacked by a wolf [7]. DNA typing showed conclusively that the man was attacked by a guard dog and not a wolf, or wolf/dog hybrid, as claim; the male later confessed that this was the case [7].

The International Society for Animal Genetics (ISAG) had published a list of putative dog STRs: these comprised 21 dinucleotide loci and 3 tetra repeats. Due to the issues of increased stutters with dinucleotide repeats, and that tetra repeats were recommended by the ISFG [**1**], a group at UC Davies developed a canine STR test that used 15 unlinked STR loci combined into one multiplex, entitled DogFiler [**8**]. A full validation was performed in accordance with the recommendations of the Scientific Working Group for DNA Analysis Methods (SGDAM). The authors of this study sequenced alleles to characterise fully the repeat motifs and also created allelic ladders to allow genotyping. The publication of DogFiler set a precedent as to how to create an STR multiplex that meets the same standards as commercially available kits used in human identification.

Often only shed dog hairs are available for analyses. In such instances, amplification of all the loci to generate a full STR profile might not be possible. To overcome this problem, the same group developed three mini multiplexes by moving the primers closer to the amplicons, thus shortening the length of any allele amplified [**9**]. The result is that no locus is greater than 205 bases in length. Therefore, called Mini-DogFiler met the same standards as the full multiplex.

The CaDNAP group based at the Medical University of Innsbruck separately developed 13 hypervariable microsatellite loci into a multiplex and analysed 1184 dogs [**10**]. All the dogs were from either Germany, Austria or Switzerland (the so called DACH countries). CaDNAP is a working group of the ISFG and members of the CaDNAP group have extensive experience in human identification and very familiar with the requirements for full validation prior to publication and use in the criminal justice system. The equipment required is also that used in any operational forensic science laboratory performing human identification. The inclusion of such a large number of individual dogs from many breeds allowed the construction of a dog population sample database. The chance of two dogs sharing an allele identical by decent could be calculated allowing the same statistics to be used as performed in human identification.

3.3. Livestock

Cats and dogs are the most prevalent domesticated animals. Animals such as cattle, horses, sheep, and camels are occasionally the focus of forensic inquiries. The ISAG plays a key role in establishing standards for genetic testing used to determine parentage in animal breeding (such as stud or pedigree studies). These tests can also be utilized in criminal investigations if necessary. Below are two instances of published case reports.

There are currently 16 cattle (Bos taurus) STR loci listed on a prominent website (**https://strbase.nist.gov//cattleSTRs.htm** (accessed on 15 March 2021)), all of which are dinucleotide repeats. There is a StockMarks® available from ThermoFisher Scientific (Waltham, MA, USA) that includes 11 loci. A recent report extended the panel of STRs to 30 [**11**]. This is largely for parentage studies where many loci are needed for confidence in associating a bull with calves, but also highly useful in confirming meat in the food industry.

Sheep (Ovis aries) are the most commonly grazed species and breeds such as merino and mouflon are either highly prized, or protected. A case report used 16 STR loci, that there amplified in four separate multiplex reactions, to link a carcass of a mouflon to items sized from a vehicle [**12**]. This case occurred on the island of

Sardinia, used Bayesian assignment modelling to support this genetic linkage.

3.4. Wildlife STR Typing

The ivory trade is causing the extinction of elephants in numerous African countries. An elephant tusk is an enlarged tooth and hence a possible reservoir of trace DNA. The utilization of DNA typing on the genetic material obtained from ivory seizures allows for the correlation of these seizures, enabling the determination of the number of elephants that have been killed in each instance. This information will prove valuable in forensic investigations, or at the at least, in shedding light on the magnitude of the illicit trade. Professor Sam Wasser and his team at the University of Washington created a set of Short Tandem Repeats (STRs) specifically for two types of African elephants: the savannah species (Loxodonta Africana) and the forest dwelling species (Loxodonta cyclotis) [13,14]. The objective of the investigation was to ascertain the precise geographical origin of the poached elephants. Elephants that have shared recent ancestors, meaning distant family groups, are likely to have a higher number of common alleles at the examined STR loci compared to elephants with a more distant genetic history. Understanding the distribution of STR alleles across a wide geographic area can be enhanced by studying the movement patterns of matriarchal herds in African savannahs and forests. This groundbreaking research faced the challenge of developing a multiplex of STR loci and extracting high-quality DNA from tusks. This was particularly difficult when the tusks had been stored in unfavorable conditions, potentially leading to degradation of the small amount of DNA available due to bacterial activity.

RhODIS® is a comparable system for the linkage of rhino horns to that of elephants [**15**]. The RhODIS® test is promoted by the University of Pretoria and is comprised of 12 STR loci plus a gender test. It was developed for the two species of rhino that still live in Africa: the white rhino (Ceratotheriumsimum) and the black rhino (Dicerosbicornis). A potential for RhODIS® is that samples from members of the last remaining white and black rhino in wildlife parks such as Kruger can be collected and then later matched to seized horns taken from poached rhino. The author of this review was a guest of a World Bank and TRAFFIC supported visit to Kruger national park in eastern South Africa to witness RhODIS® in action. **Figure 2** is an image of the author attending the poaching of a mother rhino, nearby was the corpse of the offspring; both killed for their horns.

A panel of STR markers have also been created for the one horned Indian rhino (Rhinocerosunicornis) [**16**], as this species has also suffered extreme loss of numbers due to poaching for their horns. This work is part of the official RhODIS-India program. The authors of this paper used 14 STR markers—these were all dinucleotide repeats and far from ideal but had been characterised previously and therefore saved time and resources rather than trying to find and characterise new tetra-repeats [16].

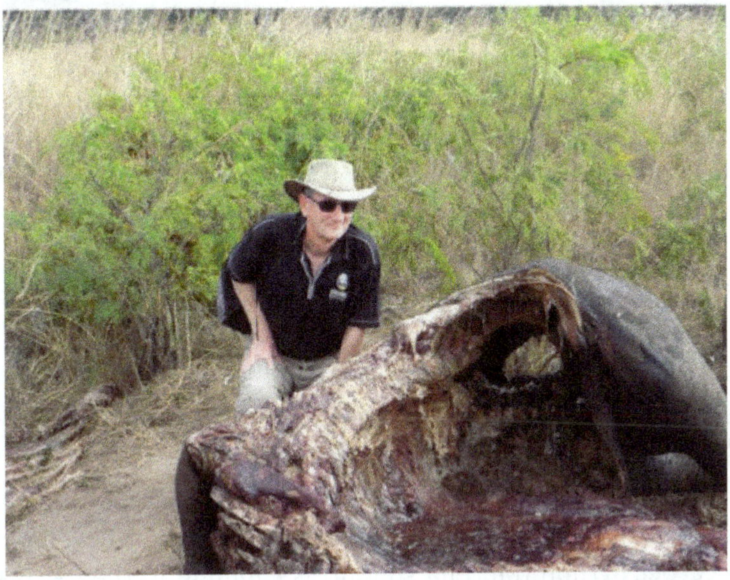

Figure 2. Showing the author at the site of a recently (within 4 days of taking the image) poached mother rhino. The rhino had been shot and then the horn removed with a chain saw. The image was taken in Kruger National Park, South Africa, and is one of around 34 poached rhino recorded in the park every month.

As is likely to be the case for any species that has suffered a loss in numbers and is now breeding from a small set of individuals, the frequency of some alleles starts to either increase as homozygosity increases, and conversely some alleles will decrease or be lost. As reported in the paper on the Indian rhino, many of the STR loci only have 3 or 4 alleles. Despite this, a power of discrimination was reported as 1.4×10^{-9} [16].

Elephant and rhino are iconic mammalian species whose body parts are highly traded internationally. Other mammalian species for which STR multiplexes have been developed include bears, wolves and badgers. As populations increase in the USA there is greater encroachment onto territories of the American black bear (Ursus americanus). Such human bear interactions can lead to injury, and on very rare occasions, death of the human, so tracking down the bear responsible is needed so that an innocent bear is not shot. Eleven tetra-nucleotide repeats were selected along with a sex test and made into one multiplex [17]. The test worked on trace amounts of DNA, down to 78 pg, so it is possible using this method to generate profiles from hairs and scat. A further example is that of STR typing for the European badger (Meles meles) [18]. Badgers are still hunted illegally and therefore the need to link samples from dead badgers or badger parts to items found in the cars, homes or persons of interest is needed.

Bird species are traded illegally for their use in the pet trade, i.e., parrots and cockatoos, or persecuted as perceived threats to livestock, i.e., eagles, harriers and hawks. Cockatoos can be brightly coloured and are also known to be birds that can be caged and then kept as pets. As so happens, a criminal case spurred this research as there was a need to analyse the parentage of seized cockatoos, resulting in the application of 20 STR loci to aid in resolving a dispute as to whether eggs in possession of a person of interest had been taken from a nest illegally [**19**]. Hen harriers (Circus cyaneus) were once a very common sight over northern European moorlands, but now they are extremely rare due to habitat loss and being shot or poisoned as a perceived threat to grouse and other game birds. In response to the need to link carcasses of dead birds to biological material (blood and feathers) on seized items (such as traps and snares) a multiplex of 8 STR markers was created (tetra-repeats with one tri-repeat locus) and validated for use [**20**]. A sex test based on the CHD 1 gene (male birds are Z,Z and females are W,Z) was included and an allelic ladder created.

Reptiles and amphibians have also been the subject of development of STR panels. The carpet python (Morelia spilota) is common in the pet trade and can be kept in captivity if bred from pairs that were also captive (i.e., not taken from the wild). However, the number of known captive snakes appears greater than the expected captive bred population and therefore it is likely that snakes are collected illegally from the wild. In response to a need to test this, three separate multiplexes that covered a total of 24 loci, plus allelic ladders for each locus, was created and called OzPythonPlex [**21**].

The illegal collection of animals from the wild to fuel the pet trade extends to tortoise. The slow-moving reptiles are commonly kept as pets as they are easy to look after. A result, along with habitat loss, is that the number of tortoises in the wild has fallen dramatically. An example is Herman's tortoise (Testudo hermanni), that used to span much of the northern Mediterranean countries. To ensure that seized tortoise are correctly relocated to their correct geographical range, a panel of STR markers were applied for geographical provenance [**22**].

3.5. Finding, Characterising and Applying Short Tandem Repeat LociDiscovering, Describing, and Utilizing Short Tandem Repeat Loci

The aforementioned results utilizing Short Tandem Repeats (STRs) need a substantial amount of research to formulate a multifaceted STR test. Individuals from the forensic community who have only worked in the field of human identification are unlikely to be familiar with the complex process involved in developing a multiplex assay. The reviewer originates from a period when the initial STR test was documented, employing four STR loci [23]. Subsequently, the test advanced to include six STRs together with amelogenin, referred to as the 'second generation multiplex' (or SGM) [24]. The SGM test was developed internally by the UK Forensic Science Service.

The use of STRs from dogs, elephant, rhino and hen harriers as examples, is based on previously reported putative loci. More recently, such as from pythons, the entire genome of the animal was sequenced using massively parallel DNA sequencing (MPS) technology [**21**]. From the mass of genetic sequence data, there are software programs to locate repetitive DNA, then provide a list of putative primers [**25**]. Having ordered primer sequences, these need to be tested on DNA from multiple members of the species to ensure reproducibility and variability at the locus. If still suitable, then homozygotes at each locus need to be sequenced to confirm the repeat motif. Ideally the primers should have similar binding temperatures (termed TMs) so that they can all the amplified in the same reaction. By characterising the loci, an allelic window can be created to determine the smallest and largest alleles likely to be encountered; this is needed to ensure that the alleles do not overlap and fit within a size limit using up to 5 dyes. Sampling many members of the population leads to the creation of allelic ladders, essential for accurate genotyping. This sample set might form the basis of a frequency data set (typically need up to 200 individuals from a population). Standard population genetic calculations need to be undertaken: examining loci for Hardy–Weinberg equilibrium, checking if there is any genetic linkage, and examining for power of discrimination. Validation steps, akin to those provided by SGDAM, include: specificity testing to ensure the primers only amplify from the species/genus for which they were designed; sensitivity tests to determine the limit of detection and effect of adding sub-optimal mass of DNA; stability to see the effects of environmental factors; reproducibility to see the effect of running multiple samples for instance down a column by capillary electrophoresis; interlaboratory testing to ensure the test works on varying equipment and by different operators; blind trial testing to ensure the results are not biased by the inadvertent selection of samples; and perhaps finally publishing the data, as was the case for so many of the papers cited in this review. It is clear reading the above, that this is not something achieved in a matter of weeks and also the reason why so few complex multiplex assays exist for species other than humans and domesticated species such as dogs and cats.

4. CLASSIFICATION OF SPECIES IN THE FIELD OF WILDLIFE FORENSIC SCIENCE

A question raised in wildlife forensic science is 'which species is this?'. This is because legislation at a national level is many countries prohibits the trade or ownership products originating from legally protected species. The illegal trade in protected species is central to much of wildlife forensic science as tools employed by forensic practitioners can be applied when called on to determine whether something is, or is not, legal to trade or own.

Interpol recognized wildlife crime as the second most prevalent crime worldwide after drug trafficking [**26**]. The value of the trade is often quoted as $20 billion (USD) per year [**26,27**] although the exact figure is unknown as very little illegal trade is ever detected. It is only from intercepting seizures that the true scale be estimated. Furthermore, the low penalties and potential large financial gain lead to extensive and lucrative trade in endangered species [**28,29,30**]. This figure of USD 20 billion is also only the estimated illegal revenue from international trade and does not include the illegal trade within countries.

The scope and range of wildlife crime is wide and encompasses a variety of criminal activities such as poaching and illegal hunting of mammals [**31,32**], birds [**20,33**] and reptiles [**21,34,35**], and the use of animal derivatives in traditional medicines [**36,37**].

Forensic investigations can only be undertaken if it is alleged that legislation has been breached. Further, the willingness to conduct DNA profiling of suspected illegally traded/owned samples requires: Approval from prosecuting authorities, availability of persons competent to conduct the work, and funds to compensate that laboratory performing any wildlife investigation.

4.1. Legislation pertaining to the trade of wildlife

The international trade in endangered species is monitored and regulated through recommendations made by Convention on International Trade in Endangered Species of Wild Fauna and Flora (CITES) [**38**]. These recommendations are enforced at a national level by legislation. Normally, this legislation stipulates the names of the species that are protected. It is for these reasons that much interest at a research level has focused on methods of species identification [**38,39**].

Many countries have legislation covering the collection from the wild, breeding, ownership or international trade in animal parts or whole organisms. An example repository of information detailing the federal law in the USA can be found at **https://www.animallaw.info/article/federal-wildlife-law-20th-century** (accessed on 15 March 2021). The US Endangered Species Act (ESA) of 1973 is a key piece of legislation for both domestic (USA), and international conservation. The act aims to provide a framework to conserve and protect endangered and threatened species and their habitats. Additionally, in the USA, the Lacey Act is central to conservation of wildlife and dates from 1900 when it became the first federal law protecting wildlife. The Act makes it unlawful to import, export, sell, acquire, or purchase fish, wildlife or plants that are taken, possessed, transported, or sold: 1) in violation of U.S. or Indian law, or 2) in interstate or foreign commerce involving any fish, wildlife, or plants taken possessed or sold in violation of State or foreign law. The Lacey Act covers all fish and wildlife and their parts or products, plants protected by CITES and those protected by State law; thus regulating international trade of protected species.

The EU, comprised currently of 27 countries, has the free movement of goods across internal borders as a core value. It is only therefore trade across the first border of a member state that is an issue. The EU Council Regulation (EC) No 338/97 deals with the protection of species of wild fauna and flora by regulating trade of any species covered by this regulation. It lays down the provisions for import, export and re-export as well as internal EU trade in specimens of species listed in its four Annexes.

In the UK, the Wildlife and Countryside act of 1981 gave protection to native species, controlled the release of non-native species, protected sites of special scientific interest, and made provision for rights-of-way. A devolved Scotland and separately administered Northern Ireland and Wales resulted in local legislation to protect the environment.

4.2. mtDNA in Species Testing

It may be that the seized material has been processed to create a sculpture, ornament, item of clothing, food, or supposed medicinal product. DNA can be obtained at trace levels from ivory **[40]** where ivory is made into statues, or rhino horn is proceesed into knife handles **[32]**. The most traded mammalian species currently is one of the members of the pangolin family. Pangolins are the only mammals to have scales on the outer surface and are one of eight species: three of which are critically endangered (Manis culionensis, Manis pentadactyla and Manis javanica), three are endangered (Phataginustricuspis, Manis crassicaudata and Smutsia gigantea) and two (Phataginus tetradactyla and Smutsiatemminckii) are recorded as being 'vulnerable' on the Red List of Threatened Species of the International Union for Conservation of Nature. The threat to pangolins is their misguided use in traditional medicines, specifically when the scales are used as bogus remedies. DNA can be obtained from pangolin scales, even when processed as a soup **[41,42]**. Performing mtDNA sequencing can link seizures of pangolins, but also indicates the geographical origin from where they were taken from the wild to inform authorities about hotspots of poaching.

Ivory, rhino horn and pangolin scales are examples of evidential material where DNA is at trace levels. This is typical of much of the seizures encountered in the illegal wildlife trade such that mtDNA is the only genetic material available **[28]**. Human identification has centered on a small section of mtDNA that does not encode; termed the hypervariable regions that constitute less than 1000 of the

16,569 bases that make up the human mitochondrial genome. Vertebrate mtDNA has two strands of different densities: the heavy (or H-strand) and the light (or L-strand). The mitochondrial genome in eukaryotes encodes a total of 37 genes, 22 of which encode tRNA molecules, two encode rRNA molecules, and the other 13 encode proteins involved primarily with the process of oxidative respiration [**39**]. While the number of these genes on the mitochondrial genome does not vary within all vertebrate mitochondrial genomes decoded to-date, the order of the genes may alter [**39**]. As an example, the order is different between avian and mammalian mitochondrial genomes.

Although the use of mitochondrial loci in species testing has many benefits, there are a few disadvantages as well. Part of the benefit of mitochondrial loci is that they are inherited maternally and as a haplotype with no recombination. Maternal inheritance can be a problem if hybrid species occur, particularly if the mother is from a nonprotected species and the father is from a species that is protected [**43,44**] (see **Section 4.5**).

4.3. Identification of species using loci on the mitochondrial genome.

A classic characteristic for a locus used in species identification is that it should exhibit very little variation for any member of the same species such that all members of that species have the same, or very nearly the same, sequence; this is referred to as intraspecies variation. The second characteristic is that this same locus should exhibit sufficient differences from any member of the next closest species, being interspecies DNA sequence variation.

The main locus used in taxonomic and phylogenetic studies until recently was cytochrome b (cyt b) [**45,46**]. This occurs between bases 14,747 and 15,887 in human mtDNA and encodes a protein 380 amino acids in length. The cyt b locus has been used extensively in taxonomic and forensic studies [**32,34,35,47**].

The cytochrome c oxidase I (COI) mitochondrial gene locus was adopted by the Barcode for Life Consortium (BOLD) (**www.boldsystems.org** (accessed on 15 March 2021)) [**48,49,50**]. COI is found between bases 5904 and 7445 in human mtDNA and at a similar position for all other mammals. COI was used initially in the identification of invertebrate species [**51,52**] and became the locus of choice in forensic entomology [**53**] before being adopted by BOLD.

Currently, there is no standardized locus in species testing, hence a divergence between cyt b, COI and other locus such as ND5. The Commission for the International Society for Forensic Genetics (ISFG) recommended that there should be some rationale behind the choice of the locus used in any analysis [**1**]. It is most likely that different loci will exhibit varying inter- and intraspecies similarity depending on whether examining insects, other invertebrates, fish, reptiles, birds, or mammals. Mammals are the only taxonomic group where a detailed study has been performed to determine whether cyt b or COI have fewer false positive and false negative identifications [**54**]; in this study, cyt b was found to outperform COI.

It may often be the case, such as for ivory and rhino horn, that the DNA is highly fragmented and therefore not possible to examine the entire locus of either COI or cyt b; rather, sections of the loci are used. The first 400 bases section of the cyt b gene is typically used [**46**]. For the COI the first 645 bp are used as part of BOLD [**48**]. The use of either section of the cyt b or COI loci is aided by the design of universal primers; these are primers that can be used in PCR to amplify a section of a gene from all the species from which the specific primers are designed. For instance, up-stream from the cyt b gene is a gene for a tRNA molecule, and this sequence is highly conserved such that the primers will bind to any mammalian species. This is a real benefit if the material is single source and not contaminated with DNA from another species; as an example, it is all too easy to amplify human DNA due to external contamination.

4.4. Analysis of Mitochondrial Sequences

The standard workflow for species identification is to: (1) isolate DNA; (2) then quantify the amount of DNA isolated; (3) amplify the section of mtDNA chosen; (4) confirm that a PCR product has been generated; (5) purify the PCR amplicon; (6) DNA sequence the amplicon (in both directions); (7) compare the sequence data to a reference data base such as GenBank or ForCyt [**55**]. ForCyt was established to remove errors that do exist in GenBank [**56**]. When publishing the reference DNA sequence from a species to which comparisons of unknown material can be made, it is essential that this known sample comes from a voucher specimen; this is recommended by the ISFG Commission [**1**]. Software such as the Basic Local Alignment Search Tool (BLAST) compares the target sequence fragment to the data deposited on the database (GenBank) and produces a similarity score of the 100 most closely matched sequences. These are listed with the closest similarity at the top of the list. The ideal is a similarity score of 100% to a known species, with the next closest being less than a similarity of 95%. This situation rarely occurs with a similarity score of 98% between the sequence tested and the nearest sequence being more typical. There is no consensus on how many differences and over what number of bases is either due to intra- or interspecies variation. It was reported that one base variation per 400 bp sequence is acceptable intraspecies variation [**39**].

4.5. SNP Testing

Performing a complete DNA sequence analysis from a section of DNA provides the maximum amount of genetic information. It may be that only a few DNA bases that differ (are polymorphic), and that much of the DNA sequence is of little value as the species being considered share much of their DNA. In such instances, if the polymorphic DNA bases are known, these bases can be targeted specifically. A recent example of this is the identification of SNPs within the mitochondrial genome of tigers [**57**]. In this instance, small parts of the tiger mitochondrial genome are amplified in one reaction using primers specific for the genus Panthera. The assay is based on SNaPshot®, a process used in ancestry assignments of human populations [**58,59,60**]. As the sections amplified in the first instance are short, no more than 300 bases, this type of DNA testing works very effectively on highly degraded DNA, with a recent example being the species assignment from ivory [**61**]. In this paper the authors were able to differentiate ivory taken from Asian elephants (Elephas maximus) compared to either of the African elephants with a 99.92% reported accuracy based on an impressive 140 samples of ivory. The paper targeted SNPs in either the cyt b gene or ND5 gene. Additionally, because the SNP detection can be species-specific, the test works well even when there is a complex mixture of other species. An example was to identify up to 18 European mammalian species by using universal primers in the cyt b gene in combination with species specific primers [**62**]. The size of the resulting species-specific amplicon is itself specific for each species and with 3 amplicons per species there is redundancy to cope with one of the tests not working.

4.6. Hybrids

Sequence comparison using regions of the mitochondrial genome has a tremendous advantage over nuclear markers for sensitivity; this is due to the multiple copy number of mitochondrial genomes per cell. A potential disadvantage in species testing is the maternal inheritance of mitochondrial DNA. When the male is from a protected species, but the female is from species not protected, and viable young are produced, due to the maternal of inheritance of mtDNA, the offspring will not be recognised as a protected species. This issue was highlighted in a recent report [**43**], which is based on a talk at the ISFG congress in 2019 in Prague. There are in reality only a few examples where hybrids are the result of this type of mating as the majority of examples include species that are geographically isolated, or of little forensic relevance: examples of geographical separation are mating between an African lion (Panthera leo) and Indian tiger (Panthera tigristigris) resulting in either a tigon or liger; and of limited forensic relevance between a horse (Equus caballus) and a donkey (Equus asinus) to produce a hinny or mule.

An example where hybrids are an issue was highlighted in a case report on the alleged poaching of protected South American camelids: llamas (Lama glama), vicuñas (Vicugna vicugna), alpacas (Vicugna pacos) and guanaco (Lama guanicoe) [**44**]. Wild (vicuña and guanaco) and domesticated (llama and alpaca) animals roam within Chile freely and can mate to produce viable young capable of themselves producing young. In Chile it is illegal to hunt and kill guanaco and llama but hybrids are not protected; this leads to the potential to sell meat from protected species as from a legally killed animal. The colour of the coats of the domestic and hybrids are different and specific to the variants. This led to the group in Chile, who were faced with this problem, to use in addition to cyt b sequence data, a diagnostic base in the melanocortin 1 receptor (MC1R). The combination of species assignment with a marker for coat colour resolved this case.

4.7. Traditional Medicines

Seizures of rhino horn, ivory and pangolins usually are of either identifiable using morphology or by DNA as will be from only one species. An example where multiple protected species are found in a complex mix, along with other plant and animal derivatives, is the trade in traditional medicines. Here, the ingredients might not be listed, rather the spurious cure for while they are taken can be prominent. An example is shown in **Figure 3**.

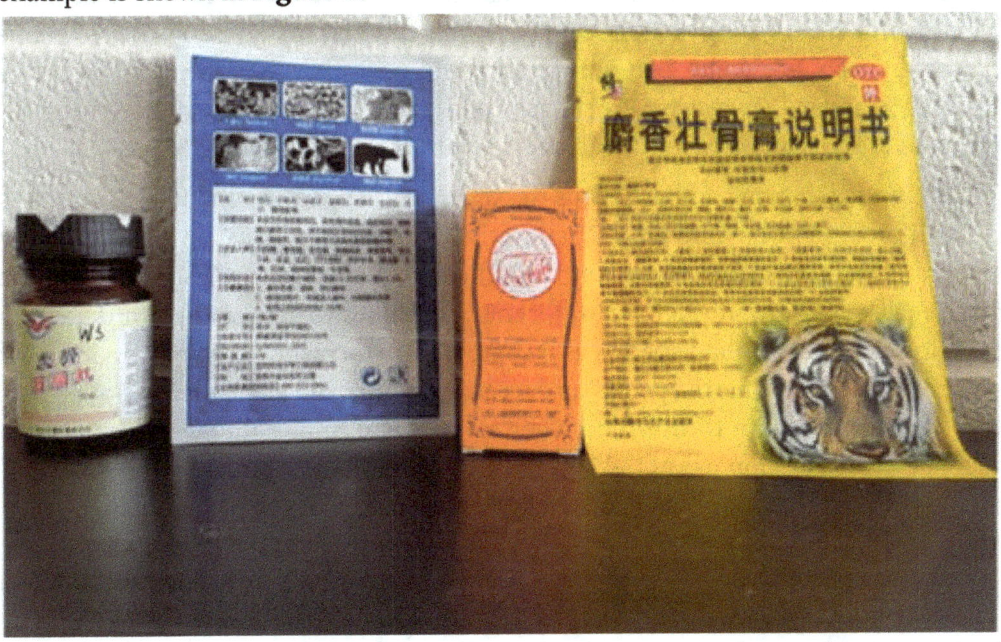

Figure 3. Showing examples of a traditional east Asian medicine that was seized by Border Force officials. The items were later show to contain traces of DNA from endangered species.

These plasters and pills list bear and tiger on the packaging, which is an offence in many countries, breaching CITES agreements, even if there is no tiger or bear present. It is likely that the amounts of any genetic material would be at extremely low amounts, and in a complex mix with potentially other species. This makes standard species testing problematic. Using universal primers and then amplifying using standard Sanger sequencing of part of the mtDNA will result in unreadable DNA sequence data. Undoubtedly the application of massively parallel DNA sequence technology overcomes the issue of any complex mixtures. The first example of this work on seized traditional medicines identified a number of protected species along with large numbers of other plant and animal species not listed on the packaging but with poor health outcomes [**37**]. A more recent study found protected species in traditional medicine products that could be bought in Australia [**36**], yet no prosecutions were undertaken even though there is clear evidence of breaching federal law.

5. ANIMAL FORENSIC PROFILING: AT A GLANCE

This review clearly identifies the need, and the growing use of, non-human animal DNA for a range of forensic applications. There are a few laboratories dedicated to this type of analyses and can demonstrate that they work to the same exacting standards required in human identification. More such facilities are needed and, when it comes to wildlife forensic science, in countries closer to where seizures happen. The STR typing of non-human animals, with cats and dogs being prime examples, uses the same equipment as in human identification and therefore creating Standard Operating Procedures and adopting the STR typing of dog for example into use in mainstream accredited laboratories is therefore possible.

There remains no standard locus for species testing. A wealth of data exists on GenBank for sections of cyt b, COI and other mtDNA regions such as ND5 from a wide range of animal species. It may be that one locus has fewer false negatives and false positives than another for different taxonomic Orders, although data only exist in some mammalian species as a comparison. Intraspecies variation needs to be known for many more species as currently there are very little data available. One answer would be to use the power of MPS and analyse multiple loci in one reaction. The common use of MPS is on the near horizon as prices for consumables and the use of this equipment decreases. MPS is also seeing acceptance in other areas of non-human DNA typing such as in analyses of bacteria for post mortem interval [**63,64**] and now in tracking microbiomes [**65,66**] and was the subject of a recent review [**67**]. If the use of MPS is growing a profile in bacterial work, then there is every reason to expect the same acceptance and profile from eukaryotic and in particular vertebrate species.The application of non-human DNA, now with examples of now bacterial DNA typing, can add an extra dimension to a forensic investigation. The use of DNA from species other than humans can add a further dimension to a forensic investigation. It is for those working in the non-human arena to ensure that their standards meet those expected and can provide a valuable service to the criminal justice system.

6. SUMMARY

The field of animal forensic genetics primarily focuses on non-human species and can be broadly categorized into two main areas: domestic species and wildlife. When there are indications of a domestic animal species that are significant to a forensic inquiry, the issue of identifying the species becomes less crucial. This is because the material might originate from either a dog or a cat, for example. However, what becomes more vital is identifying the specific pet involved. The identification of a particular animal relies on employing comparable techniques to those utilized in human identification, specifically by utilizing microsatellite markers. The utilization of feline short tandem repeats to establish a connection between a feline hair and a specific feline has facilitated the development of analogous methods for identifying canines. The field of wildlife forensic science is gaining recognition as an established discipline. Increasing recognition exists regarding the detrimental impact of the illicit wildlife trafficking on the populations of renowned species. Genetic markers on the mitochondrial genome are employed to determine the most probable species that are present. If it is possible to target certain nucleotides, sequencing the entire locus may not be necessary. Utilizing mitochondrial loci for species testing can yield advantages in terms of heightened sensitivity. However, the presence of hybrids might occasionally pose a challenge. Massively parallel DNA sequencing plays a crucial role in identifying the components of traditional remedies. Through investigations, it has been discovered that protected species are often present in these medicines. Additionally, this technology has the potential to be used in the future for assigning species. Non-human animal forensic testing can be crucial in investigations, as long as it adheres to the same rigorous requirements as other DNA profiling procedures.

REFERENCES

1. Linacre, A.; Gusmão, L.; Hecht, W.; Hellmann, A.; Mayr, W.; Parson, W.; Prinz, M.; Schneider, P.; Morling, N. ISFG: Recommendations regarding the use of non-human (animal) DNA in forensic genetic investigations. Forensic Sci. Int. Genet. **2011**, 5, 501–505. **[Google Scholar] [CrossRef] [PubMed]**
2. Menotti-Raymond, M.A.; David, V.A.; O'Brien, S.J. Pet car hair implicates murder suspect. Nature **1997**, 386, 774. **[Google Scholar] [CrossRef] [PubMed] [Green Version]**
3. Menotti-Raymond, M.; David, V.A.; Stephens, J.C.; Lyons, L.A.; O'Brien, S.J. Genetic individualization of domestic cats using feline STR loci for forensic applications. J. Forensic Sci. **1997**, 42, 14258J. **[Google Scholar] [CrossRef]**
4. Schury, N.; Schleenbecker, U.; Hellmann, A. Forensic animal DNA typing: Allele nomenclature and standardization of 14 feline STR markers. Forensic Sci. Int. Genet. **2014**, 12, 42–59. **[Google Scholar] [CrossRef]**

5. van Asch, B.; Alves, C.; Gusmão, L.; Pereira, V.; Pereira, F.; Amorim, A. A new autosomal STR nineplex for canine identification and parentage testing. Electrophoresis **2009**, 30, 417–423. **[Google Scholar]** **[CrossRef]**
6. van Asch, B.; Alves, C.; Santos, L.; Pinheiro, R.; Pereira, F.; Gusmão, L.; Amorim, A. Genetic profiles and sex identification of found-dead wolves determined by the use of an 11-loci PCR multiplex. Forensic Sci. Int. Genet. **2010**, 4, 68–72. **[Google Scholar]** **[CrossRef]**
7. Caniglia, R.; Galaverni, M.; Delogu, M.; Fabbri, E.; Musto, C.; Randi, E. Big bad wolf or man's best friend? Unmasking a false wolf aggression on humans. Forensic Sci. Int. Genet. **2016**, 24, e4–e6. **[Google Scholar]** **[CrossRef]**
8. Wictum, E.J.; Kun, T.; Lindquist, C.; Malvick, J.; Vankan, D.; Sacks, B. Developmental validation of DogFiler, a novel multiplex for canine DNA profiling in forensic casework. Forensic Sci. Int. Genet. **2013**, 7, 82–91. **[Google Scholar]** **[CrossRef]**
9. Kun, T.; Lyons, L.A.; Sacks, B.N.; Ballard, R.E.; Lindquist, C.; Wictum, E.J. Developmental validation of Mini-DogFiler for degraded canine DNA. Forensic Sci. Int. Genet. **2013**, 7, 151–158. **[Google Scholar]** **[CrossRef]**
10. Berger, B.; Heinrich, J.; Niederstätter, H.; Hecht, W.; Morf, N.; Hellmann, A.; Rohleder, U.; Schleenbecker, U.; Berger, C.; Parson, W. Forensic characterization and statistical considerations of the CaDNAP 13-STR panel in 1184 domestic dogs from Germany, Austria, and Switzerland. Forensic Sci. Int. Genet. **2019**, 42, 90–98. **[Google Scholar]** **[CrossRef]**
11. Gamarra, D.; Taniguchi, M.; Aldai, N.; Arakawa, A.; Lopez-Oceja, A.; De Pancorbo, M.M. Genetic Characterization of the Local Pirenaica Cattle for Parentage and Traceability Purposes. Animals **2020**, 10, 1584. **[Google Scholar]** **[CrossRef]**
12. Lorenzini, R.; Cabras, P.; Fanelli, R.; Carboni, G.L. Wildlife molecular forensics: Identification of the Sardinian mouflon using STR profiling and the Bayesian assignment test. Forensic Sci. Int. Genet. **2011**, 5, 345–349. **[Google Scholar]** **[CrossRef]**
13. Wasser, S.K.; Mailand, C.; Booth, R.; Mutayoba, B.; Kisamo, E.; Clark, B.; Stephens, M. Using DNA to track the origin of the largest ivory seizure since the 1989 trade ban. Proc. Natl. Acad. Sci. USA **2007**, 104, 4228–4233. **[Google Scholar]** **[CrossRef]** **[Green Version]**
14. Wasser, S.K.; Shedlock, A.M.; Comstock, K.; Ostrander, E.A.; Mutayoba, B.; Stephens, M. Assigning African elephant DNA to geographic region of origin: Applications to the ivory trade. Proc. Natl. Acad. Sci. USA **2004**, 101, 14847–14852. **[Google Scholar]** **[CrossRef]** **[Green Version]**
15. Harper, C.K.; Vermeulen, G.J.; Clarke, A.B.; de Wet, J.I.; Guthrie, A.J. Extraction of nuclear DNA from rhinoceros horn and characterization of DNA profiling

systems for white (Ceratotheriumsimum) and black (Dicerosbicornis) rhinoceros. Forensic Sci. Int. Genet. **2013**, 7, 428–433. **[Google Scholar] [CrossRef]**

16. Ghosh, T.; Sharma, A.; Mondol, S. Optimisation and application of a forensic microsatellite panel to combat Greater-one horned rhinoceros (Rhinoceros unicornis) poaching in India. Forensic Sci. Int. Genet. **2021**, 52, 102472. **[Google Scholar] [CrossRef]**
17. Meredith, E.P.; Adkins, J.K.; Rodzen, J.A. UrsaPlex: An STR multiplex for forensic identification of North American black bear (Ursus americanus). Forensic Sci. Int. Genet. **2020**, 44, 102161. **[Google Scholar] [CrossRef] [Green Version]**
18. Dawnay, N.; Ogden, R.; Thorpe, R.S.; Pope, L.C.; Dawson, D.A.; McEwing, R. A forensic STR profiling system for the Eurasian badger: A framework for developing profiling systems for wildlife species. Forensic Sci. Int. Genet. **2008**, 2, 47–53. **[Google Scholar] [CrossRef]**
19. White, N.E.; Dawson, R.; Coghlan, M.L.; Tridico, S.R.; Mawson, P.R.; Haile, J.; Bunce, M. Application of STR markers in wildlife forensic casework involving Australian black-cockatoos (Calyptorhynchus spp.). Forensic Sci. Int. Genet. **2012**, 6, 664–670. **[Google Scholar] [CrossRef] [Green Version]**
20. van Hoppe, M.J.C.; Dy, M.A.V.; van den Einden, M.; Iyenga, A. SkydancerPlex: A novel STR multiplex validated for forensic use in the hen harrier (Circus cyaneus). Forensic Sci. Int. Genet. **2016**, 22, 100–109. **[Google Scholar] [CrossRef]**
21. Ciavaglia, S.; Linacre, A. OzPythonPlex: An optimised forensic STR multiplex assay set for the Australasian carpet python (Morelia spilota). Forensic Sci. Int. Genet. **2018**, 34, 231–248. **[Google Scholar] [CrossRef] [PubMed] [Green Version]**
22. Biello, R.; Zampiglia, M.; Corti, C.; Deli, G.; Biaggini, M.; Crestanello, B.; Delaugerre, M.; Di Tizio, L.; Francesco, L.L.; Stefano, C.; et al. Mapping the geographic origin of captive and confiscated Hermann's tortoises: A genetic toolkit for conservation and forensic analyses. Forensic Sci. Int. Genet. **2021**, 51, 102447. **[Google Scholar] [CrossRef]**
23. Kimpton, C.; Fisher, D.; Watson, S.; Adams, M.; Urquhart, A.; Lygo, J.; Gill, P. Evaluation of an automated DNA profiling system employing multiplex amplification of four tetrameric STR loci. Int. J. Leg. Med. **1994**, 106, 302–311. **[Google Scholar] [CrossRef]**
24. Sparkes, R.; Kimpton, C.; Gilbard, S.; Carne, P.; Andersen, J.; Oldroyd, N.; Thomas, D.; Urquhart, A.; Gill, P. The validation of a 7-locus multiplex STR

test for use in forensic casework. (II), Artefacts, casework studies and success rates. Int. J. Legal Med. **1996**, 109, 195–204. **[Google Scholar] [CrossRef] [PubMed]**

25. Lee, J.C.-I.; Tseng, B.; Ho, B.-C.; Linacre, A. pSTR Finder: A rapid method to discover polymorphic short tandem repeat markers from whole-genome sequences. Investig. Genet. **2015**, 6, 10. **[Google Scholar] [CrossRef] [PubMed] [Green Version]**
26. Linacre, A. Wildlife crime in Australia. Emerg. Top. Life Sci. **2021**. **[Google Scholar] [CrossRef] [PubMed]**
27. Alacs, E.; Georges, A. Wildlife across our borders: A review of the illegal trade in Australia. Aust. J. Forensic Sci. **2008**, 40, 147–160. **[Google Scholar] [CrossRef]**
28. Linacre, A.; Ciavaglia, S.A. Wildlife Forensic Science. In Handbook of Forensic Genetics; Amorin, A., Budowle, B., Eds.; World Scientific Publishing: London, UK, 2017; pp. 449–772. **[Google Scholar]**
29. Wilson-Wilde, L.; Norman, J.; Robertson, J.; Sarre, S.; Georges, A. Current issues in species identification for forensic science and the validity of using the cytochrome oxidase I (COI) gene. Forensic Sci. Med. Pathol. **2010**, 6, 233–241. **[Google Scholar] [CrossRef]**
30. Johnson, R.N.; Wilson-Wilde, L.; Linacre, A. Current and future directions of DNA in wildlife forensic science. Forensic Sci. Int. Genet. **2014**, 10, 1–11. **[Google Scholar] [CrossRef]**
31. Zhang, H.; Ades, G.; Miller, M.P.; Yang, F.; Lai, K.-W.; Fischer, G.A. Genetic identification of African pangolins and their origin in illegal trade. Glob. Ecol. Conserv. **2020**, 23, e01119. **[Google Scholar] [CrossRef]**
32. Ewart, K.M.; Frankham, G.J.; McEwing, R.; Webster, L.M.; Ciavaglia, S.A.; Linacre, A.M.; The, D.T.; Ovouthan, K.; Johnson, R.N. An internationally standardized species identification test for use on suspected seized rhinoceros horn in the illegal wildlife trade. Forensic Sci. Int. Genet. **2018**, 32, 33–39. **[Google Scholar] [CrossRef] [Green Version]**
33. Coghlan, M.L.; White, N.E.; Parkinson, L.; Haile, J.; Spencer, P.B.; Bunce, M. Egg forensics: An appraisal of DNA sequencing to assist in species identification of illegally smuggled eggs. Forensic Sci. Int. Genet. **2012**, 6, 268–273. **[Google Scholar] [CrossRef]**
34. Meganathan, P.R.; Dubey, B.; Jogayya, K.N.; Whitaker, N.; Haque, I. A novel multiplex PCR assay for the identification of Indian crocodiles. Mol. Ecol. Resour. **2010**, 10, 744–747. **[Google Scholar] [CrossRef]**

35. Lee, J.C.-I.; Tsai, L.-C.; Liao, S.-P.; Linacre, A.; Hsieh, H.-M. Species identification using the cytochrome b gene of commercial turtle shells. Forensic Sci. Int. Genet. **2009**, 3, 67–73. **[Google Scholar] [CrossRef]**

36. Byard, R.W. Traditional medicines and species extinction: Another side to forensic wildlife investigation. Forensic Sci. Med. Pathol. **2016**, 12, 125–127. **[Google Scholar] [CrossRef] [Green Version]**

37. Coghlan, M.L.; Haile, J.; Houston, J.; Murray, D.C.; White, N.E.; Moolhuijzen, P.; Bellgard, M.I.; Bunce, M. Deep Sequencing of Plant and Animal DNA Contained within Traditional Chinese Medicines Reveals Legality Issues and Health Safety Concerns. PLoS Genet. **2012**, 8, e1002657. **[Google Scholar] [CrossRef]**

38. Sellar, J. Illegal Trade and the Convention on International Trade in Endangered Wild Species of Fauna and Flora. In Forensic Science in Wildlife Investigations; Linacre, A., Ed.; CRC Press, Taylor Francis Group: Boca Raton, FL, USA, 2009; pp. 11–18. **[Google Scholar]**

39. Linacre, A.; Tobe, S. Wildlife DNA Analysis: Applications in Forensic Science; John Wiley & Co.: Chichester, UK, 2013. **[Google Scholar]**

40. Ewart, K.M.; Lightson, A.L.; Sitam, F.T.; Rovie-Ryan, J.J.; Mather, N.; McEwing, R. Expediting the sampling, decalcification, and forensic DNA analysis of large elephant ivory seizures to aid investigations and prosecutions. Forensic Sci. Int. Genet. **2020**, 44, 102187. **[Google Scholar] [CrossRef] [Green Version]**

41. Mwale, M.; Dalton, D.L.; Jansen, R.; De Bruyn, M.; Pietersen, D.; Mokgokong, P.S.; Kotzé, A. Forensic application of DNA barcoding for identification of illegally traded African pangolin scales. Genome **2017**, 60, 272–284. **[Google Scholar] [CrossRef]**

42. Hsieh, H.-M.; Lee, J.C.-I.; Wu, J.-H.; Chen, C.-A.; Chen, Y.-J.; Wang, G.-B.; Chin, S.-C.; Wang, L.-C.; Linacre, A.; Tsai, L.-C. Establishing the pangolin mitochondrial D-loop sequences from the confiscated scales. Forensic Sci. Int. Genet. **2011**, 5, 303–307. **[Google Scholar] [CrossRef]**

43. Amorim, A.; Pereira, F.; Alves, C.; García, O. Species assignment in forensics and the challenge of hybrids. Forensic Sci. Int. Genet. **2020**, 48, 102333. **[Google Scholar] [CrossRef]**

44. González, B.A.; Agapito, A.M.; Novoa-Muñoz, F.; Vianna, J.; Johnson, W.E.; Marín, J.C. Utility of genetic variation in coat color genes to distinguish wild, domestic and hybrid South American camelids for forensic and judicial applications. Forensic Sci. Int. Genet. **2020**, 45, 102226. **[Google Scholar] [CrossRef] [PubMed]**

45. Kocher, T.D.; Thomas, W.K.; Meyer, A.; Edwards, S.V.; Paabo, S.; Villablanca, F.X.; Wilson, A.C. Dynamics of mitochondrial DNA evolution in animals: Amplification and sequencing with conserved primers. Proc. Natl. Acad. Sci. USA **1989**, 86, 6196–6200. **[Google Scholar] [CrossRef] [PubMed] [Green Version]**

46. Hsieh, H.-M.; Chiang, H.-L.; Tsai, L.-C.; Lai, S.-Y.; Huang, N.-E.; Linacre, A.; Lee, J.C.-I. Cytochrome b gene for species identification of the conservation animals. Forensic Sci. Int. **2001**, 122, 7–18. **[Google Scholar] [CrossRef]**

47. Lee, J.C.-I.; Tsai, L.-C.; Yang, C.-Y.; Liu, C.-L.; Huang, L.-H.; Linacre, A.; Hsieh, H.-M. DNA profiling of Shahtoosh. Electrophoresis **2006**, 27, 3359–3362. **[Google Scholar] [CrossRef] [PubMed]**

48. Hebert, P.D.N.; Gregory, T.R. The Promise of DNA Barcoding for Taxonomy. Syst. Biol. **2005**, 54, 852–859. **[Google Scholar] [CrossRef]**

49. Hebert, P.D.N.; Stoeckle, M.Y.; Zemlak, T.S.; Francis, C.M. Identification of Birds through DNA Barcodes. PLoS Biol. **2004**, 2, e312. **[Google Scholar] [CrossRef] [Green Version]**

50. Ratnasingham, S.; Hebert, P.D.N. BARCODING: Bold: The Barcode of Life Data System (http://www.barcodinglife.org). Mol. Ecol. Notes **2007**, 7, 355–364. **[Google Scholar] [CrossRef] [Green Version]**

51. Ball, S.L.; Hebert, P.D.N.; Burian, S.K.; Webb, J.M. Biological identifications of mayflies (Ephemeroptera) using DNA barcodes. J. North Am. Benthol. Soc. **2005**, 24, 508. **[Google Scholar] [CrossRef]**

52. Hajibabaei, M.; Janzen, D.H.; Burns, J.M.; Hallwachs, W.; Hebert, P.D.N. DNA barcodes distinguish species of tropical Lepidoptera. Proc. Natl. Acad. Sci. USA **2006**, 103, 968–971. **[Google Scholar] [CrossRef] [Green Version]**

53. Nelson, K.; Melton, T. Forensic Mitochondrial DNA Analysis of 116 Casework Skeletal Samples. J. Forensic Sci. **2007**, 52, 557–561. **[Google Scholar] [CrossRef]**

54. Tobe, S.S.; Kitchener, A.C.; Linacre, A.M.T. Reconstructing Mammalian Phylogenies: A Detailed Comparison of the Cytochrome b and Cytochrome Oxidase Subunit I Mitochondrial Genes. PLoS ONE **2010**, 5, e14156. **[Google Scholar] [CrossRef] [Green Version]**

55. Ahlers, N.; Creecy, J.; Frankham, G.; Johnson, R.N.; Kotze, A.; Linacre, A.; McEwing, R.; Mwale, M.; Rovie-Ryan, J.J.; Sitam, F.; et al. 'ForCyt' DNA database of wildlife species. Forensic Sci. Int. Genet. Suppl. Series **2017**, 6, e466–e468. **[Google Scholar] [CrossRef] [Green Version]**

56. Pentinsaari, M.; Ratnasingham, S.; Miller, S.E.; Hebert, P.D.N. BOLD and GenBank revisited—Do identification errors arise in the lab or in the sequence libraries? PLoS ONE **2020**, 15, e0231814. **[Google Scholar] [CrossRef]**

57. Kitpipit, T.; Tobe, S.S.; Kitchener, A.C.; Gill, P.; Linacre, A. The development and validation of a single SNaPshot multiplex for tiger species and subspecies identification—Implications for forensic purposes. Forensic Sci. Int. Genet. **2012**, 6, 250–257. **[Google Scholar] [CrossRef] [Green Version]**

58. Santos, C.; Fondevila, M.; Ballard, D.; Banemann, R.; Bento, A.; Børsting, C.; Branicki, W.; Brisighelli, F.; Burrington, M.; Capal, T.; et al. Forensic ancestry analysis with two capillary electrophoresis ancestry informative marker (AIM) panels: Results of a collaborative EDNAP exercise. Forensic Sci. Int. Genet. **2015**, 19, 56–67. **[Google Scholar] [CrossRef] [Green Version]**

59. Gettings, K.B.; Lai, R.; Johnson, J.L.; Peck, M.A.; Hart, J.A.; Gordish-Dressman, H.; Schanfield, M.S.; Podini, D.S. A 50-SNP assay for biogeographic ancestry and phenotype prediction in the U.S. population. Forensic Sci. Int. Genet. **2014**, 8, 101–108. **[Google Scholar] [CrossRef]**

60. De La Puente, M.; Santos, C.; Fondevila, M.; Manzo, L.; Carracedo, Á.; Lareu, M.; Phillips, C. The Global AIMs Nano set: A 31-plex SNaPshot assay of ancestry-informative SNPs. Forensic Sci. Int. Genet. **2016**, 22, 81–88. **[Google Scholar] [CrossRef]**

61. Kitpipit, T.; Thongjued, K.; Penchart, K.; Ouithavon, K.; Chotigeat, W. Mini-SNaPshot multiplex assays authenticate elephant ivory and simultaneously identify the species origin. Forensic Sci Int Genet. **2017**, 27, 106–115. **[Google Scholar] [CrossRef]**

62. Tobe, S.S.; Linacre, A.M.T. A multiplex assay to identify 18 European mammal species from mixtures using the mitochondrial cytochrome b gene. Electrophoresis **2008**, 29, 340–347. **[Google Scholar] [CrossRef]**

63. Zhang, J.; Wang, M.; Qi, X.; Shi, L.; Zhang, J.; Zhang, X.; Yang, T.; Ren, J.; Liu, F.; Zhang, G.; et al. Predicting the postmortem interval of burial cadavers based on microbial community succession. Forensic Sci. Int. Genet. **2021**, 52, 8. **[Google Scholar] [CrossRef]**

64. Forger, L.V.; Woolf, M.S.; Simmons, T.L.; Swall, J.L.; Singh, B. A eukaryotic community succession based method for postmortem interval (PMI) estimation of decomposing porcine remains. Forensic Sci. Int. **2019**, 302, 109838. **[Google Scholar] [CrossRef] [PubMed]**

65. López, C.D.; González, D.M.; Haas, C.; Vidaki, A.; Kayser, M. Microbiome-based body site of origin classification of forensically relevant blood traces. Forensic Sci. Int. Genet. **2020**, 47, 102280. **[Google Scholar] [CrossRef] [PubMed]**

66. Williams, D.W.; Gibson, G. Classification of individuals and the potential to detect sexual contact using the microbiome of the pubic region. Forensic Sci. Int. Genet. **2019**, 41, 177–187. **[Google Scholar] [CrossRef] [PubMed]**

67. Young, J.; Linacre, A. Massively parallel sequencing is unlocking the potential of environmental trace evidence. Forensic Sci. Int. Genet. **2021**, 50, 102393. **[Google Scholar] [CrossRef]**

07 ADVANCEMENTS IN DNA TRANSFER FOR FORENSIC SCIENCE: RECENT ACHIEVEMENTS IN ADDRESSING CHALLENGES

1. INTRODUCTION: AN OVERVIEW

Forensic scientists have recognized the growing importance of comprehending and acknowledging the transfer, persistence, prevalence, and recovery of DNA (DNA-TPPR). They also require access to pertinent data on these matters to aid in assigning probabilities. This knowledge is crucial in assisting investigations of suspected criminal activities and providing guidance to decision-makers [1,2]. The motivation to employ DNA profiling techniques stems from their significant discriminatory capability in generating profiles, which enables them to either exonerate or implicate an individual [3,4,5]. In addition, the high sensitivity of these approaches enables the creation of profiles from very small amounts of biological material [6,7,8]. The understanding that profiles can be easily obtained from objects that have been touched by hands [9,10] or worn [11,12,13,14] has greatly expanded the range of objects and surfaces that are subject to DNA sample for investigative purposes [15]. These items may encompass a variety of objects such as weapons, tools, containers, bags, bottles, personal belongings, appliances, computers, phones, tie-wraps, ropes and cords, clothing items, glasses, tape, documents, handles, steering wheels, chairs, tables and benches, windows, cartridge cases, circuit boards, stones, etc. These objects can be linked to various criminal activities including robberies, sex offenses, assaults, homicides, drug manufacturing and trafficking, and a range of other serious offenses. Additionally, they can also be associated with cases involving missing persons [6,15,16,17,18,19,20,21,22,23]. In numerous legal countries, samples obtained from these specific items constitute a significant proportion of the samples gathered for profiling purposes and are widely depended upon to aid investigations [16,20,24]. However, two elements have meant that increasingly, the question of relevance to the trier of fact has shifted from who the DNA is from, to how and when it got to the area from which it was collected [**2,25,26,27**]. The first is the knowledge that DNA can not only be deposited by a person contacting an object but can also be readily transferred by various other modes, including (a) from person to person to object; (b) from person to object to person to object; (c) from person to object to object [**1,9**]. The second is that many of the samples collected from touched objects and worn clothing [**13,28,29,30**], as well as samples of small stains of various biological materials such as blood, saliva and semen collected from various surfaces with pre-existing levels of background DNA [**31,32,33,34**], provide mixed profiles. **Figure 1** depicts a general overview of the many potential sources (including who, what, when and how) that may contribute to a recovered sample and the DNA profile generated from it, as well as the many factors that could potentially impact the levels of transfer, persistence, prevalence and recovery of these contributions.

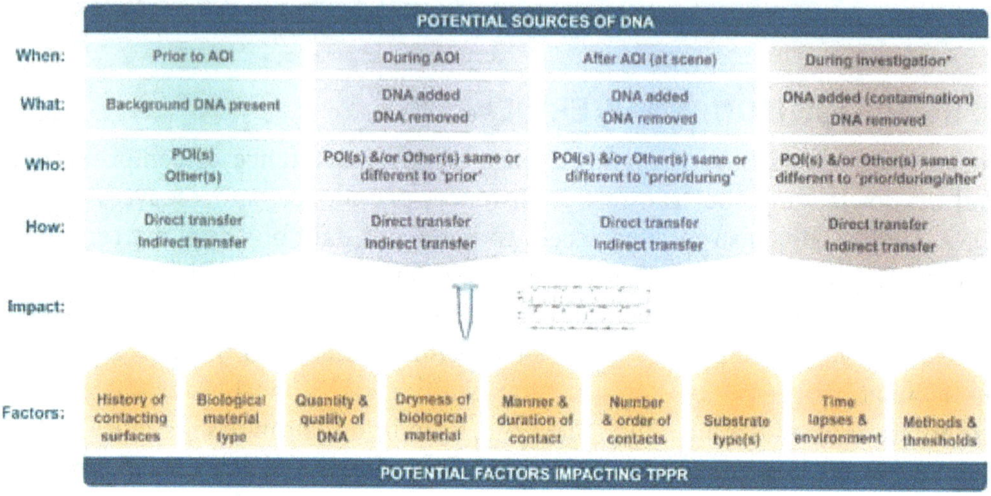

Figure 1. Potential sources contributing to, and factors impacting, the sample recovered and the DNA profile generated from it. The variable shading within each box represents that each source and factor can vary in relative contribution and impact. AOI = Action of Interest. POI = Person of Interest. * Apart from contamination of evidence by DNA from investigators and their associates during the investigation process, detection of AOI-related DNA could be due to cross contamination with another area of the same item or other item of the same case due to direct transfer events (for example, within packaging) or indirect transfer events (for example, via reused, uncleaned, or inadequately cleaned, tools, bench and/or gloves).

To provide guidance on the likelihood of DNA findings given competing propositions of interest with respect to the activities performed requires a thorough understanding of the factors and variables impacting DNA-TPPR, the availability of data in order to generate probabilities of particular types of profiles given specific sets of circumstances, and the knowledge of potential impact of the methodologies, processes and thresholds applied to generate the available data. In late 2018 and early 2019, three major reviews were published on elements of these, with each advocating the need for further research and other actions to support the conduct of DNA-related activity level evaluations. Firstly, van Oorschot et al. [**1**] conducted a review of the state of play with respect to DNA transfer in forensic science and highlighted areas requiring further attention. This was soon followed by two additional major reviews relating to DNA-TPPR: Burrill et al. [**35**] and Gosch and Courts [**36**].

In their review, van Oorschot et al. [**1**] provided a brief history of aspects relating to the transfer of DNA, indicated why understanding aspects of DNA-TPPR and availability of related data are important to the forensic and legal fraternity, plus gave a detailed summary of the many aspects pertaining to the transfer of DNA within the forensic science context. These included:

- What was known about DNA-TPPR at the time, including in relation to:
    - Potential means and complexities of transfer.
    - Core factors impacting transfer.
    - Prevalence and origins of non-self DNA on various surfaces.
    - Persistence of deposited DNA in various circumstances.
    - Potential relevance of activities performed between activities of interest.
    - Impact of using different recovery and processing methodologies on quantities of DNA retrieved and the profile types generated.
- Consideration of associated elements, including in relation to:
    - Contamination risks.
    - Type of sources of information, and tools, to utilise when addressing activity level questions.
    - Readiness of those addressing transfer-related questions, and the adequacies of training, competency/proficiency testing and accreditation programs.
    - Means of creating, gathering, sharing and using data.

The authors also highlighted several areas that could benefit from more attention/investment, including:

- Research to better understand the effect of the many variables impacting DNA-TPPR, and build the data necessary to facilitate more accurate probability assignments of generating particular types of profiles in a wide range of relevant casework situations. Specific areas of research include:

- Impacts of physical and chemical differences of contacting surfaces, including those relating to their topography, chemical compositions, fibre type, weave, thickness, electrical charge, etc.
- Assessment of transfer of primary touch deposits after long time periods.
- Drying patterns and transfer rates of various relevant biological materials, such as semen, and the impact different substrates may have.
- Effect of duration and/or frequency of use on the accumulation of DNA, and subsequent changes to profiles, for objects of different types and substrates.
- Awareness of general levels of background DNA (including quantity, origin and quality), and the impact of factors such as a person's shedder status and frequency of item use.
- Understanding of the influence of any background DNA on the interpretation of mixed profiles.
- Acquisition of more accurate probabilities of finding non-self DNA, and of the different relative mixture proportions within a deposit made by a hand, by collecting more samples from random individuals in a wide range of situations.
- Prevalence of non-self DNA on the bodies of both children and adults.
- The quantity and quality of DNA from donors and other individuals in fingernail samples after various known contact activities; acquisition of non-self DNA during regular social interaction; indirect transfer by occupying another person's space for a certain amount of time; the effects of personal habits; and an individual's shedder status, on detection of donor and foreign DNA.
- Awareness of contributors to the non-self component of DNA retrieved from personal objects and occupied spaces.
- Persistence of the temporary user of an item after use by the original owner has resumed.
- Probabilities of detection, and relative contribution, of individuals to profiles retrieved from a wider array of shared objects and surfaces within confined shared spaces (e.g., homes, offices, cars) and public spaces, given known histories.
- Impact of handwashing on the amount and quality of DNA deposited from hands, including factors such as: different methods of washing hands, the natural accumulation of DNA on hands post-handwashing,

and the different personal habits of individuals, and their effect on the accumulation of self and non-self DNA on hands.

- Impacts of genetic factors and various non-genetic factors (e.g., behavioural traits, health situation, and/or environmental conditions), and their potential interactions, on shedder status, as well as identifying and understanding their underlying properties.
- Understanding the impact of the absence/presence of the types of information one relies on that may be gathered by the crime scene attending officer, and to consider means of improving the gathering of relevant information in an efficient and consistent manner.
- Studies to help establish more accurate probability distributions for relevant factors impacting transfer.
- Determining the accuracy of 'experiential' assessment (i.e., based on experiences) relative to 'experimental' assessment (i.e., based on data from experiments).
- Enhancement of access to relevant data, including specific areas such as:
- Availability of a quality controlled open access depository of relevant DNA-TPPR information that can be easily mined for various purposes.
- Inclusion of relevant details of the methods, protocols and thresholds applied to generate the DNA-TPPR data presented.
- Recognition of DNA activity-associated expertise to be distinct and supported by dedicated training, competency testing, authorisation and ongoing proficiency testing.

In the review by Gosch and Courts [**36**], an excellent summary of the existing literature as of October 2018 was also provided with respect to our knowledge of the core variables influencing DNA-TPPR. They highlighted the limitations of much of the DNA transfer-related research studies conducted to date in terms of:

- Underestimating the complexities and multitude of factors needing to be considered.
- Recording relevant information to allow comparisons and appropriate use.
- Identifying the relative weight of different impacting variables.

Regarding the latter, they pointed out that factors such as casework-relevant persistence scenarios or the impact of inter-individual differences in handling an item are among those receiving limited attention. The authors further highlighted deficiencies in overall research study designs and documentation, lamented on the lack of agreement on the DNA analysis output parameters most appropriate to be utilised when comparing studies and addressing activity level questions and standardisation of recording these, and indicated a disequilibrium in the degree of studies relating to pertinent factors. Furthermore, they described and launched a new database ('DNA-TrAC') [**37**] to assist the accessibility of relevant DNA-TPPR information to aid addressing of activity level questions.

Around the same period, Burrill et al. [**35**] also provided a review of published research on aspects of transfer and persistence relating to 'touch DNA', including on:

- How much DNA can be recovered from handled items.
- Whether trace DNA can be detected under certain scenarios including varying degrees of indirect transfer.
- Factors which may influence these results.

Whilst the authors pointed to similar issues raised by the two above mentioned reviews, they also explored deeper the current knowledge in relation to the composition of touch deposits. They concluded that "Further exploration of relative contributions of hand-endogenous and -exogenous DNA contributions to touch deposits is warranted, along with more specific localization of DNA sources inside and outside a cellular infrastructure", and that "A more comprehensive picture of where the DNA in 'touch DNA' comes from will provide valuable information to practitioners seeking to utilize touch DNA typing results in a courtroom context, and will contribute to the ongoing effort to understand and predict the circumstances of DNA transfer in a forensic context more reliably".

A year prior to the three reviews mentioned above, in their Appendix B, Taylor et al. [**38**] identified 17 study areas that, if acted on, would improve our knowledge base and assist evaluations of evidence in light of propositions that suggest differing DNA transfer mechanisms. These specific studies related to areas including: efficiencies of different extraction methods, substrate considerations, environmental conditions, persistence of DNA in various situations, shedder consistency and shedder propensity determination, duration and manner of handling/contact, objects used habitually, accumulation of DNA from multiple contacts, levels of primary user's DNA on regularly used items, levels of background DNA, and value of profile degradation information.

Collectively, the aforementioned three reviews [**1,35,36**] and the research paper by Taylor et al. [**38**] acknowledged the importance of DNA-TPPR in investigations of criminal activity, highlighted the many limitations in our current knowledge and availability of required data, and provided some guidance on improvement opportunities. In this paper, we assess the extent to which we are meeting these challenges. This is achieved primarily by providing a synopsis of publications relevant to DNA-TPPR that have been published since these reviews. We then reflect on this and some of the actions taken by industry stakeholders in support of addressing identified gaps. Finally, we provide a general conclusion in relation to progress towards improving the guidance that experts are able to provide the courts in relation to the transfer of DNA.

2. IDENTIFICATION AND REPORTING OF RECENT DNA-TPPR PUBLICATIONS

A systematic review was conducted to identify recent and relevant publications. The search was performed on March 30, 2021, covering the time frame from 2018 to the present, using Scopus and Web of Science databases. Utilizing the Preferred Reporting Items for Systematic Reviews and Meta-Analyses (PRISMA) standards [39]. The search began by implementing the following:

> TITLE-ABS-KEY ((DNA OR "deoxyribonucleic acid") AND (transfer* OR deposit* OR contact* OR persist* OR prevalen* OR background OR shedder) AND (human OR participant OR donor OR volunteer) AND (forensic* OR crim*)) AND (LIMIT-TO (PUBYEAR, 2021) OR LIMIT-TO (PUBYEAR, 2020) OR LIMIT-TO (PUBYEAR, 2019) OR LIMIT-TO (PUBYEAR, 2018)).

One hundred and forty-four papers were identified for inclusion in the synopsis of relevant publications within the given period presented in **Section 3** (**Figure 2**). As we may not have captured some relevant publications, or inadvertently excluded some from further consideration, we advise those seeking publications relating to specific core topics to conduct additional searches relating to their narrower area of focus.

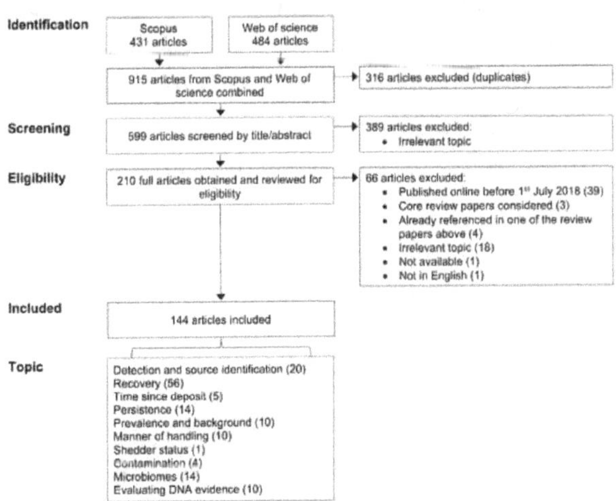

Figure 2. Process and outcome of review to identify articles to be included in synopsis. Topic categorisation of articles was based on their primary area of DNA-TPPR-related focus. Numbers of articles included/excluded are indicated in parentheses after each topic/exclusion criterion.

Based on the primary DNA-TPPR-related focus and content of the 144 included articles, each was assigned to one of the following topic categories: detection and source identification, recovery, time since deposit, persistence, prevalence and background, manner of handling, shedder status, contamination, microbiomes, evaluating DNA evidence. Where a paper was deemed to also contain information of relevance to an additional topic area, this information was also conveyed within the other topic subsection.

A synopsis is provided that gives a general overview of the focus areas and some general findings of the articles reviewed. The articles included in the synopsis were from many different journals, with Forensic Science International: Genetics (54) and Forensic Science International (23) providing the most articles. The majority of papers focused primarily on various aspects of DNA detection and recovery, with fewer concentrating on various elements of transfer, prevalence and persistence (**Figure 2**). The degrees of relevance of the publications identified vary, yet each is incorporated and referred to in the synopsis. The scope and depth of some of the presented publications are very limited. Further, some of the experimental designs within the studies conducted have limitations and while some acknowledge this, others do not. However, we have refrained from drawing attention to these and, instead, urge readers to delve fuller into the papers of interest to make their own assessment of such matters.

The reported findings of conducted research are those determined by the authors of the research and not our extrapolations. While in general we concur and/or are supportive of the vast majority of findings, conclusions and recommendations reported in the publications listed, their inclusion does not necessarily imply that we concur, and we do not make systematic comparisons of studies to inform a further judgement. For more details of the experimental designs, methodologies utilised, analyses employed, results obtained, and associated interpretations and discussion of the studies referred to, we recommend that the relevant specified references are consulted.

Several of the reported findings are new and broaden our understanding and/or improve the availability of relevant data and some produce findings verifying existing understandings/knowledge with or without making reference to relevant prior studies. We have chosen not to point out connections to prior studies here, but urge interested parties to consult the details of the publication of interest as well as any others on the relevant topic that were published prior to the period of publications bookending in this review to gain a fuller appreciation of the available knowledge and data. References within the papers of interest listed here and those listed within the aforementioned review articles can be a good start in such situations. Further, we are aware of some interesting and relevant papers that have been published since the cut-off date for inclusion within this review, and thus, are not included here. A selection of these more recent articles will be highlighted in the discussion section.

3. SUMMARY OF RECENT PUBLICATIONS ON DNA-TPPR

3.1. Detection and Source Identification

Twenty papers were identified that primarily addressed detection of biological sources and/or their identification (**Figure 2**), plus one additional study that also addressed this issue but was primarily focussed on another topic. Several studies investigated the visualisation and detection of biological materials. In addition to readily visualising biological stains, Yano et al. [**40**] demonstrated the ability of an acid-free p-dimethylaminocinnamaldehyde solution sprayed on glass slides and clothing and irradiated with blue-light-emitting diode light to visualise relatively fresh deposited finger and palm prints on clothing. This study also demonstrated that this technique does not adversely affect STR analyses, thus providing potentially useful methodology to localise areas on items of interest to assist better targeting for sampling. A number of other studies also demonstrated the ability of various treatments to potentially enhance detection of biological materials, including the use of:

- Trypan blue to improve visibility of shed skin flakes collected by adhesive film [**41**].
- Diamond™ Nucleic Acid Dye (DD) (Promega, Madison, WI, USA) to detect cellular material in lip-prints [**42**].
- DD to detect DNA on used swabs to potentially assess if further processing for DNA profiling is warranted [**43**].
- Ethidium Bromide to detect small amounts of DNA on swabs to possibly provide similar pre-screening benefits [**44**].
- Immunohistochemical staining of skin-expressed proteins to identify exfoliated epidermal cells to screen samples taken from handled/touched objects [**45**].
- NIR hyperspectral imaging to localise invisible traces of blood, urine and semen on various substrates [**46**].
- A test based on the click reaction between serum albumin and tetraphenylethene maleimide (TPE-MI) to visualise invisible blood stains (and showing that it may perform better than luminol) [**47**].
- Fluorescence spectroscopy to localise the presence of saliva stains [**48**] or detection of saliva on swab samples of human skin that had been licked [**49**].

Furthermore, Butler et al. [**50**] compared four methods that have been previously used as presumptive tests for the detection of traces of blood on dark materials, finding that luminol was, overall, the most effective method.

To explore source differences and gain insight into associations with DNA content, Burrill et al. [**51**] used flow cytometry and microscopic examination to generate granularity, size and nucleic acid fluorescence data of washed and unwashed hands, as well as saliva, nasal and eye wash that could be sources of transferred DNA onto hands. They found that hand rinses consisted mainly of anucleate corneocytes, many of which also stained positive for nucleic acids, and suggested the need for further research on the recovery and analysis of corneocyte DNA, which they report was previously assumed to be negligible.

The potential of a software tool for the automated detection and characterisation of epithelial cells from fingerprints based on fluorescence intensity across the cell surface and size/morphology was demonstrated by Olsen et al. [**52**]. This study also observed that trace cell populations from certain individuals may have distinct morphological and/or structural properties. The authors pointed out that this technique can, therefore, facilitate investigations into the deposit, transfer, and persistence of both cellular material and DNA in trace biological samples.

Tests for the detection of human PSA and human α-amylase for the identification of seminal fluid and saliva, respectively, in forensic samples are commonly used as presumptive tests in sexual assault-related cases to aid decisions on further testing procedures. It is relevant to know how frequent PSA and amylase are detectable by these tests in vaginal swabs that are void of seminal fluid and saliva. A study by Kishbaugh et al. [**53**] of 50 vaginal swabs from unique donors over the age of 18 years and relevant history, and a study by Sari et al. [**54**] of 20 pre-pubescent (3–9 years), 20 post-pubescent (16–45 years) and 20 post-menopausal (50–75 years) females, help fill this knowledge gap, and thus, assist the accuracy of interpretation of immunochromatographic testing results. In addition, a review of current methods of sperm detection, factors affecting sperm detection, and recent advances in sperm detection utilising alternative methodologies is provided by Suttipasit [**55**].

Traditional identification methods for the nature of the body fluids or tissues present in a sample collectively cater for a narrow range of biological materials tend to require one test per target fluid or tissue and may consume material compromising attaining a DNA profile. New methodologies, especially those utilising mRNA and proteomics approaches, have shown opportunities to identify a wider range of biological materials that may enhance forensic examination capacities. Molecular biology techniques continue to be explored to enhance the capacity to improve source identification. Abbas et al. [**56**] reported on the development of a protein microarray chip with enhanced fluorescence for sensitive identification of semen and vaginal fluid and pointed to the value of further development of highly sensitive chips for the identification of other biological body fluids. O'Leary and Glynn [**57**] highlighted the potential of a selection of miRNAs to identify forensically relevant body fluids. Hanson et al. [**58**], using cSNPs in body fluid-specific mRNA transcripts, demonstrated the ability to identify forensically relevant body fluids and skin, as well as differentiate blood, semen and saliva transcripts from different individuals. Those authors also indicated that, with further development, one may in the future be able to assign body fluids to DNA donors, which, in many instances, may provide additional probative value. Kamanna et al. [**59**] demonstrated the potential of proteomic analysis, using mass spectrometry-based approaches, MALDI-ToF MS/MS and n-LC-ESI-qToF MS/MS, to identify vaginal fluid and blood from only a few fibres plucked from a microswab used to collect a sample from underneath fingernails. In addition, Watanabe et al. [**60**] explored the simultaneous analyses of semen-specific methylated (or unmethylated) CpG markers and adjacent single nucleotide polymorphisms. By combining methylation-specific polymerase chain reaction and pyrosequencing technology, the authors developed a method to detect three semen-specific methylated/unmethylated regions that was able to identify semen-derived alleles from mixed stains. The authors suggested that this type of methodology may be a useful approach for genotyping from a mixture of body fluids.

3.2. Recovery

This section includes studies that investigated various aspects of DNA recovery, specifically sampling, storage, extraction, preferential recovery from mixed samples, profiling, and differences in the methodologies employed. Fifty-six papers are reported (**Figure 2**), along with some others that were primarily included in other topics.

3.2.1. Sampling

Several studies continue to elucidate the ability to generate DNA profiles from samples taken from touched objects [**61,62,63,64**]. Additional studies evaluated means of generating human DNA profiles from traces of biological material left on various items, including hair [**65**], bricks [**66**], dogs [**67**], bite marks in food [**68**], paper documents [**69**], eye wear [**70**], superabsorbent polymer-containing products (commonly found in nappies and sanitary towels) [**71**], improvised explosive devices [**72**], rifle magazines [**73**] and bullet cartridges [**74,75,76,77,78**]. Further, Gray et al. [**79**] demonstrated that STR DNA profiles can be generated from human blood found in Anopheles mosquitoes, from one or multiple individuals, and that the quality of the profiles declined as the duration between mosquito blood meal and sample collection increased.

The performance of different swabs on the collection and profiling of DNA continues to be explored. When considering touch DNA recovery, two studies compared the performance of different swabs, with each finding that a specific type of swab performed better than others [**80,81**]. A further study indicated that the use of pieces of absorbing paper moistened with 70% ethanol recovered epithelial cells/touch DNA from various surface types better than a cotton swab moistened with water [**82**]. In addition, Sherier et al. [**83**] illustrated the potential benefits of using the microFLOQ® Direct Swab (Copan, Brescia, Italy) for collecting DNA from minute stains, and possibly using it as a pre-screening methodology (i.e., sampling a small portion of a stain for initial screening and testing for expeditious processing) while saving the remainder of the stain for later testing. They also demonstrated that swabbing the centre of stains of blood, semen and saliva provided more DNA and complete profiles than swabbing the edge of stains.

Investigation also continues into the use of adhesives, such as tapes and gels, for DNA sampling. Kanokwongnuwut et al. [**84**] compared the efficiencies of different types of tape on collecting DNA from fingermarks and the effect of different numbers of applications, illustrating that particular tapes performed better than others and the benefits of ten applications compared to just one or two applications. Damsteeg-van Berkel et al. [**85**] showed that collection efficiency from textile substrates increased with increasing stubbing force in a concave down increasing function to a threshold depending on the substrate material. Zorbo and Jeuniaux [**86**] illustrated that DNA profiles can also be generated from cells, particularly those deposited by skin contact, collected using 1:1 tapings that are conventionally used to obtain microtraces of fibres and hairs prior to sampling for DNA from a body or clothing. However, the authors recommended taking additional samples from an area of interest post 1:1 taping using other techniques such as swabbing. Dierig et al. [**41**] compared DNA yields and profiles of single skin cells recovered from adhesive tape versus processing of 1 × 1 cm areas of adhesive tape after the adhesive tape had been applied to external areas of T-shirts after a period of wearing and where they had been vigorously grappled for 10 sec to mimic a physical assault. They found the approach of sampling 1 × 1 cm areas to be superior in regard to DNA yield, profile completeness and identification of the offender profile. Finally, gels have also been shown to be efficient methods for the recovery of DNA from fingermarks [**87,88,89,90**].

A few studies point to the potential benefits of applying different collection methods depending on the type of substrate [**91**], especially with respect to metal surfaces [**80,92**]. In addition, Sessa et al. [**93**] compared three sampling techniques (adhesive tape, cutting out, dry swab) for the detection of touch DNA from wearers and handlers of brassieres, and found no difference in the recovery of the handler's DNA among the three techniques, even though the cutting out technique showed the greatest recovery. However, recovery of the wearer's DNA was best achieved using adhesive tape. Overall, for their sets of samples, use of the dry swab collection method performed worst. However, for the subset of samples where in the experimental design the period of contact was shortest, out of the three techniques, samples collected using the dry swab technique yielded the highest number of handler profiles. The authors also demonstrated that when targeting for foreign DNA, the sample area should be narrowed as much as practicable to the smallest area possible to maximise target DNA recovery.

In addition to its use in visualising areas of cellular deposits, DD has also been used to determine how many cells are required to generate an informative DNA profile, either by direct PCR or conventional DNA profiling methodologies [**94**]. This study found that, when using direct PCR, ≥40 buccal cells collected from a saliva sample by either a swab or tapelift were required, whereas, from a touch sample, ≥800 corneocytes collected by swabbing or ≥4000 corneocytes collected by tapelift were required. However, more cells were required for the same DNA profile result when samples were processed through a DNA extraction workflow: ≥80 buccal cells from a swab and tapelift, ≥4000 corneocytes collected by a swab, >8000 corneocytes collected by a tapelift, illustrating that the use of direct PCR can be more efficient. The authors also concluded that cell-free DNA forms a major component of the DNA collected from touched deposits, and that tapelifting is not as efficient as swabbing in co-collecting this component of the total DNA deposited. Miller et al. [**95**] and Burrill et al. [**96**] also provided evidence that extracellular DNA can represent a substantial proportion of total DNA recovered from handled substrates. Additionally, Burrill et al. [**96**] determined a suitable technique to separate cellular and cell-free fractions of hand deposits (i.e., one that maintains the representative fraction of cell-free DNA at the time of collection) and the best of three methods tested to purify the cell-free DNA for DNA profiling. A separate study by Burrill et al. [**97**] demonstrated that enhanced lysis methods using a reducing agent and longer incubation may be valuable for the extraction of DNA from corneocytes, which make up the majority of the cellular material left in touch deposits by hands. The authors also showed that the corneocyte DNA is fragmented. The authors suggested that use of methods that extract the DNA from corneocytes more efficiently than standard methodologies, and application of profiling techniques more suitable to fragmented DNA, could enhance the ability to obtain useful profiles from touch DNA samples.

3.2.2. Storage

Three studies investigated the impact of storage conditions on the preservation of DNA in biological materials. Kaur et al. [**98**] looked at the degradation (using UV-visible spectroscopic profiles) of various types of forensic blood-related casework samples preserved under various conditions and different durations. They found that the preservation techniques had a greater impact on the quality of DNA than the aging of the sample, but not to the degree that STR profiles could not be generated. Badu-Boateng et al. [**99**] examined various storage conditions to determine the most appropriate means of storing crime scene soil–blood mixed samples prior to analysis at the laboratory, based on DNA quantification, DNA degradation and DNA profile parameters. They found that storage at -20 °C was the best for this sample type, followed by room temperature and 4 °C, respectively. Corradini et al. [**100**] showed that buccal cells collected directly on to FTA mini cards (GE Healthcare) and stored for 11 years still provided good quantities of DNA and good-quality DNA profiles. In addition to these studies, Suttipasit [**55**] emphasised the need for appropriate long-term specimen preservation in order to be able to take advantage of potential future methodological advances to interrogate samples beyond current abilities.

3.2.3. Extraction

Several studies reported the benefits of using direct PCR methods over processes that include a magnetic bead extraction step for the generation of DNA profiles from touched objects, including Kanokwongnuwut et al. [**94**]. Dierig et al. [**41**], comparing different DNA extraction methods, found that direct lysis methods (a Chelex solution method, Casework Direct Kit (Promega, Mannheim, Germany), Investigator Casework GO! Kit (Qiagen, Hilden, Germany)) were more suitable than a magnetic bead-based method (Maxwell RSC Blood DNA Kit (Promega)) for low template traces due to the limited loss of DNA. Meanwhile, de Oliveira Francisco et al. [**101**] found that the Casework Direct Kit (Promega) was much more efficient for processing touch DNA samples than the DNA IQ™ System (Promega), another magnetic bead-based DNA extraction method.

A couple of studies looked toward the future, considering how we might better understand and improve extraction efficiencies. LeSassier et al. [**102**] described means of developing artificial fingerprint samples and advocated their use to assist future studies on the efficiencies of various methods of collection and extraction of DNA from fingerprints. Liu et al. [**103**] summarised the recent development of magnetic solid-phase extraction in forensic science applications, including DNA extraction, and pointed out that modifications of functional materials on the surface of magnetic particles that could lead to potential improvements (e.g., to better cope with negative impacts of some pre-processing tools, such as fingerprint powder and tapes) and broadening of their application (e.g., detection of biomarkers, such as amino acids, peptides, hormones, etc.).

Two studies considered the extraction of non-DNA elements of biological samples for forensic applications. O'Leary and Glynn [**57**] identified the best of three methods investigated for the extraction of miRNAs from body fluids for the purpose of using miRNAs for body fluid identification. A study to support the potential future application of genetically variable peptide analysis of touched samples for forensic identification [**104**] considered a workflow for the collection, enrichment and fractionation of DNA and protein in latent fingerprint samples. The authors demonstrated that the workflow provided sufficient DNA and protein from touch samples for further analysis. Further, the authors observed that the quantity and quality of protein remained robust, regardless of fingerprint age, and that the proteomic content of the touch samples was consistent across donors and fingerprint age.

3.2.4. Preferential Recovery from Mixed Samples

Some studies considered the impact of different sampling and pre-sampling methods on preferential recovery of DNA from particular donor(s) in mixed samples. Hayden and Wallin [**105**], investigating the effectiveness of different methods of sampling from fingernails to minimise the collected amount of endogenous (female) DNA and maximise the amount of exogenous (male) DNA, concluded that their swabbing method did this better than two alternative methods tested. One study compared an automated procedure to a manual procedure for standard differential extraction of sperm-cell fractions, and found that similar levels of semen separation efficiency were achieved for sperm-cell fractions using both automated and manual procedures [**106**]. Three studies continue to look at novel means of separating sperm cells from other cells to assist the interpretation of DNA profiles generated downstream. These include the application of optical tweezers [**107**], acoustic differential extraction technologies [**108**], and capillary zone electrophoresis [**109**]. Furthermore, using DEPArray™ technology (Menarini Silicon Biosystems, Bologna, Italy), Anslinger et al. [**110**] demonstrated the ability to obtain complete DNA profiles from isolated single white cells from each of the two or three known contributors to mixed stains. They concluded that this technology opens up new possibilities with respect to mixture deconvolution, especially for mixtures composed of cells of the same type. However, as touch samples can contain a substantial proportion of extracellular DNA, Miller et al. [**95**] pointed out potential challenges for front-end cell sorting approaches to recovering DNA from touch samples, which necessitate the presence of cells with sufficient amounts of intracellular DNA.

3.2.5. Profiling

Two studies demonstrated improvements in the abilities to generate Y-STR profiles from non-semen sexual assault samples. Henry and Scandrett [**111**] showed that the Yfiler® Plus kit (Thermo Fisher Scientific, Melbourne, Australia) significantly outperformed AmpFlSTRYfiler® (Thermo Fisher Scientific) in the ability to generate useful profiles from semen negative sexual assault samples, i.e., swabs that gave negative results to a screening test for acid phosphatase or ABAcard® p30 antigen test (Abacus Diagnostics, West Hills, CA, USA) in combination with the absence of spermatozoa by microscopy, and excluding samples that tested positive for the presence of human salivary amylase using the RSID™ Saliva test (Independent Forensics, Lombard, IL, USA). In contrast, Owers et al. **[112]** showed that Powerplex® Y23 (Promega, Madison, WI, USA) significantly outperformed Yfiler (Thermo Fisher Scientific, Waltham, MA, USA) in the quality of profiles generated from vaginal swabs of alleged penetration where no semen was detected.

Two studies also investigated the use of non-traditional DNA profiling systems, specifically field-based systems and Massive Parallel Sequencing (MPS). While rapid field-based DNA identification systems have their benefits, Dawnay et al. **[113]** illustrated the limitations of the ParaDNA Field Instrument and Intelligence Test Chemistry (LGC) to collect viable DNA samples and produce profiles from the surfaces of the skin, exposed tissue or carrion larvae. The use of MPS in comparison to traditional Capillary Electrophoresis (CE) techniques to generate DNA profiles from real casework samples obtained from semen, saliva, blood, and epithelial material on various surfaces, as well as reference oral swabs, was evaluated by Avila et al. **[114]**. They found that the biological nature of the samples impacted various relevant MPS sequencing, and base-calling quality metrics associated with producing a DNA profile, not apparent when generating DNA profiles using CE; this was especially so for epithelial samples. The authors advocated for further research on MPS genotyping of forensic casework samples, including evaluation of DNA transfer effects, impact of the substrate or deposition surface for each sample and other aspects of the nature of individual samples.Interpretation of DNA profiles and mixture deconvolution requires use of software and laboratory-specific interpretation methods. Mortera **[115]** reviewed the different methods and software available to assist in determining whether or not the DNA of a given individual is present in a sample. The author provided details on a quantitative method that used Bayesian Networks as a computational device for efficiently computing likelihoods. This method also allowed the combination of evidence from multiple samples to make inferences about relationships from DNA mixtures and other more complex scenarios **[115]**. Furthermore, Buckleton et al. **[116]** revisited a previously conducted interlaboratory exercise (comprising five mock cases, with each case consisting of an electropherogram file and typed reference profiles from individuals described as victims, consensual partners, or suspects) (NIST MIX13) to re-evaluate DNA mixture interpretation using currently available methods, especially several modern probabilistic genotyping systems. Their analyses demonstrated the benefits of utilising ‘probabilistic genotyping’ over ‘combined probability of inclusion’ methodology.

3.2.6. Methodology Differences

In the studies by Szkuta et al. [**117**] and Szkuta et al. [**118**] of DNA quantities and profiles generated from samples collected from clothing, and by Goray et al. [**119**] of DNA quantities and profiles generated from samples collected from items/surfaces within office spaces, similar sets of samples were processed by different laboratories using different suites of processing, from sample collection through to the generation and analyses of DNA. These studies showed that differences in methodologies applied between the laboratories appeared to impact the quantity of DNA recovered and the composition of the profiles produced. When determining probabilities using data from various studies, Gill et al. [**120**] stressed the need to consider the differences in methodologies used by different studies to generate the available data.

3.3. Time since Deposition

Five studies were identified that considered how one might determine time since deposition (TSD) of biological materials (**Figure 2**), specifically blood, semen and saliva. Weber and Lednev [**121**] provided an overview of what is known about the biochemical mechanisms of blood aging, how these are used to determine the age of a bloodstain, the current techniques for bloodstain age determination, emerging spectroscopic techniques and technology, and the limitations of all these methodologies. Stotesbury et al. [**122**] and Cossette et al. [**123**] presented further research on using visible absorbance spectroscopy and DNA degradation to explore their use in determining TSD of blood, with the latter publication focusing on the impact of temperature. Bird et al. [**124**] considered degradation patterns of semen-specific mRNA genes to assist with determining TSD of semen. Meanwhile, Asaghiar and Williams [**125**] evaluated the use of changes in the expression of a hypoxia-sensitive marker for determining the age of deposited samples of blood, semen and saliva. Each of these studies demonstrated scope for potential use of the methodologies they investigated in TSD determination. They also noted the limitations in the scope of sample types analysed and the accuracy of TSD analyses, and recommended further research. Additionally, Weber and Ladnev [**121**] pointed out the need of any methodology being considered for use in forensic casework to be validated and that this would require further research into the impacts of environmental and substrate effects.

3.4. Persistence

This section summarises the fourteen papers identified that investigated the persistence of DNA from various biological materials (**Figure 2**), plus one additional study that also provided comment on persistence but was primarily categorised in another topic. Whilst it is possible to generate DNA STR profiles from a 100 year old semen stain [**126**] and from fingerprints archived for several years [**127**], when considering persistence of DNA in fingermarks left at room temperature for up to just one week, Alketbi and Goodwin [**128**] indicated that the quantity of DNA recovered was not influenced by the duration that the fingermarks were left before sampling, but was influenced by the environmental conditions (temperature and humidity) and type of substrate on which they were deposited.When investigating the persistence of DNA from blood and keratinocytes deposited on a variety of porous and non-porous substrates, as well as a range of mock exhibits with natural deposits of touch DNA and saliva, under various environmental conditions (indoor temperature controlled, indoors ambient temperature, outdoors forest area in Singapore where rainfall is abundant and relative humidity is high) for a duration up to 85 weeks, Lee et al. [**129**] found that degradation and persistence of DNA are highly dependent on the environment. DNA on articles left outdoors degraded rapidly, but most samples collected from the items kept within indoor environments were less affected and provided good profiles for long periods after deposition, similar to trends observed in studies performed in temperate countries.Several studies investigated the persistence of DNA on surfaces of the body (skin, beneath fingernails and hands) when immersed or washed in water under varying conditions. Meixner et al. [**130**] found that DNA profiles can still be generated from blood stains and 'touch' deposits on skin specimens after several days of being immersed in water (cold, room-temperature or warm water as well as in a stream and a pond). The duration of persistence was dependent on the temperature and aquatic environment and was longest when immersed in cold water. Hayden and Wallin [**105**] demonstrated that DNA can remain under fingernails (female fingernail donor's consensual partner) and on the skin (male sweat donor's consensual partner) after showering. While Romero-García et al. [**131**] noted that samples taken from towels used once to dry hands immediately after having washed them with neutral pH soap only provided partial profiles of the person drying their hands. This was the case both after the individual's hand performed various daily activities and in separate tests where individuals had held hands with someone else for 5 min prior to washing their hands.

Other studies looked at the persistence of DNA and biological fluids on various non-porous and porous items after cleaning or washing. Helmus et al. [**132**] investigated whether DNA traces (blood, saliva, epithelial cells) on different objects (knives, plates, glasses, and plastic lids) can persist on the surface despite cleaning by different methods (such as washing by hand or use of a dishwasher). They found that small deposits of biological material often still provided sufficient DNA to generate full profiles after the item they were on was rinsed or washed by hand, while profiles were not able to be generated after cleaning in a dishwasher. Further studies showed that sufficient DNA for STR profiling could be recovered from cuttings of semen stains on polyester and/or cotton fabric after washing, with the amount of DNA dependent on the type of washing applied [**133,134,135**]. Noël et al. [**133**] showed that this was possible even after multiple washings, and that more DNA was recovered from cuttings than swabbing of stained cotton bedsheets. Both Noël et al. [**133**] and Karadayi et al. [**134**] also showed that the washed stains were able to be visually detected using a light source and provided positive prostate-specific antigen test results. Similarly, Hofmann et al. [**136**] showed that washed blood stains can generally also be detected using luminol, but the quality of the bloodstains is dependent on a number of factors including the type of washing machine, the washing temperature, the filling degree of the washing machine, and the drying conditions of the blood stain (temperature, duration).

To provide a dataset that may help guide sample targeting and prioritisation, as well as manage expectations of stakeholders regarding observing positive or negative results, Fonneløp et al. [**137**] performed a retrospective study on the transfer, persistence and recovery of sperm (from internal vaginal swabs, external vaginal swabs, rectal swabs, oral swabs and skin surfaces) and epithelial cells (from external genital swabs, hand swabs, skin swabs, penile swabs, internal vaginal swabs, rectal swabs and oral swabs) collected in sexual assault casework. The samples collected from different areas of the skin to assess the presence of the person of interest (POI)-derived epithelial DNA included face, lips and around the mouth, neck/throat, breast/chest, arm, leg, seat, thigh, rest of body. The authors found that sperm cells had the highest persistence rate in internal vaginal swabs, and were detected up to 72 h post assault, but the majority of the positive samples (i.e., case specific POI DNA profile detected) were collected within 48 h. Analysis of skin and penile swabs demonstrated the persistence of case-specific POI DNA from epithelial cells up to 48 h, and the majority of positive samples were within 24 h. The authors also found that POI-derived epithelial cells were not detected in external genital swabs when collected beyond 12 h post assault.

In addition to DNA, the persistence of mRNA and miRNA in laundered or cleaned biological fluid stains has also been investigated. Mayes et al. [**138**] showed that mRNA and miRNA markers were able to detect blood and semen from stains exposed to various laundering conditions. They also tested blood and semen stains exposed to various environmental conditions relating to temperature, humidity and light for six months, and found that mRNA targets were observed through six months for some conditions but undetectable after 30 days for other conditions, whereas their miRNA targets persisted under all test conditions for the duration of the study. Furthermore, when investigating the level of blood-derived DNA and miRNA inside firearm barrels after cleaning with DNA-ExitusPlus™ (AppliChem GmbH, Darmstadt, Germany), Schyma et al. [**139**] found that while the DNA had been removed, the blood-specific miRNA was still detectable.

3.5. *Incidence and Context*

This section provides a concise overview of the ten publications that were found to examine the occurrence of DNA and the existence of background DNA (as shown in Figure 2). Additionally, one extra study is included that also offers insights on this topic, but it is largely classified under a different subject. Three studies [140,141,142] have investigated the occurrence of DNA from drivers, passengers, and other individuals in various areas of vehicles that are typically driven by a single person. The experiments revealed that DNA could be successfully obtained from all designated locations, and the yields and composition of profiles differed between the sites, with comparatively higher yields obtained from steering wheels and seats. The study revealed that the driver consistently appeared as a contributor in DNA profiles obtained from locations on the driver's side. In many cases, the driver was the only or primary contributor. Additionally, the driver was also identified as the only or primary contributor at many locations on the passenger side. Additionally, it was discovered that DNA profiles belonging to passengers who were recently identified, those closely connected to the driver, and unidentified individuals were detected on numerous locations on both the passenger and driver sides.

The prevalence of DNA from users in an office space was considered by Goray et al. [**119**]. They investigated the extent to which DNA, left by a temporary user of the office space that had been occupied by a regular user for an extended period, is detectable when the duration of their temporary occupancy and their general activities are known, as well as how readily the DNA of the regular user is still detectable after a known period of occupancy by another person. From samples collected from several items/surfaces within single use office spaces that had been used temporarily by another occupant for 2.5–7 h, the authors found that sufficient DNA for profiling was recovered from nearly all areas sampled. They found that the regular user of the office space was the major or majority contributor (as defined by the authors) to profiles from most items within the space, even after temporary use by another person. It was reported that detectability of the temporary occupier varied among offices and items tested, and whilst the temporary occupier was not observed on all items they touched, in most instances when detected, it was known that they had touched the surface at some stage. The authors also observed profiles from other individuals, including colleagues, family members and unknowns, that were present on several items, mostly as minor contributors.

The study by Szkuta et al. [**143**] considered background levels of DNA on common entry points to homes (rarely contacted external and internal windowsills and edges, and frequently contacted entrance door handles) occupied by known individuals with some general knowledge on the history of use. They found that interpretable DNA profiles were able to be generated from nearly all door handles (all mixed profiles) and internal windowsills and edges (mostly mixed profiles), but the majority of external windowsills and edges yielded limited to no DNA profile information. The authors reported that the individuals living in the house tended to be main contributors to the profiles, and that the last person to make contact with a door handle was observed as a contributor in most but not all profiles. The authors also observed unknown contributors in the profiles of many of the door handle, internal windowsill and edge samples, and in most situations, but not all, they were a minor contributor.

The study by Albani et al. [**144**] investigated the extent of male-derived DNA presence on unused feminine sanitary products (tampons, pads, liners). The authors postulated, but did not test, that if such DNA was present, it could possibly be transferred onto the wearer and subsequently be detected in samples taken from intimate areas during a medical examination. However, the authors found no to very little background DNA present, with only 4 of the 52 items (1 tampon and 3 liners) exhibiting one or two Y-STR alleles and 1 additional item (pad) exhibiting two alleles using an autosomal STR kit, with all alleles appearing with low RFU signals.

To elucidate the level and origins of background DNA on worn upper garments, Szkuta et al. [**117**] and Szkuta et al. [**118**] collected samples from several areas (two internal and six external) of two garments (both owned and previously worn by the participant) each worn on separate occasions, for 6 to 15 h on a work day and a non-work day, after being washed. They also recorded details of the history of the garment, and the interactions and activities during wearing, and collected samples for reference DNA profiles from participants and their close associates. They found variation in the DNA quantity, profile composition and inclusion/exclusion of the wearer and their associates, among participants, garments worn on different occasions and the garment areas sampled. The authors reported that DNA from the wearer of a garment was found on all internal and external areas sampled, with the best quality profiles corresponding to the wearer obtained from internal collars followed by internal cuffs. They also found that DNA from individuals living or sharing a space with the wearer was frequently detected in samples from external areas of the garment. In such samples, the contribution of the wearer to the DNA profile was occasionally absent or minor relative to the presence of the close associate; this was most frequently observed in samples taken from the external back of the garment.

A further study by Murphy et al. [**145**] examined the background levels of male DNA on the inside front of clean, but not new, pairs of underpants worn for a day by a female who was asked to abstain from sexual intercourse for 48 h prior to taking part in the study. The authors reported that, of the 103 samples taken after a day of wearing, 83 showed the presence of male DNA to varying quantities (as detected by the Quantifiler Trio DNA quantification kit (Thermo Fisher Scientific, Warrington, UK)) and 24 contained sufficient DNA to proceed to profiling. Of those 24 profiled samples, 12 samples showed the detection of the Y chromosome and varying numbers of minor alleles (not from the female wearer) using the autosomal NGM SElect kit (Thermo Fisher Scientific, Warrington, UK), 5 gave a complete Y-STR profile, and 18 gave incomplete Y-STR profiles. Each of the samples that gave a complete Y-STR profile was from a female who cohabited with a male partner and the profile matched that of the partner where a reference profile was available (four of five). Based on the results of their study, the authors concluded that the finding of a Y-filer profile on the inside front of underpants worn by a female is not expected in the absence of sexual contact. Further, in the absence of sexual contact, a Y-STR profile, if present, is more likely to be obtained from a cohabitating male rather than from a non-cohabitating male in social contact with a female.

Two studies included investigation of the impact of cleaning on levels and composition of background DNA on various surfaces. Reither et al. [**146**] found that domestic cleaning methods (e.g., vacuuming, mopping with cleaning agents that did not contain cholic acid) had limited impact on the quantity of DNA recovered from various types of flooring (e.g., carpet, tiles), but often altered the DNA profile composition of the samples collected when comparing the profile from the post-cleaned area with the profile from the corresponding pre-cleaned area. Similarly, in experiments to determine the impact of a range of cleaning agents and cleaning actions using DNA-free towel pieces and sponges on small blood stains, saliva stains and fingermarks on plastic table tops and fabric surfaces, Helmus et al. [**147**] found that the DNA was redistributed to other areas of the item by the cleaning action. They also found that the cleaning agent had little impact on the ability to generate DNA profiles of the sample collected, with the exception of chloric agents, which the authors asserted rendered almost everything DNA-free.

3.6. Manner of Handling

This section reports ten studies that investigated manner of handling (**Figure 2**). We have broken down this section into further subtopics to categorise the studies into elements of handling, including time, pressure, and testing of various scenarios. We have also included studies on non-contact DNA transfer in this section.

3.6.1. Handling Time

In their study of the impact of handling time by a non-wearer of a worn brassiere, Sessa et al. [**93**] found that the contact duration does not appear to have an effect on the amount of DNA deposited and when a major contributor is detected on a garment. Outcomes of their experiments (which included small specific target areas of known contact by the 'handler') also showed that the person handling the garment last contributed the most to the recovered DNA, even though they may have touched the garment for only a few seconds.

3.6.2. Pressure

Examining the effect of deposition pressure (using weights from 0.1 to 10 kg) applied by fingers on the quality of latent fingermarks and DNA STR profiles, Hefetz et al. [**148**] found that as deposition pressure increased, so did the length and width of fingermarks and the efficiency of DNA profiling from the fingermarks. The latter was based on increases in the amount of DNA recovered, number of amplified loci, and number of forensically useful DNA profiles, which were observed for each of the substrates tested (glass, polythene, paper).

3.6.3. Scenario Testing

The transfer of DNA to clothing under a number of case-relevant scenarios was investigated by Szkuta et al. [**118**] and De Wolff et al. [**149**]. Szkuta et al. [**118**] examined whether an 'activity partner' was discernible on clothing worn by another individual after specific interactions: 'contact' where the final action during the wearing of the garment was an embrace with a known other individual; 'close proximity' where the final action during the wearing of the garment was to travel to and from a nearby café to have a meal with a known other individual; 'physical absence' where the wearer of the garment spent most of a working day in an office of a known other individual, in the absence of the other individual. The study did not find any DNA from the activity partner on the garments after the wearer had gone on an outing, even though they had been in close proximity with each other for a while. However, the study did observe DNA from the activity partner on several areas of the garments following the embrace and after temporarily occupying another person's office. It was reported that particular areas of the garment were more prone to acquiring DNA from the hugging partner or the office owner than others, and their detection as a major or minor component was deemed activity dependent. When investigating DNA transfer to clothing within vehicles, De Wolff et al. [**149**] found that in many instances, DNA from a regular driver of a vehicle could be recovered from samples collected from the external back of the upper garment, and from the seat of the trousers pants, worn by an incidental driver (30 min) of that vehicle soon after departing the vehicle. This highlighted a potential avenue of indirect transfer that may be relevant during investigations of particular types of offences.

DNA transfer within specific scenarios that can occur during sexual assaults was investigated by Ramos et al. [**150**]. Their study recorded where underwear was contacted and how much DNA was transferred by volunteer 'offenders' during six types of mock sexual assault scenarios: removing underwear; removing brassiere; digital penetration of the vagina from the front; grabbing breasts over the top of the brassiere; digital penetration of the vagina from the rear; grabbing the breasts under the brassiere from the rear. The authors found that the pattern of contact varied for different activities and identified the areas of underwear most commonly contacted from various sexual assault activities. They demonstrated that some areas corresponded to areas typically sampled during casework and others less so, thus providing information to help improve sample targeting. They too observed several instances of a colleague or cohabitating partner of mock offenders being detected within a DNA sample.

A study by Gosch et al. **[151]** considered trace DNA characteristics (including DNA yield, number of contributors, relative profile contribution for known and unknown contributors, LRs) of samples recovered from various surfaces of two types of firearms handled in four realistic casework-relevant scenarios. In each scenario, the firearm had background DNA deposited over four days by the mock owner. The four different activities then undertaken with the firearms included: the mock owner performed a shooting scenario; a second individual performed the same shooting scenario as the mock owner; a second individual imitated a longer and more intensive contact with the firearm; a second individual performed the same shooting scenario as the mock owner, then wiped the firearm using a dry cotton towel for 15 s simulating fingerprint removal. The authors observed a large variability of trace characteristics that was partly attributable to the way the firearms were handled, the firearm surface types sampled, and factors of inter- as well as intra-individual variability.

When considering DNA transfer to knife handles, particularly within opportunistic crimes, Butcher et al. **[152]** conducted experiments to generate data to help address consideration of questions relating to whether the DNA obtained comes from the regular user, the last user (ostensibly, the user at the time of the crime) or from indirect transfer events. The authors found that regularly used knives that were then used for just 2–60 s by a second person, performing a stabbing action, resulted for three of the four participant pairings in a decrease in contribution from the regular user's DNA with simultaneous increase in contribution from the second user's DNA. They reported that the trend appeared to be due to a decrease in regular user DNA via transfer to the second user's hands, rather than an increase in DNA deposited from the second user, but a deviation from this general trend was observed for the fourth participant pairing. While they found a low level contribution of the non-handler's DNA on most knife handles, one volunteer deposited a similar amount of DNA through regular use as the amount of indirectly transferred unknown DNA deposited by another volunteer's hands, leading the authors to indicate that caution should be taken when relying solely on absolute quantities of DNA to inform evaluative interpretations and that other parameters, such as profile quality and relative contributions to mixed profiles, should also be taken into account. However, when also considering DNA transfer within stabbing scenarios, Samie et al. [**153**] observed that the quantity of DNA generally reduced when moving from hand (the quantity collected when sampling directly from a hand) to primary transfer (the quantity collected from a surface handled by a hand) and, subsequently, to secondary transfer.

To assist activity level evaluation, Euteneuer et al. [**154**] investigated the correlation between shooting distance and the amount of blood backspatter in/on a used firearm. The authors could not establish any meaningful correlation between backspatter distribution and DNA yields, the shooting distance and the condition of the wound channel.

3.6.4. Non-Contact Transfer

The first study to consider non-contact transfer with dried biological materials was published by Thornbury et al. [**155**]. They investigated the possibility of indirect DNA transfer without contact from various substrates (two different non-porous hard substrates and two different porous, soft substrates) after various biological materials (blood, saliva, semen, vaginal fluid, touch DNA) deposited on them had dried and after applying two types of agitation (tapping—all substrates; stretching—all fabric substrates). The authors found that detectable levels of indirect transfer of DNA without contact were possible. They also demonstrated that the type of biological material and substrate affected the drying time and characteristics of deposits, and that the rate and percentage transfer appeared to be dependent on the type of agitation, substrate, biological material and its drying properties.

3.7. Shedder Status

This section summarises the one paper where shedder status was deemed the most relevant DNA-TPPR aspect (**Figure 2**), plus seven additional studies that also provided comment on this subject matter but were primarily categorised in other topics. When investigating shedder status as a possible factor influencing the extent of secondary DNA transfer to a crime scene when the offender wears working gloves, Otten et al. [**156**] initially determined the shedder status of a group of individuals, finding that good shedders deposited higher amounts and quality of DNA onto objects compared to bad shedders. The authors then conducted experiments where participants were paired into groups of various combinations of good and bad shedders, with the first participant of each pair wearing working gloves to pack and carry boxes, and then, two days later, the same gloves were worn by the second participant to break-in using a screwdriver. The study reported that good shedders, overall, deposited more DNA than bad shedders, both onto the outside and inside of the gloves regardless of being the first or second wearer and user of the gloves. The authors also found that a DNA profile of the first wearer was found on the screwdriver in several instances, and in each of the situations where this was observed, the first user had been a designated good shedder, confirming the possibility of a person's DNA profile being found on an object they never handled.

Several other papers demonstrated or alluded to observing differences in the quantities of DNA deposited, which was attributed to differences in shedder status, for example [**51**,**78**,**150**,**152**]. However, Miller et al. [**95**] found that individuals who deposited extremely large amounts of DNA by touch one day may deposit no detectable DNA on another day despite a restriction on handwashing close in time to deposition, leading the authors to question the concept that there are consistently good shedders, at least through the palms of hands. Similarly, Samie et al. [**153**] noted that while a person could be judged as a good shedder overall, when considering a single experiment, that same person could be a very poor shedder. They suggest that when assessing the probability of observing a given quantity of DNA, for a given donor, the whole distribution should be accounted for and not only its mean value. The authors also showed that the 'transfer proportion' (quantity of DNA transferred onto a surface over the initial quantity on the hand) may vary between participants and will depend on the type of transfer (primary versus secondary), indicating that the quantification of DNA on one hand cannot be used to infer the shedder status and asses what will be transferred onto a surface.

Like shedder status determination from finger/hand marks, a study by Kanokwongnuwut et al. [**42**] found that the amounts of cellular material deposited by lip-prints is consistent for individuals, but different among individuals. The authors were able to categorise lip shedder status from heavy to light, but they did not observe a correlation between lip-print shedder status and the shedder status of the individual determined from thumb prints.

3.8. Contamination

The potential unwanted transfer of DNA during a forensic examination (or contamination) can also be relevant and has been considered in four of the studies identified (**Figure 2**). Three of these studies looked at the potential of DNA contamination via items used during an examination in the laboratory, specifically gloves and fingerprint brushes [**157**,**158**,**159**]. In the study by Goray et al. [**157**], a number of laboratory-based evidence recovery personnel were videoed performing a range of examinations and several factors were assessed to evaluate the risks of DNA loss, addition and redistribution via gloves. The factors included: what each glove touched and in what sequence; the number, duration and type of contact made by each glove with the item under examination, tools used and other surfaces;

when gloves were replaced; DNA profiles of samples taken from worn gloves at the time of replacement against those relating to the item under investigation, the examiner, and other staff members. The authors observed that many different surface areas are touched by gloves during examinations, and differences exist among examiners in what they touch and when they change gloves. They reported that, in many instances, the case-associated person of interest was observed within the profile generated from DNA retrieved from outer surfaces of most gloves sampled at time of replacement. They also observed DNA profiles of the examiner, or other staff members, predominantly in samples taken from the first and last gloves used during the examination, which were associated with removing the exhibit from the packaging and repackaging it. Their evaluation deemed that several of the observed contacts made by the gloves were a high contamination risk event. Furthermore, Van den Berge et al. [**158**] performed tests showing that DNA from hands transferred to various parts of the external side of laboratory gloves while being donned. With respect to used fingerprint brushes, the study by Nontiapirom et al. [**159**] produced results verifying findings that human DNA can persist on fingerprint brushes after use, such that fingerprint brushes can be a potential contamination risk when reused.

Two of the identified studies also considered the effectiveness of contamination-minimisation procedures within the laboratory [**158,160**]. In the above study by Van den Berge et al. [**158**], they also performed tests providing outcomes supporting the use of 0.3% sodium hypochlorite solution or commercially available RNase AWAY™ (Thermo Fisher Scientific, Waltham, MA, USA) as decontamination reagents to clean and subsequently dry the exterior of donned gloves prior to entering the laboratory and/or handling items of evidence. The authors reported that the results precipitated an update to their laboratory's contamination risk reduction strategy. The study by Basset and Castella [**160**] compared the number of DNA contamination events by laboratory staff before and after the implementation of additional contamination minimisation procedures (that included: physical separation between living environments (e.g., offices, cafeteria) and laboratory zones; personal objects prohibited from laboratory zones; double gloving; use of different disposable lab coats within different laboratory rooms; lab coats changed daily; stain collection split among different operators so that the person in contact with the swab does not touch other surfaces; automation of DNA extraction for standard traces) and found that the number of such contamination events declined by more than 70% after implementation of the procedures.

3.9. Microbiomes

Fourteen studies (**Figure 2**) delve into the opportunities to identify individuals, or associate them with a location or an activity, that may be offered from analysing microbiomes in the absence of and/or in addition to traditional DNA evidence. These include investigations into:

- Classification of individuals and the potential to detect sexual contact using the microbiome of the pubic region [**161**].
- Bacterial communities associated with cell phones and shoes of the same person [**162**].
- Microbial communities of a wide range of known body sites and the detection of the source of different microbial contributions in mixtures of different body sites or with soil [**163**].
- Distinguishing microbiome communities of saliva, skin and mixtures of both as a potential tool for identifying samples of single and mixed biological materials [**164**].
- Correlations between the presence of certain bacterial species on a donor's hands and personal characteristics [**165**].
- The direct and indirect transfer of microbiomes between individuals [**166**].
- The ability of several commercial kits to recover sufficient bacterial DNA from fingerprints to generate a microbiome profile [**167**].
- Generating both STR profiles and microbial population profiles from the same DNA extract of each sample to evaluate the sub-source and source questions, respectively in two forensic cases [**168**].
- The usefulness of the likelihood ratio approach for the evaluation of source attribution in microbial forensic cases to facilitate the interpretation of evidence in legal proceedings [**169**].

In addition, Young and Linacre [**170**] provided a review of studies on the potential and limitations of utilising microbiome analyses in forensic science, especially in relation to skin microbiome. Meanwhile, Jurkevitch and Pasternal [**171**] provided a review on the use of soil bacterial community comparisons to assist investigation of alleged crimes. Each of these studies and reviews, as well as a review by Neckovic et al. [**172**], indicated some positive results and potential useful applications, but also highlighted a range of limitations of their applicability and the challenges of microbial profiling for forensic science casework applications. These challenges are further illustrated by investigations of the presence of microbiomes within forensic evidence recovery laboratories, and the potential for microbiomes to transfer during examinations [**173,174**].

3.10. Evaluating DNA Evidence

This final section of the synopsis reports papers that consider the evaluation of DNA evidence given propositions at different levels within the Hierarchy of

Propositions. Ten papers with a primary focus on this subject matter are included (**Figure 2**), along with one other that was primarily included in another topic, and are reported within two subsections: setting propositions and use of Bayesian Networks, and other activity level assessment-related matters.

3.10.1. Setting Propositions and Use of Bayesian Networks

When evaluating the value of biological evidence, it is important that the propositions are formulated appropriately. Gill et al. [**120**] presented guidelines from the DNA Commission of the International Society for Forensic Genetics (ISFG) on determining and formulating the propositions for the evaluation of biological traces, given activity level propositions. This paper included eleven specific recommendations and provided examples to illustrate the principles espoused. The authors also noted that suitable propositions are ideally set before knowledge of the trace DNA evidence, that data relevant to the case in question be gathered to assign probabilities, and that Bayesian Networks (BNs) are useful to help consider all relevant possibilities. Taylor et al. [**175**] also stressed the importance of properly constructing the propositions. The authors indicated the need for a clear summary of propositions representing the views of the prosecution and defence, accompanied with details on the agreed and contested information and assumptions by the scientist, to assist in carrying out an evaluation and in understanding by the courts. Furthermore, Buckleton et al. [**176**] showed an example where considerations of DNA-TPPR are required to inform sub-source level proposition setting, specifically to condition the calculation on the presence of DNA of an assumed contributor. The authors showed this in relation to the number of contributors, as this is likely to impact on the LR at the sub-source level.

Several studies focussed on the use of BNs to evaluate DNA results given competing propositions, including Taylor et al. [**177**], Gill et al. [**120**], Volgin [**178**], De March and Tarino [**179**], and Samie et al. [**180**]. Examples of the use of BNs to evaluate biological traces given activity level propositions are provided in: the supplementary material within the article of Gill et al. [**120**] (that is accessible in the online version); and by Volgin [**178**] involving the use of a T-shirt as a balaclava. Further, De March and Tarino [**179**] provided an insight into the application of BNs to real criminal cases through the assessment of the probative value of different analyses related to some biological material retrieved from an object of interest.

Two studies went further to consider the applicability of BNs to the complexities of issues of DNA transfer. Taylor et al. [**177**] showed the value of an Object-Oriented Bayesian Network (OOBN) to tackle cases involving repeating elements of complex and various DNA transfer mechanisms and indicated that, as new data on DNA-TPPR factors become available, these can be readily accommodated by the general overall OOBN architecture. Further, Samie et al. [**180**] showed that BNs can handle the complexity of variables associated with DNA-TPPR to inform activity level assessments. Their study demonstrated the uses of BNs and simulation methods to identify the variables impacting the value of evidence assessed under activity level propositions. The authors did so by focussing on trace DNA evidence recovered from knife handles allegedly involved in stabbing instances, showing that some variables had greater bearing on the variation of the LR than others. In the situation they investigated, the authors reported that the identified key variables were associated with the sampling, the extraction efficiency, the background and the quantity of DNA on hands, and they asserted that data acquisition should focus mainly on those variables with the greatest impact.

3.10.2. Other Activity Level Assessment-Related Matters

In his commentary, Gill [**181**] pointed out that the increased sensitivity of modern DNA profiling techniques means that DNA may be recovered that is irrelevant to the crime and stressed the importance of scientists, lawyers and judges to be aware of the limitations of DNA profiling evidence. This was echoed by Sessa et al. [**93**], who also pointed out the need for everyone in the medico-legal community to know the power of touch DNA and understand the potential limitations associated with it. Gill [**181**] went on to note that the presence of DNA does not tell us when or how it got there, so additional context is needed from other non-DNA evidence, which if ignored could result in miscarriages of justice. He provided several real case examples to highlight how ignorance of key aspects, such as background DNA, secondary transfer, and laboratory contamination, can influence case outcomes. Similarly, Perepechina [**182**] referred to a retrospective analysis of a case where consideration of transfer issues was pertinent. Given these issues, he [**181**] also pointed out the need to educate stakeholders, including all parties engaged in the criminal justice system, with respect to the various facets relating to activity level assessments.

An additional concern highlighted by Gill [**181**] is the occurrence of carryover of the strength of evidence associated with a DNA 'match' to weight of evidence associated with activity level propositions. He reported that this cannot be done; activity level assessments are to be undertaken separately using different information and generating a different statistic. This point is also made by the DNA Commission of the ISFG [**120**].

Apart from the few calls for specific further research noted above, many of the other publications incorporated in this synopsis, in their discussion sections, also incorporate suggestions/recommendations/advocacy for further research to enlighten our understandings and advance the acquisition of relevant data to improve our abilities to provide activity level assessments. From challenges encountered in their study, Dunhill and Chapman [**183**] encouraged authors to publish results of studies on indirect transfer of DNA in a more streamlined fashion to allow for systematic analysis of data across studies. Further, De March and Tarino [**179**] indicated that while the data available to inform probabilities are limited and extrapolation from published data for practical use in a case analysis can be troublesome, this should not prevent the forensic scientist from providing a statement at the activity level when the circumstances of a case require it.

4. REFLECTIONS ON THE RESEARCH EFFORTS TO MEET THE CHALLENGES

Based on the focus, scope and depth of the research activities published over the last few years, we reflect that overall, some progress has been made to meet the many challenges, but much of the challenges noted in the introduction remain and require more effort to address them. While several of the recent studies have provided means of improving the detection and recovery of DNA and DNA profiles of relevance from crime-related items, more effort will be required to determine the best practices given the specific circumstances encountered. Of the 144 articles included in the synopsis, relatively few (35) primarily focus on aspects of persistence, DNA prevalence and background DNA, manner of handling and shedder status (**Figure 2**). Of these, few provide the highly desired data to help assign probabilities of obtaining profile types given particular sets of circumstances, especially those that are relatively commonly encountered. The latter is partly due to the relatively recent and increasing need for such data, and the requirement for sufficient repeats to be conducted to generate robust frequency data, which may place this type of research beyond the scope of some research groups. The multitude of situations and associated variables for which probabilities are desired provides scope for conducting many future research projects to provide welcomed outputs.

Some additional research efforts have been directed at determining and mitigating risks of contamination of evidence (see **Section 3.8**). Further research may highlight additional risk factors and means of mitigating these, thus providing opportunities to enhance the integrity of the evidence throughout the forensic process and the interpretation thereof.

Some research has been conducted on other elements of information that may be gleaned from deposits of biological materials to facilitate activity level evaluations (see **Section 3.1**, **Section 3.3**, **Section 3.9**). Further studies towards improving abilities to accurately determine the TSD of various types of biological material in various circumstances (preferably even of different components within mixed samples), and into microbiome profiles that inform on the environment that a sample is associated with, and/or its source, and/or provide an avenue for identity determination in the absence of human DNA, may assist future activity level evaluations.

To assist with activity level evaluations, BNs are starting to be utilised more (see **Section 3.10.1**), such that any developments towards making BN-related software packages even more user friendly for forensic practitioners may further facilitate their utilisation and the standard of the guidance provided to the court. However, there appears to be little recent human factors-related research effort directed towards facilitating the development of competencies of those tasked with providing activity level-related guidance and how to best convey this guidance to other stakeholders. Such research, as well as human factors research relating to individuals and processes associated with the collection of evidence and maintaining its integrity, would be welcomed as they may identify improvement opportunities in the means of training experts and the quality of tasks undertaken and the services provided.

Encouragingly, very recent publications (i.e., articles published after conducting the systematic search, or during the search period but not captured) demonstrate the realisation of the need for, and the efforts supporting, ongoing research activity towards meeting the broad range of outstanding challenges. Examples of such publications of studies addressing identified knowledge and data gaps include:

- DNA profile success of samples from casework-related items [**24**].
- Impacts of surface roughness and physicochemical interactions on deposits of biological materials [**184**].
- Impacts of chewing gum on drying properties of saliva [**185**].
- Prevalence and persistence of saliva in vehicles [**186**].
- Exploring means of determining an individual's shedder status.
- Consideration of distance and time with respect to accumulation of DNA within offices on surfaces that are not touched [**187**].
- Evaluation of profiles retrieved from the outside of gloves after simulating transfer scenarios related to breaking and entering [**188**].
- Findings indicating that cities around the globe have distinct microbial taxonomic signatures [**189**].
- Development of an LR framework incorporating sensitivity analysis to model multiple direct and secondary transfer events on skin surfaces [**190**].
- Highlighting the importance/value of considering common sources of unknown DNA [**191**].
- Assigning weight of cell type testing results [**192**] when evaluating findings given activity level propositions.

These studies demonstrate the realisation of the need for, and the efforts supporting, ongoing research activity towards meeting the broad range of outstanding challenges.

5. INDUSTRY ACTIONS TOWARDS ADDRESSING CHALLENGES

5.1. Research

Many of the reviews and research papers referenced in the previous sections note the need for more research to better inform our understanding of variables affecting DNA-TPPR and supplying relevant data to determine probabilities given a set of circumstances. Meakin et al. [**193**], apart from also advocating this, urged for better designed research studies to cater for this need. In particular, they expanded on the recommendation of Gosch and Courts [**36**] for different experimental designs to be employed when generating probabilities for activity level evaluations as opposed to investigating DNA transfer mechanisms. They recommended that the former requires iterations of realistic experiments (e.g., a casework-relevant scenario performed once by multiple participants), whereas the latter require repetitions of highly controlled and potentially unrealistic experiments (e.g., a single participant performing the same action multiple times). Meakin et al. [**193**] also directed readers to the ISFG recommendations [**120**], which provide further advice for designing experiments to generate activity level probabilities.

Evident from the authorships and their affiliations, forensic laboratories, alone or in collaboration with other forensic laboratories and/or academic institutions, are major contributors to much of the published DNA-TPPR-related research. Much of this is being funded by internal resources. Major research funding bodies are also increasingly supporting DNA-TPPR-related research. For example, the National Institute of Justice (NIJ) in the United States of America has funded over 60 DNA-related projects to the value in excess of USD 42 million during 2018–2020 [**194,195**], which include a wide range of DNA-TPPR-related research projects, and the European Network of Forensic Institutes (ENSFI) has recently funded a large multi-institutional collaborative project to generate accessible DNA transfer rate data [**196**].

5.2. Education and Training

Apart from the need for research to improve our understanding and generate data to allow the assignment of probabilities given a set of circumstances, there are other challenges to be met by relevant industry stakeholders. These include aspects relating to the education and training of those tasked with providing expert evidence on DNA-TPPR-related matters, building of awareness of aspects associated with DNA-TPPR among crime scene attendees and those within the legal fraternity, availability and utility of published data, and setting of standards associated with DNA-related activity level evaluative reporting. Steps are being taken to address these challenges.

DNA-TPPR-related research findings, including unpublished findings, are being presented and discussed within dedicated sessions and workshops at international forensic conferences attended by forensic, policing and legal practitioners as well as academia. For example, Congresses of the International Society of Forensic Genetics [**197**]; Gordon Research Conferences: Forensic Analysis of Human DNA [**198**]; American Academy of Forensic Sciences (AAFS) conferences [**199**]; the International Symposium on Human Identification ((ISHI) [**200**]; and the symposium on Recent Progress on Forensic Sciences and DNA Transfer organised by Laboratoired'Hématologie Médico-Légale [**201**].

Further education/upskilling of stakeholders on the topic of DNA-TPPR and the associated activity level evaluative reporting is also being made possible through the development and availability of dedicated programs such as summer schools on various aspects of forensic genetics organised by the International Society of Forensic Genetics [**202**] and university-based courses such as the Certificate of Advanced Studies on 'Statistics and the evaluation of forensic evidence' run by the University of Lausanne [**203**]. Freely accessible courses and webinars have also been produced, such as that on 'Challenging Forensic Science: How Science Should Speak to Court' made available by the University of Lausanne [**204**] and the series of webinars on DNA mixture interpretation and probabilistic genotyping organised by the Federal Bureau of Investigation (FBI) Laboratory and NIJ's Forensic Technology Center of Excellence [**205**].

The skill set required to become expert at the provision of guidance on DNA-TPPR at the activity level is distinct from those required to provide guidance at the DNA sub-source level, biological material source level or non-DNA activity level. Recognition of this can be an important first step for laboratories to help define the necessary enrichments and changes to a suite of methodologies, protocols, training units and authorisations. Introduction of these is then to be managed, such that the increasing demands for such services can be met at the expected standards. Most forensic DNA experts trained over the last twenty years have been trained to provide statements at the sub-source level. A forensic expert solely trained and competent at providing DNA evidence at the sub-source level should not provide opinion at the activity level without also being trained and authorised to do so.

An example of a jurisdiction with a competency testing program specific to evaluation of forensic biology findings given activity level propositions can be found in the Netherlands [**206**]. Experts can submit an application for registration as an expert in the field to the Netherlands Register of Court Experts (**www.nrgd.nl**). They are subsequently assessed by a committee of both scientific experts and legal professionals against a standard that has been developed by a group of international experts in the field. The standards demarcate the field of 'DNA activity' from 'DNA source' and 'DNA kinship' and list the minimum requirements for experts in these fields. These requirements cover training, experience, methodology, reporting, and knowledge of the Dutch legal system [**207**]. Registered individuals must demonstrate their ongoing competency to the Board on a regular (five year) basis.

5.3. Availability and Sharing of Data

Kokshoorn et al. [**208**] and Gosch and Courts [**36**] advocated the need for sharing of research data associated with DNA-TPPR. They also indicated the type of information that is relevant when interpreting the generated data and should be made available when publishing DNA-TPPR-related research (or making it available on sharing platforms). These included information on: item (type of item, construction and surface composition, etc.); item history (handling, packaging, etc.); sampling (surface area targeted, sampling method, etc.); analysis (DNA extraction, amplification, CE, etc.); and interpretation (allele calling, statistical model, parameter settings, proposition setting, NoC determination, etc.). Kokshoorn et al. [**208**] also advocated for harmonisation and standardisation in how some of this information should be recorded, to further assist utilisation of the data. Gosch and Courts [**36**] constructed a database for entry and accessibility of such data, added the data from relevant publications and requested researchers to submit the relevant data to DNA-TrAC [**37**]. DNA-TrAC contains 311 entries of relevant research articles published in the period 1993–2017. Detailed information is provided per publication covering a wide range of aspects relevant to understanding DNA-TPPR and utilising data for activity level evaluations. It also provides the ability to sort information based on various parameters including general details of the publications, questions being addressed by the studies, transfer scenarios in the context of a specific type of activity, categories of study object (e.g., primary deposit, further transfer, background DNA, persistence, recovery), and variables affecting DNA-TPPR. The website also includes a list of 17 review articles published in the period 2002–2020 with a summary of the topics addressed by each as well as a file listing 33 articles relevant to DNA-TPPR published during the period 2018–2020 for which the details have not yet been entered into the DNA-TrAC database. The last version fully and actively curated by the Gosch and Courts was uploaded in December 2019 and a request is issued for others to assist with the maintenance of the database. DNA-TrAC is a useful portal to source DNA-TPPR information and data that may be relevant to a range of stakeholders. Maintenance and upkeep of this database, or the creation of something similar, would be an asset to the forensic community and thus desirable.

A separate relevant database ('BDATT-TTADB'), constructed with funding support from research grants from the Social Sciences and Humanities Research Council of Canada, has recently become available [**209,210**]. The database was built with the aim of being relevant for practitioners to interpret transfer traces at activity level, integrating transfer experiments in an operational situation [**209**]. It provides information for a wide range of trace types, including DNA and biological fluids. It allows for easy searching according to type of trace, type of study (including transfer, persistence, recovery, background, contamination), key words (as determined by the database custodians, not the ones listed in the associated publication) as well as aspects such as authors. Apart from the general information regarding the publication (i.e., title, authors, journal), it provides a copy of the published abstract, a summary statement regarding the studies' experimental conditions and results, a summary statement regarding the relevancy of the study for the Canadian environment, and a link to the publication. The database includes several hundred papers relating to DNA-TPPR and is updated regularly [**209,210**]. This database resource provides an excellent means for any interested parties to identify potentially relevant studies. However, those seeking some of the finer details often required when conducting activity level evaluations, as described above, will need to examine the identified literature more closely. An additional source of relevant data will also be made available in early 2022, when the UK Body Fluid Forum launches a digital collection of casework-informed research and case reports to facilitate sharing of experiences and data specifically relevant to informing evaluation of biological findings given activity level propositions. When available, these articles will be accessible here: **https://www.sciencedirect.com/journal/science-and-justice/special-issues**. Further development and maintenance of databases containing all the relevant information that allow easy mining of desired finer details, and further efforts towards harmonisation and standardisation of the data generated and shared as suggested by Kokshoorn et al. [**208**], would be welcomed.

5.4. Standards and Guidance

Many standards and guidance on how to conduct DNA-related activity level evaluative reporting are being provided by governing bodies. For example, the Forensic Science Regulator in England and Wales [**211**] and the DNA Commission of the ISFG [**120,212**]; there is also an ISO standard relating to forensic science reporting currently under development [**213**]. Additionally, some of the fallacies associated with the reporting of DNA-TPPR matters, that forensic practitioners need be cognisant of and avoid when providing guidance to the triers of fact, are highlighted by Meakin et al. [**193**].

Forensic laboratories are also investing in developing in-house methods, procedures and training modules to facilitate the conduct of DNA-related activity level evaluations and the training of their staff to do so. However, unlike many other forensic disciplines, independent ongoing proficiency testing in all the relevant elements associated with DNA-related activity level evaluations for those authorised to provide expert opinion to assist triers of fact is not readily available. Creation of a good fit for purpose internationally available proficiency testing program would facilitate the provision of high-quality guidance by forensic practitioners.

The National Institute of Standards and Technology (NIST) in the USA has very recently (June 2021) published a draft of a scientific foundation review in relation to the interpretation of DNA mixtures [**214**]. It also contemplates several of the points we raised earlier. It is a wide ranging comprehensive in-depth review that provides an overview of the past, present and future of DNA mixture interpretation and identifies challenges and pathways to deal with them. It includes a general introduction; principles and practices relating to DNA mixture interpretation; sources of data and information; delving into the issues pertaining to the reliability of DNA mixture measurements and interpretation as well as the context and relevance of DNA mixture interpretation (with details on various factors associated with DNA transfer); consideration of the potential and limitations of new technologies to provide solutions to existing problems. The chapters and appendices are accompanied with highlighted key takeaways, principal points and/or future considerations. Takeaways that directly relate to DNA transfer and activity level reporting, presented in chapter 5 of the review [**214**], include:

- #5.1: DNA can be transferred from one surface or person to another, and this can potentially happen multiple times. Therefore, the DNA present on an evidence item may be unrelated (irrelevant) to the crime being investigated.
- #5.2: Highly sensitive DNA methods increase the likelihood of detecting irrelevant DNA. When assessing evidence that involves very small quantities of DNA, it is especially important to consider relevance.
- #5.3: Highly sensitive methods increase the likelihood of detecting contaminating DNA that might affect an investigation. Contamination avoidance procedures should be robust both at the crime scene and in the laboratory.
- #5.4: DNA statistical results such as a sub-source likelihood ratio do not provide information about how or when DNA was transferred, or whether it is relevant to a case. Therefore, using the likelihood ratio as a standalone number without context can be misleading.

- #5.5: The fact that DNA transfers easily between objects does not negate the value of DNA evidence. However, the value of DNA evidence depends on the circumstances of the case.
- #5.6: There is a growing body of knowledge about DNA transfer and persistence, but significant knowledge gaps remain.

5.5. *Collaboration with other scientific disciplines, the legal community, and law enforcement agencies*

The compartmentalised nature of the scientific disciplines in many modern forensic laboratories hampers the proper evaluation of forensic findings [**215**]. Interdisciplinary assessments of traces increase the impact of the forensic sciences on the criminal justice system (CJS), both improving efficiency by reducing unnecessary examinations and improving understanding of the combined weight of the findings given case-relevant propositions at the activity level [**216**].

Case-relevant information is structured in propositions, assumptions, and other, undisputed case information [**175**]. For any evaluation of findings given activity level propositions that a scientist is asked to perform, it is crucial that all parties in the CJS are in a position to share task-relevant information with the scientist.

Education and training of stakeholders in the CJS is a crucial step to reduce common misconceptions of what evaluations given propositions at the activity level are, as well as to achieve the desired communication and collaboration between the scientist and the other actors in the CJS. Efforts are being made in several jurisdictions, for instance, by providing guidance documents for legal professionals [**217,218,219,220**].

6. AT A GLANCE

Much progress has been made recently towards addressing identified challenges concerning the provision of expert guidance in relation to DNA-TPPR-associated activity level evaluations sought to facilitate just outcomes during legal proceedings. However, many challenges remain. These include in relation to:

- Quantity and quality of research directed at informing our understanding of DNA-TPPR and building the data needed to assign probabilities to DNA quantities and profile types being obtained given a vast range of circumstances.
- Harmonisation, standardisation, and accessibility of available data.
- Development of validated standardised methodologies and protocols to perform DNA-related activity level evaluations.

- Training and authorisation of experts to perform such evaluations and provide the guidance when needed as well as recognition of this expertise as a separate discipline.
- Education and cooperation of stakeholders within the legal fraternity.

Continued investment in addressing these challenges will improve the value and understanding of the data and the guidance given to the triers of fact.

7. SUMMARY

Gaining a comprehensive understanding of the factors that can influence the transfer, persistence, prevalence, and recovery of DNA (DNA-TPPR), as well as having access to data that can determine the likelihood of obtaining specific DNA quantities and profile types in different scenarios and circumstances, is crucial when conducting evaluations of DNA findings based on activity level propositions (activity level evaluations). Between late 2018 and early 2019, three significant reviews were released about various parts of DNA-TPPR. Each review emphasized the necessity for additional research and other measures to facilitate the assessment of activity levels associated to DNA. In this analysis, we examine the strategies employed to overcome obstacles, focusing on summarizing papers relating to DNA-TPPR that have been published following the completion of these evaluations. Additionally, we briefly explore the measures taken by industry stakeholders to solve the gaps that have been found. Considerable progress has been made in recent years, and ongoing attempts are being made, to enhance the ability of forensic professionals to effectively assist the judiciary in regards to the transfer of DNA.

REFERENCES

1. Van Oorschot, R.A.H.; Szkuta, B.; Meakin, G.E.; Kokshoorn, B.; Goray, M. DNA transfer in forensic science: A review. Forensic Sci. Int. Genet. **2019**, 38, 140–166. **[Google Scholar] [CrossRef] [PubMed]**
2. Taylor, D.; Kokshoorn, B.; Biedermann, A. Evaluation of forensic genetics findings given activity level propositions: A review. Forensic Sci. Int. Genet. **2018**, 36, 34–49. **[Google Scholar] [CrossRef] [PubMed] [Green Version]**
3. Gill, P.; Haned, H.; Bleka, O.; Hansson, O.; Dørum, G.; Egeland, T. Genotyping and interpretation of STR-DNA: Low-template, mixtures and database matches—Twenty years of research and development. Forensic Sci. Int. Genet. **2015**, 18, 100–117. **[Google Scholar] [CrossRef] [PubMed]**
4. Børsting, C.; Morling, N. Next generation sequencing and its applications in forensic genetics. Forensic Sci. Int. Genet. **2015**, 18, 78–89. **[Google Scholar] [CrossRef] [PubMed]**

5. Butler, J.M. Advanced Topics in Forensic DNA Typing: Methodology; Academic Press: San Diego, CA, USA, 2012. **[Google Scholar]**

6. Van Oorschot, R.A.H.; Ballantyne, K.N.; Mitchell, J.R. Forensic trace DNA: A review. Investig. Genet. **2010**, 1, 1–17. **[Google Scholar] [CrossRef] [PubMed] [Green Version]**

7. Ballantyne, K.N.; Poy, A.L.; van Oorschot, R.A.H. Environmental DNA monitoring: Beware of the transition to more sensitive typing methodologies. Aust. J. Forensic Sci. **2013**, 45, 323–340. **[Google Scholar] [CrossRef]**

8. Farash, K.; Hanson, E.K.; Ballantyne, J. Single source DNA profile recovery from single cells isolated from skin and fabric from touch DNA mixtures in mock physical assaults. Sci. Justice **2018**, 58, 191–199. **[Google Scholar] [CrossRef] [PubMed]**

9. Van Oorschot, R.A.H.; Jones, M.K. DNA fingerprints from fingerprints. Nature **1997**, 387, 767. **[Google Scholar] [CrossRef]**

10. Lowe, A.; Murray, C.; Whitaker, J.; Tully, G.; Gill, P. The propensity of individuals to deposit DNA and secondary transfer of low level DNA from individuals to inert surfaces. Forensic Sci. Int. **2002**, 129, 25–34. **[Google Scholar] [CrossRef]**

11. Van Oorschot, R.A.H.; Glavich, G.; Mitchell, R.J. Persistence of DNA deposited by the original user on objects after subsequent use by a second person. Forensic Sci. Int. Genet. **2014**, 8, 219–225. **[Google Scholar] [CrossRef] [PubMed]**

12. Breathnach, M.; Williams, L.; McKenna, L.; Moore, E. Probability of detection of DNA deposited by habitual wearer and/or the second individual who touched the garment. Forensic Sci. Int. Genet. **2016**, 20, 53–60. **[Google Scholar] [CrossRef] [PubMed]**

13. Magee, A.M.; Breathnach, M.; Doak, S.; Thornton, F.; Noone, C.; McKenna, L.G. Wearer and non-wearer DNA on the collars and cuffs of upper garments of worn clothing. Forensic Sci. Int. Genet. **2018**, 34, 152–161. **[Google Scholar] [CrossRef] [PubMed]**

14. Poetsch, M.; Pfeifer, M.; Konrad, H.; Bajanowski, T.; Helmus, J. Impact of several wearers on the persistence of DNA on clothes—A study with experimental scenarios. Int. J. Legal Med. **2018**, 132, 117–123. **[Google Scholar] [CrossRef] [PubMed]**

15. Wickenheiser, R.A. Trace DNA: A review, discussion of theory, and application of the transfer of trace quantities of DNA through skin contact. J. Forensic Sci. **2002**, 47, 442–450. **[Google Scholar] [CrossRef]**

16. Harbison, S.-A.; Fallow, M.; Bushell, D. An analysis of the success rate of 908 trace DNA samples submitted to the Crime Sample Database Unit in New Zealand. Aust. J. Forensic Sci. **2008**, 40, 49–53. **[Google Scholar] [CrossRef]**

17. Castella, V.; Mangin, P. DNA profiling success and relevance of 1739 contact stains from caseworks. Forensic Sci. Int. Genet. Suppl. Ser. **2008**, 1, 405–407. **[Google Scholar] [CrossRef]**

18. Raymond, J.J.; van Oorschot, R.A.H.; Walsh, S.J.; Roux, C.; Gunn, P.R. Trace DNA and street robbery: A criminalistic approach to DNA evidence. Forensic Sci. Int. Genet. Suppl. Ser. **2009**, 2, 544–546. **[Google Scholar] [CrossRef]**

19. Mapes, A.A.; Kloosterman, A.D.; de Poot, C.J.; van Marion, V. Objective data on DNA success rates can aid the selection process of crime samples for analysis by rapid mobile DNA technologies. Forensic Sci. Int. **2016**, 264, 28–33. **[Google Scholar] [CrossRef] [PubMed]**

20. Mapes, A.A.; Kloosterman, A.D.; van Marion, V.; de Poot, C.J. Knowledge on DNA success rates to optimize the DNA analysis process: From crime scene to laboratory. J. Forensic Sci. **2016**, 61, 1055–1061. **[Google Scholar] [CrossRef] [PubMed]**

21. Dziak, R.; Peneder, A.; Buetter, A.; Hageman, C. Trace DNA sampling success from evidence items commonly encountered in forensic casework. J. Forensic Sci. **2018**, 63, 835–841. **[Google Scholar] [CrossRef]**

22. Martin, B.; Blackie, R.; Taylor, D.; Linacre, A. DNA profiles generated from a range of touched sample types. Forensic Sci. Int. Genet. **2018**, 36, 13–19. **[Google Scholar] [CrossRef] [PubMed] [Green Version]**

23. Van Oorschot, R.A.H.; Szkuta, B.; Verdon, T.J.; Mitchell, R.J.; Ballantyne, K.N. Trace DNA profiling in missing persons investigations. In Handbook of Missing Persons; Morewitz, S.J., Sturdy Colls, C., Eds.; Springer: Cham, Switzerland, 2016; pp. 353–363. **[Google Scholar]**

24. Krosch, M.N. Variation in forensic DNA profiling success among sampled items and collection methods: A Queensland perspective. Aust. J. Forensic Sci. **2020**, 53, 612–625. **[Google Scholar] [CrossRef]**

25. Taroni, F.; Biedermann, A.; Vuille, J.; Morling, N. Whose DNA is this? How relevant a question? (A note for forensic scientists). Forensic Sci. Int. Genet. **2013**, 7, 467–470. **[Google Scholar] [CrossRef] [PubMed] [Green Version]**

26. Meakin, G.; Jamieson, A. DNA transfer: Review and implications for casework. Forensic Sci. Int. Genet. **2013**, 7, 434–443. **[Google Scholar] [CrossRef] [PubMed]**

27. Gill, P. Analysis and implications of the miscarriages of justice of Amanda Knox and Raffaele Sollecito. Forensic Sci. Int. Genet. **2016**, 23, 9–18. **[Google Scholar] [CrossRef] [Green Version]**

28. Blackie, R.; Taylor, D.; Linacre, A. DNA profiles from clothing fibers using direct PCR. Forensic Sci. Med. Pathol. **2016**, 12, 331–335. **[Google Scholar] [CrossRef]**

29. Ruan, T.; Barash, M.; Gunn, P.; Bruce, D. Investigation of DNA transfer onto clothing during regular daily activities. Int. J. Leg. Med. **2018**, 132, 1035–1042. **[Google Scholar] [CrossRef]**

30. Hess, S.; Haas, C. Recovery of trace DNA on clothing: A comparison of mini-tape lifting and three other forensic evidence collection techniques. J. Forensic Sci. **2017**, 62, 187–191. **[Google Scholar] [CrossRef]**

31. Van den Berge, M.; Ozcanhan, G.; Zijlstra, S.; Lindenbergh, A.; Sijen, T. Prevalence of human cell material: DNA and RNA profiling of public and private objects and after activity scenarios. Forensic Sci. Int. Genet. **2016**, 21, 81–89. **[Google Scholar] [CrossRef]**

32. Van den Berge, M.; van de Merwe, L.; Sijen, T. DNA transfer and cell type inference to assist activity level reporting: Post-activity background samples as a control in dragging scenario. Forensic Sci. Int. Genet. Suppl. Ser. **2017**, 6, e591–e592. **[Google Scholar] [CrossRef] [Green Version]**

33. Fonneløp, A.E.; Ramse, M.; Egeland, T.; Gill, P. The implications of shedder status and background DNA on direct and secondary transfer in an attack scenario. Forensic Sci. Int. Genet. **2017**, 29, 48–60. **[Google Scholar] [CrossRef] [PubMed]**

34. Noël, S.; Lagace, K.; Rogic, A.; Granger, D.; Bourgoin, S.; Jolicoeur, C.; Séguin, D. DNA transfer during laundering may yield complete genetic profiles. Forensic Sci. Int. Genet. **2016**, 23, 240–247. **[Google Scholar] [CrossRef]**

35. Burrill, J.; Daniel, B.; Frascione, N. A review of trace "Touch DNA" deposits: Variability factors and an exploration of cellular composition. Forensic Sci. Int. Genet. **2019**, 39, 8–18. **[Google Scholar] [CrossRef] [PubMed] [Green Version]**

36. Gosch, A.; Courts, C. On DNA transfer: The lack and difficulty of systematic research and how to do it better. Forensic Sci. Int. Genet. **2019**, 40, 24–36. **[Google Scholar] [CrossRef]**

37. DNA-TrAC Database. Available online: **https://bit.ly/2R4bFgL** (accessed on 15 August 2021).

38. Taylor, D.; Biedermann, A.; Samie, L.; Pun, K.M.; Hicks, T.; Champod, C. Helping to distinguish primary from secondary transfer events for trace DNA. Forensic Sci. Int. Genet. **2017**, 28, 155–177. **[Google Scholar] [CrossRef] [PubMed] [Green Version]**

39. Moher, D.; Liberati, A.; Tetzlaff, J.; Altman, D.G. Preferred reporting items for systematic reviews and meta-analyses: The PRISMA statement. BMJ **2009**, 339, b2535. **[Google Scholar] [CrossRef] [PubMed] [Green Version]**

40. Yano, R.; Shimoda, O.; Okitsu, T.; Sakurada, M.; Ueno, Y. Development of a modified p-dimethylaminocinnamaldehyde solution for touch DNA analysis and its application to STR analysis. Forensic Sci. Int. Genet. **2019**, 38, 86–92. **[Google Scholar] [CrossRef] [PubMed]**

41. Dierig, L.; Schmidt, M.; Wiegand, P. Looking for the pinpoint: Optimizing identification, recovery and DNA extraction of micro traces in forensic casework. Forensic Sci. Int. Genet. **2020**, 44, 102191. **[Google Scholar] [CrossRef]**

42. Kanokwongnuwut, P.; Kirkbride, K.P.; Linacre, A. Detection of cellular material in lip-prints. Forensic Sci. Med. Pathol. **2019**, 15, 362–368. **[Google Scholar] [CrossRef]**

43. Kanokwongnuwut, P.; Kirkbride, P.; Linacre, A. Visualising latent DNA on swabs. Forensic Sci. Int. **2018**, 291, 115–123. **[Google Scholar] [CrossRef] [Green Version]**

44. Kitchner, E.; Chavez, J.; Ceresa, L.; Bus, M.M.; Budowle, B.; Gryczynski, Z. A novel approach for visualization and localization of small amounts of DNA on swabs to improve DNA collection and recovery process. Analyst **2021**, 146, 1198–1206. **[Google Scholar] [CrossRef] [PubMed]**

45. Akutsu, T.; Ikegaya, H.; Watanabe, K.; Miyasaka, S. Immunohistochemical staining of skin-expressed proteins to identify exfoliated epidermal cells for forensic purposes. Forensic Sci. Int. **2019**, 303, 109940. **[Google Scholar] [CrossRef]**

46. Malegori, C.; Alladio, E.; Oliveri, P.; Manis, C.; Vincenti, M.; Garofano, P.; Barni, F.; Berti, A. Identification of invisible biological traces in forensic evidences by hyperspectral NIR imaging combined with chemometrics. Talanta **2020**, 215, 120911. **[Google Scholar] [CrossRef]**

47. Wang, Z.; Zhang, P.; Liu, H.; Zhao, Z.; Xiong, L.; He, W.; Kwok, R.T.K.; Lam, J.W.Y.; Ye, R.; Tang, B.Z. Robust Serum Albumin-Responsive AIEgen Enables Latent Bloodstain Visualization in High Resolution and Reliability for Crime Scene Investigation. ACS Appl. Mater. Interfaces **2019**, 11, 17306–17312. **[Google Scholar] [CrossRef] [PubMed]**

48. Denny, S.E.; Nazeer, S.S.; Sivakumar, T.T.; Nair, B.J.; Jayasree, R.S. Forensic application of fluorescence spectroscopy: An efficient technique to predict the presence of human saliva. J. Lumin. **2018**, 203, 696–701. **[Google Scholar] [CrossRef]**

49. Raj, C.K.; Garlapati, K.; Karunakar, P.; Badam, R.; Soni, P.; Lavanya, R. Saliva as Forensic Evidence using Fluorescent Spectroscopy: A Pilot Study. J. Clin. Diagn. Res. **2018**, 12, ZC27–ZC29. **[Google Scholar] [CrossRef]**

50. Butler, J.; Chaseling, J.; Wright, K. A Comparison of Four Presumptive Tests for the Detection of Blood on Dark Materials. J. Forensic Sci. **2019**, 64, 1838–1843. **[Google Scholar] [CrossRef]**

51. Burrill, J.; Daniel, B.; Frascione, N. Illuminating touch deposits through cellular characterization of hand rinses and body fluids with nucleic acid fluorescence. Forensic Sci. Int. Genet. **2020**, 46, 102269. **[Google Scholar] [CrossRef] [PubMed]**

52. Olsen, A.; Miller, M.; Yadavalli, V.K.; Ehrhardt, C.J. Open source software tool for the automated detection and characterization of epithelial cells from trace biological samples. Forensic Sci. Int. **2020**, 312, 110300. **[Google Scholar] [CrossRef] [PubMed]**

53. Kishbaugh, J.M.; Cielski, S.; Fotusky, A.; Lighthart, S.; Maguire, K.; Quarino, L.; Conte, J. Detection of prostate specific antigen and salivary amylase in vaginal swabs using SERATEC® immunochromatographic assays. Forensic Sci. Int. **2019**, 304, 109899. **[Google Scholar] [CrossRef]**

54. Sari, D.; Hitchcock, C.; Collins, S.; Cochrane, C.; Bruce, D. Amylase testing on intimate samples from pre-pubescent, post-pubescent and post-menopausal females: Implications for forensic casework in sexual assault allegations. Aust. J. Forensic Sci. **2020**, 52, 618–625. **[Google Scholar] [CrossRef]**

55. Suttipasit, P. Forensic Spermatozoa Detection. Am. J. Forensic Med. Pathol. **2019**, 40, 304–311. **[Google Scholar] [CrossRef]**

56. Abbas, N.; Lu, X.; Badshah, M.A.; In, J.B.; Heo, W.I.; Park, K.Y.; Lee, M.-K.; Kim, C.H.; Kang, P.; Chang, W.-J.; et al. Development of a protein microarray chip with enhanced fluorescence for identification of semen and vaginal fluid. Sensors **2018**, 18, 3874. **[Google Scholar] [CrossRef] [PubMed] [Green Version]**

57. O'Leary, K.R.; Glynn, C.L. Investigating the Isolation and Amplification of microRNAs for Forensic Body Fluid Identification. MicroRNA **2018**, 7, 187–194. **[Google Scholar] [CrossRef] [PubMed] [Green Version]**

58. Hanson, E.; Ingold, S.; Dorum, G.; Haas, C.; Lagace, R.; Ballantyne, J. Assigning forensic body fluids to DNA donors in mixed samples by targeted RNA/DNA deep seqeuncing of coding region SNPs using ion torrent technology. Forensic Sci. Int. Genet. Suppl. Ser. **2019**, 7, 23–24. **[Google Scholar]** **[CrossRef]**

59. Kamanna, S.; Henry, J.; Voelcker, N.; Linacre, A.; Kirkbride, K.P. A complementary forensic 'proteo-genomic' approach for the direct identification of biological fluid traces under fingernails. Anal. Bioanal. Chem. **2018**, 410, 6165–6175. **[Google Scholar]** **[CrossRef]** **[PubMed]**

60. Watanabe, K.; Taniguchi, K.; Akutsu, T. Development of a DNA methylation-based semen-specific SNP typing method: A new approach for genotyping from a mixture of body fluids. Forensic Sci. Int. Genet. **2018**, 37, 227–234. **[Google Scholar]** **[CrossRef]**

61. Mishra, I.K.; Singh, B.; Mishra, A.; Mohapatra, B.K.; Kaushik, R.; Behera, C. Touch DNA as forensic aid: A review. Indian J. Forensic Med. Toxicol. **2020**, 14, 58–62. **[Google Scholar]**

62. Yudianto, A.; Indah Nuraini, M.; Furqoni, A.H.; ManyanzaNzilibili, S.M.; Harjanto, P. The use of touch DNA analysis in forensic identification focusing on Short Tandem Repeat-Combined DNA Index System loci THO1, CSF1PO and TPOX. Infect. Dis. Rep. **2020**, 12, 8716. **[Google Scholar]** **[CrossRef]** **[PubMed]**

63. Wong, H.Y.; Tan, J.; Lim, Z.G.; Kwok, R.; Lim, W.; Syn, C.K.C. DNA profiling success rates of commonly submitted crime scene items. Forensic Sci. Int. Genet. Suppl. Ser. **2019**, 7, 597–599. **[Google Scholar]** **[CrossRef]**

64. Ferrara, M.; Sessa, F.; Rendine, M.; Spagnolo, L.; De Simone, S.; Riezzo, I.; Ricci, P.; Pascale, N.; Salerno, M.; Bertozzi, G.; et al. A multidisciplinary approach is mandatory to solve complex crimes: A case report. Egypt. J. Forensic Sci. **2019**, 9, 11. **[Google Scholar]** **[CrossRef]**

65. Naue, J.; Sänger, T.; Lutz-Bonengel, S. Get it off, but keep it: Efficient cleaning of hair shafts with parallel DNA extraction of the surface stain. Forensic Sci. Int. Genet. **2020**, 45, 102210. **[Google Scholar]** **[CrossRef]** **[PubMed]**

66. Cahill, M.J.; Chapman, B. The novel use of a spray-on rubber coating to recover cellular material from the surface of bricks. Forensic Sci. Int. Genet. **2020**, 49, 102404. **[Google Scholar]** **[CrossRef]** **[PubMed]**

67. Brower, A.; Akridge, B.; Siemens-Bradley, N. Human DNA collection from police dogs: Technique and application. Forensic Sci. Med. Pathol. **2021**, 17, 230–234. **[Google Scholar]** **[CrossRef]**

68. Musse, J.O.; Marques, J.A.M.; Remualdo, V.; Pitlovanciv, A.K.; da Silva, C.A.L.; Corte-Real, F.; Vieira, D.N.; Vieira, W.A.; Paranhos, L.R.; Corte-Real, A.T. Deoxyribonucleic acid extraction and quantification from human saliva deposited on foods with bitemarks. J. Contemp. Dent. Pract. **2019**, 20, 548–551. **[Google Scholar] [PubMed]**

69. Thakar, M.K.; Sahajpal, V.; Bhambara, A.K.; Bhandari, D.; Sharma, A. DNA profiling of saliva traces habitually deposited on various documents: A pilot study. Egypt. J. Forensic Sci. **2020**, 10, 14. **[Google Scholar] [CrossRef]**

70. Aparna, R.; Shanti Iyer, R. Tears and Eyewear in Forensic Investigation—A Review. Forensic Sci. Int. **2020**, 306, 110055. **[Google Scholar] [CrossRef] [PubMed]**

71. O'Connor, A.M.; Watts, J.E.M. The development of a rapid and reliable method (SAPSWash): For the extraction and recovery of spermatozoa from superabsorbent polymer containing products. Forensic Sci. Int. **2020**, 316, 110501. **[Google Scholar] [CrossRef]**

72. Vanderheyden, N.; Verhoeven, E.; Vermeulen, S.; Bekaert, B. Survival of forensic trace evidence on improvised explosive devices: Perspectives on individualisation. Sci. Rep. **2020**, 10, 12813. **[Google Scholar] [CrossRef] [PubMed]**

73. Tasker, E.; Roman, M.G.; Akosile, M.; Mayes, C.; Hughes, S.; LaRue, B. Efficacy of "touch" DNA recovery and room-temperature storage from assault rifle magazines. Leg. Med. **2020**, 43, 101658. **[Google Scholar] [CrossRef] [PubMed]**

74. Booth, N.; Chapman, B. DNA recovery from fired hollow point ammunition. Aust. J. Forensic Sci. **2019**, 51, S107–S110. **[Google Scholar] [CrossRef] [Green Version]**

75. Sterling, S.A.; Mason, K.E.; Anex, D.S.; Parker, G.J.; Hart, B.; Prinz, M. Combined DNA Typing and Protein Identification from Unfired Brass Cartridges. J. Forensic Sci. **2019**, 64, 1475–1481. **[Google Scholar] [CrossRef] [PubMed]**

76. Thanakiatkrai, P.; Rerkamnuaychoke, B. Direct STR typing from fired and unfired bullet casings. Forensic Sci. Int. **2019**, 301, 182–189. **[Google Scholar] [CrossRef] [PubMed]**

77. Holland, M.M.; Bonds, R.M.; Holland, C.A.; McElhoe, J.A. Recovery of mtDNA from unfired metallic ammunition components with an assessment of sequence profile quality and DNA damage through MPS analysis. Forensic Sci. Int. Genet. **2019**, 39, 86–96. **[Google Scholar] [CrossRef]**

78. Jansson, L.; Forsberg, C.; Akel, Y.; Dufva, C.; Ansell, C.; Ansell, R.; Hedman, J. Factors affecting DNA recovery from cartridge cases. Forensic Sci. Int. Genet. **2020**, 48, 102343. **[Google Scholar] [CrossRef] [PubMed]**

79. Gray, S.L.; Tiedge, T.M.; Butkus, J.M.; Earp, T.J.; Lindner, S.E.; Roy, R. Determination of human identity from Anopheles stephensi mosquito blood meals using direct amplification and massively parallel sequencing. Forensic Sci. Int. Genet. **2020**, 48, 102347. **[Google Scholar] [CrossRef] [PubMed]**

80. Bonsu, D.O.M.; Higgins, D.; Austin, J.J. Forensic touch DNA recovery from metal surfaces—A review. Sci. Justice **2020**, 60, 206–215. **[Google Scholar] [CrossRef]**

81. Comte, J.; Baechler, S.; Gervaix, J.; Lock, E.; Milon, M.-P.; Delémont, O.; Castella, V. Touch DNA collection—Performance of four different swabs. Forensic Sci. Int. Genet. **2019**, 43, 102113. **[Google Scholar] [CrossRef]**

82. Janssen, K.; Aune, M.; Olsen, M.; Olsen, G.H.; Berg, T. Biological stain collection—Absorbing paper is superior to cotton swabs. Forensic Sci. Int. Genet. Suppl. Ser. **2019**, 7, 468–469. **[Google Scholar] [CrossRef]**

83. Sherier, A.J.; Kieser, R.E.; Novroski, N.M.M.; Wendt, F.R.; King, J.L.; Woerner, A.E.; Ambers, A.; Garofano, P.; Budowle, B. Copan microFLOQ® Direct Swab collection of bloodstains, saliva, and semen on cotton cloth. Int. J. Legal Med. **2020**, 134, 45–54. **[Google Scholar] [CrossRef]**

84. Kanokwongnuwut, P.; Kirkbride, K.P.; Linacre, A. An assessment of tape-lifts. Forensic Sci. Int. Genet. **2020**, 47, 102292. **[Google Scholar] [CrossRef] [PubMed]**

85. Damsteeg-van Berkel, S.; Beemster, F.; Dankelman, J.; Loeve, A.J. The influence of contact force on forensic trace collection efficiency when sampling textiles with adhesive tape. Forensic Sci. Int. **2019**, 298, 278–283. **[Google Scholar] [CrossRef] [PubMed]**

86. Zorbo, S.; Jeuniaux, P.P.J.M.H. DNA Recovery From Tape-Lifting Kits: Methodology and Practice. J. Forensic Sci. **2020**, 65, 641–648. **[Google Scholar] [CrossRef] [PubMed]**

87. Zieger, M.; Schneider, C.; Utz, S. DNA recovery from gelatin fingerprint lifters by direct proteolytic digestion. Forensic Sci. Int. **2019**, 295, 145–149. **[Google Scholar] [CrossRef] [PubMed]**

88. Fieldhouse, S.; Parsons, R.; Bleay, S.; Walton-Williams, L. The effect of DNA recovery on the subsequent quality of latent fingermarks: A pseudo-operational trial. Forensic Sci. Int. **2020**, 307, 110076. **[Google Scholar] [CrossRef] [PubMed]**

89. Harush-Brosh, Y.; Hefetz, I.; Hauzer, M.; Mayuoni-Kirshenbaum, L.; Mashiach, Y.; Faerman, M.; Levin-Elad, M. Clean and clear (out): A neat method for the recovery of latent fingermarks from crime-scenes. Forensic Sci. Int. **2020**, 306, 110049. **[Google Scholar] [CrossRef]**

90. Harush-Brosh, Y.; Mayuoni-Kirshenbaum, L.; Mashiach, Y.; Hauzer, M.; Hefetz, I.; Bengiat, R.; Levin-Elad, M.; Faerman, M. An efficient and eco-friendly workflow for dual fingermark processing and STR profiling. Forensic Sci. Int. Genet. **2020**, 47, 102310. **[Google Scholar] [CrossRef]**

91. Hartless, S.; Walton-Williams, L.; Williams, G. Critical evaluation of touch DNA recovery methods for forensic purposes. Forensic Sci. Int. Genet. Suppl. Ser. **2019**, 7, 379–380. **[Google Scholar] [CrossRef]**

92. Bonsu, D.O.M.; Higgins, D.; Henry, J.; Austin, J.J. Evaluation of the efficiency of Isohelix™ and Rayon swabs for recovery of DNA from metal surfaces. Forensic Sci. Med. Pathol. **2021**, 17, 199–207. **[Google Scholar] [CrossRef]**

93. Sessa, F.; Salerno, M.; Bertozzi, G.; Messina, G.; Ricci, P.; Ledda, C.; Rapisarda, V.; Cantatore, S.; Turillazzi, E.; Pomara, C. Touch DNA: Impact of handling time on touch deposit and evaluation of different recovery techniques: An experimental study. Sci. Rep. **2019**, 9, 9542. **[Google Scholar] [CrossRef] [Green Version]**

94. Kanokwongnuwut, P.; Martin, B.; Taylor, D.; Kirkbride, K.P.; Linacre, A. How many cells are required for successful DNA profiling? Forensic Sci. Int. Genet. **2021**, 51, 102453. **[Google Scholar] [CrossRef] [PubMed]**

95. Miller, M.; Philpott, M.K.; Olsen, A.; Tootham, M.; Yadavalli, V.K.; Ehrhardt, C.J. Technical note: Survey of extracellular and cell-pellet-associated DNA from 'touch'/trace samples. Forensic Sci. Int. **2021**, 318, 110557. **[Google Scholar] [CrossRef] [PubMed]**

96. Burrill, J.; Kombara, A.; Daniel, B.; Frascione, N. Exploration of cell-free DNA (cfDNA) recovery for touch deposits. Forensic Sci. Int. Genet. **2021**, 51, 102431. **[Google Scholar] [CrossRef] [PubMed]**

97. Burrill, J.; Rammenou, E.; Alawar, F.; Daniel, B.; Frascione, N. Corneocyte lysis and fragmented DNA considerations for the cellular component of forensic touch DNA. Forensic Sci. Int. Genet. **2021**, 51, 102428. **[Google Scholar] [CrossRef]**

98. Kaur, S.; Saini, V.; Dalal, R. UV-Visible spectroscopic effect on Haemoglobin& DNA degradation: A forensic approach. Forensic Sci. Int. **2020**, 307, 110078. **[Google Scholar] [PubMed]**

99. Badu-Boateng, A.; Twumasi, P.; Salifu, S.P.; Afrifah, K.A. A comparative study of different laboratory storage conditions for enhanced DNA analysis of crime scene soil-blood mixed sample. Forensic Sci. Int. **2018**, 292, 97–109. **[Google Scholar] [CrossRef]**

100. Corradini, B.; Alù, M.; Magnanini, E.; Galinier, M.E.; Silingardi, E. The importance of forensic storage support: DNA quality from 11-year-old saliva on FTA cards. Int. J. Legal Med. **2019**, 133, 1743–1750. **[Google Scholar] [CrossRef] [PubMed]**

101. Francisco, D.D.O.; Lopez, L.F.; Gonçalves, F.D.T.; Fridman, C. Casework direct kit as an alternative extraction method to enhance touch DNA samples analysis. Forensic Sci. Int. Genet. **2020**, 47, 102307. **[Google Scholar] [CrossRef]**

102. LeSassier, D.S.; Schulte, K.Q.; Manley, T.E.; Smith, A.R.; Powals, M.L.; Albright, N.C.; Ludolph, B.C.; Weber, K.L.; Woerner, A.E.; Gardner, M.W.; et al. Artificial fingerprints for cross-comparison of forensic DNA and protein recovery methods. PLoS ONE **2019**, 14, e0223170. **[Google Scholar] [CrossRef] [PubMed] [Green Version]**

103. Liu, C.; Wu, S.; Yan, Y.; Dong, Y.; Shen, X.; Huang, C. Application of magnetic particles in forensic science. TrAC Trends Anal. Chem. **2019**, 121, 115674. **[Google Scholar] [CrossRef]**

104. Schulte, K.Q.; Hewitt, F.C.; Manley, T.E.; Reed, A.J.; Baniasad, M.; Albright, N.C.; Powals, M.E.; LeSassier, D.S.; Smith, A.R.; Zhang, L.; et al. Fractionation of DNA and protein from individual latent fingerprints for forensic analysis. Forensic Sci. Int. Genet. **2021**, 50, 102405. **[Google Scholar] [CrossRef] [PubMed]**

105. Hayden, D.D.; Wallin, J.M. A comparative study for the isolation of exogenous trace DNA from fingernails. Forensic Sci. Int. Genet. **2019**, 39, 119–128. **[Google Scholar] [CrossRef] [PubMed]**

106. Timken, M.D.; Klein, S.B.; Kubala, S.; Scharnhorst, G.; Buoncristiani, M.R.; Miller, K.W.P. Automation of the standard DNA differential extraction on the Hamilton AutoLys STAR system: A proof-of-concept study. Forensic Sci. Int. Genet. **2019**, 40, 96–104. **[Google Scholar] [CrossRef] [PubMed]**

107. Auka, N.; Valle, M.; Cox, B.D.; Wilkerson, P.D.; Cruz, T.D.; Reiner, J.E.; Seashols-Williams, S.J. Optical tweezers as an effective tool for spermatozoa isolation from mixed forensic samples. PLoS ONE **2019**, 14, e0211810. **[Google Scholar] [CrossRef]**

108. Clark, C.P.; Xu, K.; Scott, O.; Hickey, J.; Tsuei, A.C.; Jackson, K.; Landers, J.P. Acoustic trapping of sperm cells from mock sexual assault samples. Forensic Sci. Int. Genet. **2019**, 41, 42–49. **[Google Scholar] [CrossRef]**

109. Wright, S.N.; Huge, B.J.; Dovichi, N.J. Capillary zone electrophoresis separation and collection of spermatozoa for the forensic analysis of sexual assault evidence. Electrophoresis **2020**, 41, 1344–1353. **[Google Scholar] [CrossRef] [PubMed]**

110. Anslinger, K.; Graw, M.; Bayer, B. Deconvolution of blood-blood mixtures using DEPArray TM separated single cell STR profiling. Rechtsmedizin **2019**, 29, 30–40. **[Google Scholar] [CrossRef] [Green Version]**

111. Henry, J.; Scandrett, L. Assessment of the Yfiler® Plus PCR amplification kit for the detection of male DNA in semen-negative sexual assault cases. Sci. Justice **2019**, 59, 480–485. **[Google Scholar] [CrossRef]**

112. Owers, R.; McDonald, A.; Montgomerie, H.; Morse, C. A casework study comparing success rates and expectations of detecting male DNA using two different Y-STR multiplexes on vaginal swabs in sexual assault investigations where no semen has been detected. Forensic Sci. Int. Genet. **2018**, 37, 1–5. **[Google Scholar] [CrossRef]**

113. Dawnay, N.; Flamson, R.; Hall, M.J.R.; Steadman, D.W. Impact of sample degradation and inhibition on field-based DNA identification of human remains. Forensic Sci. Int. Genet. **2018**, 37, 46–53. **[Google Scholar] [CrossRef]**

114. Avila, E.; Cavalheiro, C.P.; Felkl, A.B.; Graebin, P.; Kahmann, A.; Alho, C.S. Brazilian forensic casework analysis through MPS applications: Statistical weight-of-evidence and biological nature of criminal samples as an influence factor in quality metrics. Forensic Sci. Int. **2019**, 303, 109938. **[Google Scholar] [CrossRef] [PubMed]**

115. Mortera, J. DNA Mixtures in Forensic Investigations: The Statistical State of the Art. Annu. Rev. Stat. Appl **2020**, 7, 111–142. **[Google Scholar] [CrossRef]**

116. Buckleton, J.S.; Bright, J.A.; Cheng, K.; Budowle, B.; Coble, M.D. NIST interlaboratory studies involving DNA mixtures (MIX13): A modern analysis. Forensic Sci. Int. Genet. **2018**, 37, 172–179. **[Google Scholar] [CrossRef] [PubMed]**

117. Szkuta, B.; Ansell, R.; Boiso, L.; Connolly, E.; Kloosterman, A.D.; Kokshoorn, B.; McKenna, L.G.; Steensma, K.; van Oorschot, R.A.H. Assessment of the transfer, persistence, prevalence and recovery of DNA traces from clothing: An inter-laboratory study on worn upper garments. Forensic Sci. Int. Genet. **2019**, 42, 56–68. **[Google Scholar] [CrossRef] [PubMed]**

118. Szkuta, B.; Ansell, R.; Boiso, L.; Connolly, E.; Kloosterman, A.D.; Kokshoorn, B.; McKenna, L.G.; Steensma, K.; van Oorschot, R.A.H. DNA transfer to worn upper garments during different activities and contacts: An inter-laboratory study. Forensic Sci. Int. Genet. **2020**, 46, 102268. **[Google Scholar] [CrossRef] [PubMed]**

119. Goray, M.; Kokshoorn, B.; Steensma, K.; Szkuta, B.; van Oorschot, R.A.H. DNA detection of a temporary and original user of an office space. Forensic Sci. Int. Genet. **2020**, 44, 102203. **[Google Scholar] [CrossRef] [PubMed] [Green Version]**

120. Gill, P.; Hicks, T.; Butler, J.M.; Connolly, E.; Gusmão, L.; Kokshoorn, B.; Morling, N.; van Oorschot, R.A.H.; Parson, W.; Prinz, M.; et al. DNA commission of the International society for forensic genetics: Assessing the value of forensic biological evidence—Guidelines highlighting the importance of propositions. Part II: Evaluation of biological traces considering activity level propositions. Forensic Sci. Int. Genet. **2020**, 44, 102186. **[Google Scholar] [CrossRef] [PubMed] [Green Version]**

121. Weber, A.R.; Lednev, I.K. Crime clock—Analytical studies for approximating time since deposition of bloodstains. Forensic Chem. **2020**, 19, 100248. **[Google Scholar] [CrossRef]**

122. Stotesbury, T.; Cossette, M.L.; Newell-Bell, T.; Shafer, A.B.A. An Exploratory Time Since Deposition Analysis of Whole Blood Using Metrics of DNA Degradation and Visible Absorbance Spectroscopy. Pure Appl. Geophys. **2021**, 178, 735–743. **[Google Scholar] [CrossRef]**

123. Cossette, M.L.; Stotesbury, T.; Shafer, A.B.A. Quantifying visible absorbance changes and DNA degradation in aging bloodstains under extreme temperatures. Forensic Sci. Int. **2021**, 318, 110627. **[Google Scholar] [CrossRef]**

124. Bird, T.A.G.; Walton-Williams, L.; Williams, G. Time since deposition of biological fluids using RNA degradation. Forensic Sci. Int. Genet. Suppl. Ser. **2019**, 7, 401–402. **[Google Scholar] [CrossRef]**

125. Asaghiar, F.; Williams, G.A. Evaluating the use of hypoxia sensitive markers for body fluid stain age prediction. Sci. Justice **2020**, 60, 547–554. **[Google Scholar] [CrossRef] [PubMed]**

126. Mameli, A.; Scudiero, C.M.; Delogu, G.; Ghiani, M.E. Successful analysis of a 100 years old semen stain generating a complete DNA STR profile. J. Forensic Leg. Med. **2019**, 61, 78–81. **[Google Scholar] [CrossRef] [PubMed]**

127. Romano, C.G.; Mangiaracina, R.; Donato, L.; D'Angelo, R.; Scimone, C.; Sidoti, A. Aged fingerprints for DNA profile: First report of successful typing. Forensic Sci. Int. **2019**, 302, 109905. **[Google Scholar] [CrossRef] [PubMed]**

128. Alketbi, S.K.; Goodwin, W. The effect of time and environmental conditions on Touch DNA. Forensic Sci. Int. Genet. Suppl. Ser. **2019**, 7, 701–703. **[Google Scholar] [CrossRef]**

129. Lee, L.Y.C.; Wong, H.Y.; Lee, J.Y.; Waffa, Z.B.M.; Aw, Z.Q.; Fauzi, S.N.A.B.M.; Hoe, S.Y.; Lim, M.-L.; Syn, C.K.-C. Persistence of DNA in the Singapore context. Int. J. Legal Med. **2019**, 133, 1341–1349. **[Google Scholar] [CrossRef]**

130. Meixner, E.; Kallupurackal, V.; Kratzer, A.; Voegeli, P.; Thali, M.J.; Bolliger, S.A. Persistence and detection of touch DNA and blood stain DNA on pig skin exposed to water. Forensic Sci. Med. Pathol. **2020**, 16, 243–251. **[Google Scholar] [CrossRef]**

131. Romero-García, C.; Rosell-Herrera, R.; Revilla, C.J.; Baeza-Richer, C.; Gomes, C.; Palomo-Díez, S.; Arroyo-Pardo, E.; López-Parra, A.M. Effect of the activity in secondary transfer of DNA profiles. Forensic Sci. Int. Genet. Suppl. Ser. **2019**, 7, 578–579. **[Google Scholar] [CrossRef]**

132. Helmus, J.; Poetsch, J.; Pfeifer, M.; Bajanowski, T.; Poetsch, M. Cleaning a crime scene 2.0—What to do with the bloody knife after the crime? Int. J. Legal Med. **2020**, 134, 171–175. **[Google Scholar] [CrossRef]**

133. Noël, S.; Lagacé, K.; Raymond, S.; Granger, D.; Loyer, M.; Bourgoin, S.; Jolicoeur, C.; Séguin, D. Repeatedly washed semen stains: Optimal screening and sampling strategies for DNA analysis. Forensic Sci. Int. Genet. **2019**, 38, 9–14. **[Google Scholar] [CrossRef]**

134. Karadayi, S.; Moshfeghi, E.; Arasoglu, T.; Karadayi, B. Evaluating the persistence of laundered semen stains on fabric using a forensic light source system, prostate-specific antigen Semiquant test and DNA recovery-profiling. Med. Sci. Law **2020**, 60, 122–130. **[Google Scholar] [CrossRef] [PubMed]**

135. Basyoni, H.A.; Mohamed, K.M.; El-Barrany, U.M.; Rashed, L.A.; Aboubakr, H.M.; Razik, H.A.A. How possible is it to recover semen DNA from laundered cotton and polyester fabrics? Indian J. Forensic Med. Toxicol. **2020**, 14, 2941–2948. **[Google Scholar]**

136. Hofmann, M.; Adamec, J.; Anslinger, K.; Bayer, B.; Graw, M.; Peschel, O.; Schulz, M.M. Detectability of bloodstains after machine washing. Int. J. Legal Med. **2019**, 133, 3–16. **[Google Scholar] [CrossRef] [PubMed]**

137. Fonneløp, A.E.; Johannessen, H.; Heen, G.; Molland, K.; Gill, P. A retrospective study on the transfer, persistence and recovery of sperm and epithelial cells in samples collected in sexual assault casework. Forensic Sci. Int. Genet. **2019**, 43, 102153. **[Google Scholar] [CrossRef]**

138. Mayes, C.; Houston, R.; Seashols-Williams, S.; LaRue, B.; Hughes-Stamm, S. The stability and persistence of blood and semen mRNA and miRNA targets for body fluid identification in environmentally challenged and laundered samples. Leg. Med. **2019**, 38, 45–50. **[Google Scholar] [CrossRef] [PubMed] [Green Version]**

139. Schyma, C.; Madea, B.; Müller, R.; Zieger, M.; Utz, S.; Grabmüller, M. DNA-free does not mean RNA-free—The unwanted persistence of RNA. Forensic Sci. Int. **2021**, 318, 110632. **[Google Scholar] [CrossRef]**

140. Boyko, T.; Mitchell, R.J.; van Oorschot, R.A.H. DNA within cars: Prevalence of DNA from driver, passenger and others on steering wheels. Aust. J. Forensic Sci. **2019**, 51, S91–S94. **[Google Scholar] [CrossRef]**

141. Boyko, T.; Szkuta, B.; Mitchell, R.J.; van Oorschot, R.A.H. Prevalence of DNA from the driver, passengers and others within a car of an exclusive driver. Forensic Sci. Int. **2020**, 307, 110139. **[Google Scholar] [CrossRef]**

142. De Wolff, T.R.; Aarts, L.H.J.; van den Berge, M.; Boyko, T.; van Oorschot, R.A.H.; Zuidberg, M.; Kokshoorn, B. Prevalence of DNA of regular occupants in vehicles. Forensic Sci. Int. **2021**, 320, 110713. **[Google Scholar] [CrossRef]**

143. Szkuta, B.; Reither, J.B.; Conlan, X.A.; van Oorschot, R.A.H. The presence of background DNA on common entry points to homes. Forensic Sci. Int. Genet. Suppl. Ser. **2019**, 7, 784–786. **[Google Scholar] [CrossRef]**

144. Albani, P.P.; Patel, J.; Fleming, R.I. DNA on feminine sanitary products. Forensic Sci. Int. **2018**, 293, 24–26. **[Google Scholar] [CrossRef] [PubMed]**

145. Murphy, C.; Kenna, J.; Flanagan, L.; Lee Gorman, M.; Boland, C.; Ryan, J. A Study of the Background Levels of Male DNA on Underpants Worn by Females. J. Forensic Sci. **2020**, 65, 399–405. **[Google Scholar] [CrossRef] [PubMed]**

146. Reither, J.B.; Gray, E.; Durdle, A.; Conlan, X.A.; van Oorschot, R.A.H.; Szkuta, B. Background DNA on flooring: The effect of cleaning. Forensic Sci. Int. Genet. Suppl. Ser. **2019**, 7, 787–790. **[Google Scholar] [CrossRef]**

147. Helmus, J.; Pfeifer, M.; Feiner, L.-K.; Krause, L.J.; Bajanowski, T.; Poetsch, M. Unintentional effects of cleaning a crime scene—When the sponge becomes an accomplice in DNA transfer. Int. J. Legal Med. **2019**, 133, 759–765. **[Google Scholar] [CrossRef] [PubMed]**

148. Hefetz, I.; Einot, N.; Faerman, M.; Horowitz, M.; Almog, J. Touch DNA: The effect of the deposition pressure on the quality of latent fingermarks and STR profiles. Forensic Sci. Int. Genet. **2019**, 38, 105–112. **[Google Scholar] [CrossRef] [PubMed]**

149. De Wolff, T.; Aarts, L.H.J.; van den Berge, M.; Boyko, T.; van Oorschot, R.A.H.; Zuidberg, M.; Kokshoorn, B. Prevalence of DNA in vehicles: Linking clothing of a suspect to car occupancy. Aust. J. Forensic Sci. **2019**, 51, S103–S106. **[Google Scholar] [CrossRef]**

150. Ramos, P.; Handt, O.; Taylor, D. Investigating the position and level of DNA transfer to undergarments during digital sexual assault. Forensic Sci. Int. Genet. **2020**, 47, 102316. **[Google Scholar] [CrossRef]**

151. Gosch, A.; Euteneuer, J.; Preuß-Wössner, J.; Courts, C. DNA transfer to firearms in alternative realistic handling scenarios. Forensic Sci. Int. Genet. **2020**, 48, 102355. **[Google Scholar] [CrossRef]**

152. Butcher, E.V.; van Oorschot, R.A.H.; Morgan, R.M.; Meakin, G.E. Opportunistic crimes: Evaluation of DNA from regularly-used knives after a brief use by a different person. Forensic Sci. Int. Genet. **2019**, 42, 135–140. **[Google Scholar] [CrossRef]**

153. Samie, L.; Taroni, F.; Champod, C. Estimating the quantity of transferred DNA in primary and secondary transfers. Sci. Justice **2020**, 60, 128–135. **[Google Scholar] [CrossRef] [Green Version]**

154. Euteneuer, J.; Gosch, A.; Cachée, P.; Courts, C. A distant relationship?—Investigation of correlations between DNA isolated from backspatter traces recovered from firearms, wound profile characteristics, and shooting distance. Int. J. Legal Med. **2020**, 134, 1619–1628. **[Google Scholar] [CrossRef] [PubMed]**

155. Thornbury, D.; Goray, M.; van Oorschot, R.A.H. Indirect DNA transfer without contact from dried biological materials on various surfaces. Forensic Sci. Int. Genet. **2021**, 51, 102457. **[Google Scholar] [CrossRef] [PubMed]**

156. Otten, L.; Banken, S.; Schürenkamp, M.; Schulze-Johann, K.; Sibbing, U.; Pfeiffer, H.; Vennemann, M. Secondary DNA transfer by working gloves. Forensic Sci. Int. Genet. **2019**, 43, 102126. **[Google Scholar] [CrossRef]**

157. Goray, M.; Pirie, E.; van Oorschot, R.A.H. DNA transfer: DNA acquired by gloves during casework examinations. Forensic Sci. Int. Genet. **2019**, 38, 167–174. **[Google Scholar] [CrossRef]**

158. Van den Berge, M.; Wagner, S.; Meijers, E.; Kokshoorn, B.; Kloosterman, A.; van der Scheer, M.; Sijen, T. Minimizing hand-to-glove DNA contamination. Forensic Sci. Int. Genet. Suppl. Ser. **2019**, 7, 19–20. **[Google Scholar] [CrossRef]**

159. Nontiapirom, K.; Bunakkharasawat, W.; Sojikul, P.; Panvisavas, N. Assessment and prevention of forensic DNA contamination in DNA profiling from latent fingerprint. Forensic Sci. Int. Genet. Suppl. Ser. **2019**, 7, 546–548. **[Google Scholar] [CrossRef]**

160. Basset, P.; Castella, V. Positive impact of DNA contamination minimization procedures taken within the laboratory. Forensic Sci. Int. Genet. **2019**, 38, 232–235. **[Google Scholar] [CrossRef] [Green Version]**

161. Williams, D.W.; Gibson, G. Classification of individuals and the potential to detect sexual contact using the microbiome of the pubic region. Forensic Sci. Int. Genet. **2019**, 41, 177–187. **[Google Scholar] [CrossRef] [PubMed]**

162. Coil, D.A.; Neches, R.Y.; Lang, J.M.; Jospin, G.; Brown, W.E.; Cavalier, D.; Hampton-Marcell, J.; Gilbert, J.A.; Eisen, J.A. Bacterial communities associated with cell phones and shoes. PeerJ **2020**, 8, e9235. **[Google Scholar] [CrossRef] [PubMed]**

163. Tackmann, J.; Arora, N.; Schmidt, T.S.B.; Rodrigues, J.F.M.; Von Mering, C. Ecologically informed microbial biomarkers and accurate classification of mixed and unmixed samples in an extensive cross-study of human body sites. Microbiome **2018**, 6, 192. **[Google Scholar] [CrossRef]**

164. Yao, T.; Han, X.; Guan, T.; Zhai, C.; Liu, C.; Liu, C.; Zhu, B.; Chen, L. Exploration of the microbiome community for saliva, skin, and a mixture of both from a population living in Guangdong. Int. J. Legal Med. **2021**, 135, 53–62. **[Google Scholar] [CrossRef]**

165. Phan, K.; Barash, M.; Spindler, X.; Gunn, P.; Roux, C. Retrieving forensic information about the donor through bacterial profiling. Int. J. Legal Med. **2020**, 134, 21–29. **[Google Scholar] [CrossRef]**

166. Neckovic, A.; van Oorschot, R.A.H.; Szkuta, B.; Durdle, A. Investigation of direct and indirect transfer of microbiomes between individuals. Forensic Sci. Int. Genet. **2020**, 45, 102212. **[Google Scholar] [CrossRef]**

167. Assenmacher, D.M.; Fields, S.D.; Crupper, S.S. Comparison of Commercial Kits for Recovery and Analysis of Bacterial DNA From Fingerprints. J. Forensic Sci. **2020**, 65, 1310–1314. **[Google Scholar] [CrossRef] [PubMed]**

168. Quaak, F.C.A.; van de Wal, Y.; Maaskant-van Wijk, P.A.; Kuiper, I. Combining human STR and microbial population profiling: Two case reports. Forensic Sci. Int. Genet. **2018**, 37, 196–199. **[Google Scholar] [CrossRef]**

169. Lindgren, P.; Myrtennäs, K.; Forsman, M.; Johansson, A.; Stenberg, P.; Nordgaard, A.; Ahlinder, J. A likelihood ratio-based approach for improved source attribution in microbiological forensic investigations. Forensic Sci. Int. **2019**, 302, 109869. **[Google Scholar] [CrossRef]**

170. Young, J.M.; Linacre, A. Massively parallel sequencing is unlocking the potential of environmental trace evidence. Forensic Sci. Int. Genet. **2021**, 50, 102393. **[Google Scholar] [CrossRef]**

171. Jurkevitch, E.; Pasternak, Z. A walk on the dirt: Soil microbial forensics from ecological theory to the crime lab. FEMS Microbiol. Rev. **2021**, 45, fuaa053. **[Google Scholar] [CrossRef] [PubMed]**

172. Neckovic, A.; van Oorschot, R.A.H.; Szkuta, B.; Durdle, A. Challenges in Human Skin Microbial Profiling for Forensic Science: A Review. Genes **2020**, 11, 1015. **[Google Scholar] [CrossRef]**

173. Neckovic, A.; van Oorschot, R.A.H.; Szkuta, B.; Durdle, A. Investigation into the presence and transfer of microbiomes within a forensic laboratory setting. Forensic Sci. Int. Genet. **2021**, 52, 102492. **[Google Scholar] [CrossRef] [PubMed]**

174. Neckovic, A.; van Oorschot, R.A.H.; Szkuta, B.; Durdle, A. Identifying background microbiomes in an evidence recovery laboratory: A preliminary study. Sci. Justice **2021**, 61, 280–290. **[Google Scholar] [CrossRef]**

175. Taylor, D.; Kokshoorn, B.; Hicks, T. Structuring cases into propositions, assumptions, and undisputed case information. Forensic Sci. Int. Genet. **2020**, 44, 102199. **[Google Scholar] [CrossRef] [Green Version]**

176. Buckleton, J.; Taylor, D.; Bright, J.-A.; Hicks, T.; Curran, J. When evaluating DNA evidence within a likelihood ratio framework, should the propositions be exhaustive? Forensic Sci. Int. Genet. **2021**, 50, 102406. **[Google Scholar] [CrossRef]**

177. Taylor, D.; Samie, L.; Champod, C. Using Bayesian networks to track DNA movement through complex transfer scenarios. Forensic Sci. Int. Genet. **2019**, 42, 69–80. **[Google Scholar] [CrossRef]**

178. Volgin, L. The importance of evaluating findings given activity level propositions in order to avoid misleading evidence. Aust. J. Forensic Sci. **2019**, 51, S10–S13. **[Google Scholar] [CrossRef]**

179. De March, I.; Taroni, F. Bayesian networks and dissonant items of evidence: A case study. Forensic Sci. Int. Genet. **2020**, 44, 102172. **[Google Scholar] [CrossRef] [PubMed] [Green Version]**

180. Samie, L.; Champod, C.; Taylor, D.; Taroni, F. The use of Bayesian Networks and simulation methods to identify the variables impacting the value of evidence assessed under activity level propositions in stabbing cases. Forensic Sci. Int. Genet. **2020**, 48, 102334. **[Google Scholar] [CrossRef] [PubMed]**

181. Gill, P. DNA evidence and miscarriages of justice. Forensic Sci. Int. **2019**, 294, e1–e3. **[Google Scholar] [CrossRef]**

182. Perepechina, I.O. Considering DNA transfer issues in a retrospective analysis of forensic examinations. Forensic Sci. Int. Genet. Suppl. Ser. **2019**, 7, 853–855. **[Google Scholar] [CrossRef]**

183. Dunhill, T.; Chapman, B. Meta-analysis of the secondary transfer of DNA. Aust. J. Forensic Sci. **2019**, 51, S44–S47. **[Google Scholar] [CrossRef] [Green Version]**

184. Hughes, D.A.; Szkuta, B.; van Oorschot, R.A.H.; Yang, W.; Conlan, X.A. Impact of surface roughness on the deposition of saliva and fingerprint residue on non-porous substrates. Forensic Chem. **2021**, 23, 100318. **[Google Scholar] [CrossRef]**

185. Thornbury, D.; Goray, M.; van Oorschot, R.A.H. Drying properties and DNA content of saliva samples taken before, during and after chewing gum. Aust. J. Forensic Sci. **2021**, 1–10. **[Google Scholar] [CrossRef]**

186. Kelly, P.; Connolly, E. The prevalence and persistence of saliva in vehicles. Forensic Sci. Int. Genet. **2021**, 53, 102530. **[Google Scholar] [CrossRef]**

187. Puliatti, L.; Handt, O.; Taylor, D. The level of DNA an individual transfers to untouched items in their immediate surroundings. Forensic Sci. Int. Genet. **2021**, 54, 102561. **[Google Scholar] [CrossRef] [PubMed]**

188. Tanzhaus, K.; Reiß, M.-T.; Zaspel, T. "I've never been at the crime scene!"—Gloves as carriers for secondary DNA transfer. Int. J. Legal Med. **2021**, 135, 1385–1393. **[Google Scholar] [CrossRef] [PubMed]**

189. Danko, D.; Bezdan, D.; Afshin, E.E.; Ahsanuddin, S.; Bhattacharya, C.; Butler, D.J.; Chng, K.R.; Donnellan, D.; Hecht, J.; Jackson, K.; et al. A global metagenomic map of urban microbiomes and antimicrobial resistance. Cell **2021**, 184, 3376–3393.e3317. **[Google Scholar] [CrossRef]**

190. Gill, P.; Bleka, Ø.; Roseth, A.; Fonneløp, A.E. An LR framework incorporating sensitivity analysis to model multiple direct and secondary transfer events on skin surface. Forensic Sci. Int. Genet. **2021**, 53, 102509. **[Google Scholar] [CrossRef]**

191. Taylor, D.; Volgin, L.; Kokshoorn, B.; Champod, C. The importance of considering common sources of unknown DNA when evaluating findings given activity level propositions. Forensic Sci. Int. Genet. **2021**, 53, 102518. **[Google Scholar] [CrossRef] [PubMed]**

192. Ypma, R.J.F.; Maaskant van Wijk, P.A.; Gill, R.; Sjerps, M.; van den Berge, M. Calculating LRs for presence of body fluids from mRNA assay data in mixtures. Forensic Sci. Int. Genet. **2021**, 52, 102455. **[Google Scholar] [CrossRef]**

193. Meakin, G.E.; Kokshoorn, B.; van Oorschot, R.A.H.; Szkuta, B. Evaluating forensic DNA evidence: Connecting the dots. WIREs Forensic Sci. **2020**, 3, e1404. **[Google Scholar]**

194. Jones, N.S.; Fornaro, E. National Institute of Justice Forensic Science Research and Development Symposium; RTI Press: Research Triangle, NC, USA, 2021. **[Google Scholar] [CrossRef]**

195. National Institute of Justice. Available online: **https://nij.ojp.gov** (accessed on 15 August 2021).

196. European Network of Forensic Science Institutes (ENFSI). Monopoly Programmes. Available online: **https://enfsi.eu/projects** (accessed on 15 August 2021).

197. International Society of Forensic Genetics (ISFG). Conferences. Available online: **https://www.isfg.org/Meeting** (accessed on 15 August 2021).

198. Gordon Research Conferences (GRC). Forensic Analysis of Human DNA. Available online: **https://www.grc.org/forensic-analysis-of-human-dna-conference/** (accessed on 15 August 2021).

199. American Academy of Forensic Sciences (AAFS). Conference Proceedings. Available online: **https://aafs.org/aafs/Resources/Proceedings/AAFS/Resources/Proceedings.aspx?hkey=b8e1fc6b-2c69–411a-a386–7d38929ca963** (accessed on 10 October 2021).

200. Promega. International Symposium on Human Identification (ISHI). Available online: **https://www.ishinews.com** (accessed on 15 August 2021).

201. Budowle, B.; van Oorschot, R.A.H.; Morling, N.; Martinez de Pancorbo, M.; Doutremepuich, C.; Piters, A.; Esponda, A.; Monique, G. Les Progrès Récents enEmpreintesGénétiques et en ADN de Transfert (Recent Progress on Forensic Sciences and DNA Transfer); Librairie Mollat: Bordeaux, France, 2020; Available online: **https://www.expertise-adn.fr/actualites-adn/les-progres-recents-en-empreintes-genetiques-et-en-adn-de-transfert** (accessed on 15 August 2021).

202. International Society of Forensic Genetics (ISFG). Summer School. Available online:**https://isfgsummerschool.events.idloom.com/virtual-edition-2021** (accessed on 15 August 2021).

203. University of Lausanne. Statistics and the Evaluation of Forensic Evidence. Available online:**https://www.formation-continue-unil-epfl.ch/formation/statistics-evaluation-forensic-evidence-cas/** (accessed on 15 August 2021).

204. University of Lausanne. Challenging Forensic Science: How Science Should Speak to Court. Available online: **https://www.coursera.org/learn/challenging-forensic-science** (accessed on 15 August 2021).

205. Forensic Technology Center of Excellence; National Institute of Justice. Probabilistic Genotyping of Evidentiary DNA Typing Results: Online Workshop Series. Available online: **https://forensiccoe.org/online-workshop-series-probabilistic-genotyping-of-evidentiary-dna-typing-results** (accessed on 15 August 2021).

206. Netherlands Register of Court Experts (NRGD). Register Open for Applications DNA Activity Level. 2021. Available online: **https://english.nrgd.nl/news/register-open-for-applications-dna-activity-level.aspx** (accessed on 8 October 2021).

207. Netherlands Register of Court Experts (NRGD). Standards: Human DNA Analysis and Interpretation (001.1–001.3). 2021. Available online: **https://english.nrgd.nl/binaries/10321%20-%20Standards%20Human%20DNA%20Analysis%20and%20Interpretation%20v4.1_tcm40-493992.pdf** (accessed on 10 October 2021).

208. Kokshoorn, B.; Aarts, L.H.J.; Ansell, R.; Connolly, E.; Drotz, W.; Kloosterman, A.D.; McKenna, L.G.; Szkuta, B.; van Oorschot, R.A.H. Sharing data on DNA transfer, persistence, prevalence and recovery: Arguments for harmonization and standardization. Forensic Sci. Int. Genet. **2018**, 37, 260–269. [**Google Scholar**] [**CrossRef**]

209. Université Du Québec À Trois-Rivières. BDATT-TTADB (Transfer Traces Activity DataBase). Available online: **http://www.uqtr.ca/LRC/BDATT-TTADB** (accessed on 15 August 2021).

210. Cadola, L.; Charest, M.; Lavallée, C.; Crispino, F. The occurrence and genesis of transfer traces in forensic science: A structured knowledge database. J. Can. Soc. Forensic Sci **2021**, 54, 86–100. [**Google Scholar**] [**CrossRef**]

211. GOV.UK. Forensic Science Providers: Codes of Practice and Conduct. Available online: **https://www.gov.uk/government/collections/forensic-science-providers-codes-of-practice-and-conduct** (accessed on 15 August 2021).

212. Gill, P.; Hicks, T.; Butler, J.M.; Connolly, E.; Gusmão, L.; Kokshoorn, B.; Morling, N.; van Oorschot, R.A.H.; Parson, W.; Prinz, M.; et al. DNA Commission of the International Society for Forensic Genetics: Assessing the value of forensic biological evidence—Guidelines highlighting the importance of propositions: Part I: Evaluation of DNA profiling comparisons given (sub-) source propositions. Forensic Sci. Int. Genet. **2018**, 36, 189–202. **[Google Scholar] [CrossRef] [PubMed] [Green Version]**

213. International Organization for Standardization. Forensic Sciences—Part 5: Reporting. ISO/CD 21043-5. 2021. Available online: **https://www.iso.org/standard/73896.html?browse=tc** (accessed on 16 August 2021).

214. Butler, J.M.; Iyer, H.; Press, R.; Taylor, M.K.; Vallone, P.M.; Willis, S. National Institute of Standards and Technology. DNA Mixture Interpretation: A NIST Scientific Foundation Review. 2021. Available online: **https://nvlpubs.nist.gov/nistpubs/ir/2021/NIST.IR.8351-draft.pdf** (accessed on 10 October 2021).

215. Roux, C.; Willis, S.; Weyermann, C. Shifting forensic science focus from means to purpose: A path forward for the discipline? Sci. Justice **2021**, 61, 678–686. **[Google Scholar] [CrossRef]**

216. De Koeijer, J.A.; Sjerps, M.J.; Vergeer, P.; Berger, C.E.H. Combining evidence in complex cases—A practical approach to interdisciplinary casework. Sci. Justice **2020**, 60, 20–29. **[Google Scholar] [CrossRef] [PubMed]**

217. National Institute of Forensic Science Australia New Zealand. An Introductory Guide to Evaluative Reporting. 2017. Available online: **http://www.anzpaa.org.au/forensic-science/our-work/projects/evaluative-reporting** (accessed on 10 October 2021).

218. Willis, S.M.; McKenna, L.; McDermott, S.D.; O'Donnell, G.; Barrett, A.; Rasmusson, B.; Höglund, T.; Berger, C.E.H.; Sierps, M.J.; Lucena-Molina, J.J.; et al. ENFSI Guideline for Evaluative Reporting in Forensic Science. 2015. Available online: **http://enfsi.eu/wp-content/uploads/2016/09/m1_guideline.pdf** (accessed on 10 October 2021).

219. Kokshoorn, B.; Aarts, B.; De Blaeij, T.; Maaskant-van Wijk, P.; Blankers, B. Bewijskracht van onderzoeknaarbiologischesporenen DNA. Deel 3: Activiteitniveau. Expert. en Recht **2014**, 6, 213–219. **[Google Scholar]**

220. Robertson, P.; Aitken, C.; Royal Statistical Society. The Logic of Forensic Proof: Inferential Reasoning in Criminal Evidence and Forensic Science. 2014. Available online: **https://rss.org.uk/RSS/media/File-library/Publications/rss-inferential-reasoning-criminal-evidence-forensic-science.pdf** (accessed on 10 October 2021).

08 GENOMIC SOLUTIONS: PREDICTING PHYSICAL APPEARANCE USING DNA DATA

1. INTRODUCTION: AN OVERVIEW

Genomic data contains valuable information that can be utilized to produce leads for forensic investigations, thereby expediting the process of human identification when employed effectively. Forensic DNA intelligence employs diverse techniques, such as relatedness testing, ancestry inference, physical phenotype prediction, and age estimate [1,2,3,4]. Forensic science, being a field that combines multiple disciplines, may currently take advantage of the rapidly advancing techniques in genomics and machine learning. This is especially advantageous for the continued progress of forensic DNA analysis. Current studies on human genome variation, undertaken on an unprecedented scale, are elucidating the mechanisms by which genes regulate phenotypes. This knowledge is of paramount importance in comprehending the link between the genome and phenome. Significantly, the increasing understanding of variations in the human genome enables the creation of algorithms that can predict phenotypes with more accuracy. This leads to more dependable investigative leads, aiding in the identification of an unknown culprit or victim and the resolution of a case. It is important to mention that the DNA-based predictive tools created in the field of forensics are also valuable in the study of evolutionary anthropology.

This review paper aims to provide a concise overview of the advancements in comprehending the genetic structures of different human physical attributes. Additionally, it will discuss the advancements in high-throughput genotyping technologies and their integration with machine-learning techniques, which enable the accurate prediction of physical appearance traits. We will also examine the progression of the genetic prediction of physical features, which has transitioned from constructing predictive models using factors that exhibit genetic linkage to constructing models using variables that enhance predictive accuracy (Figure 1).

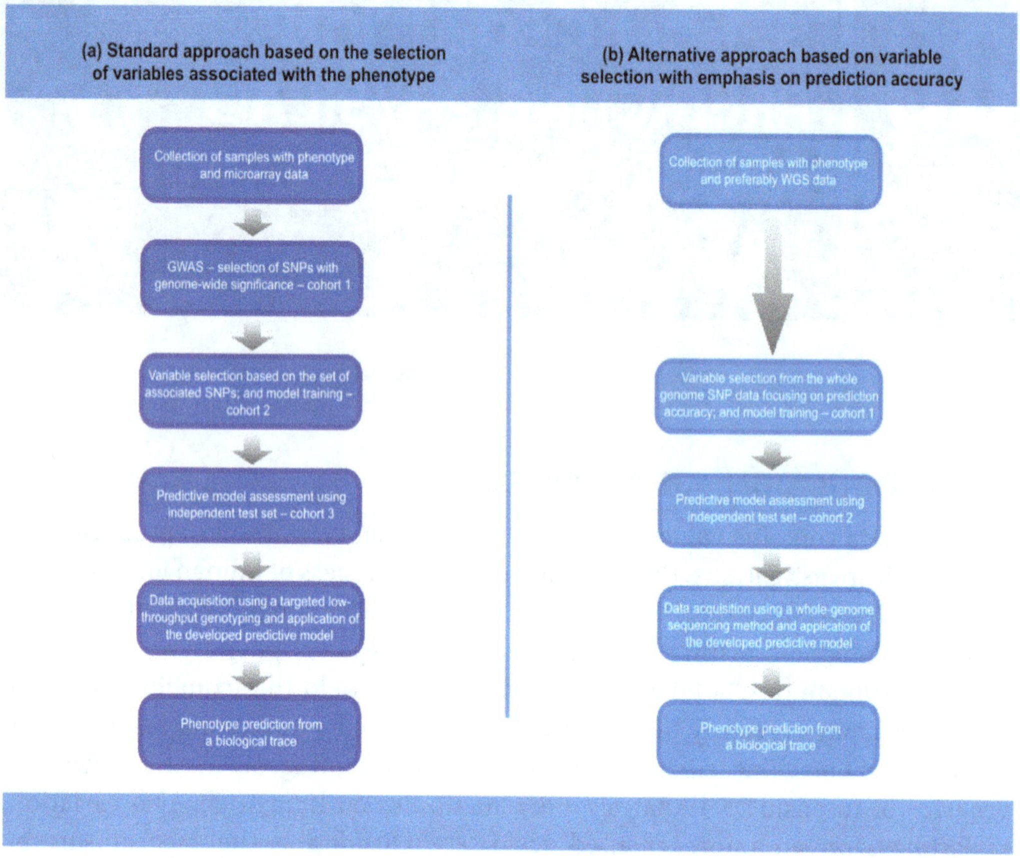

Figure 1. Procedure for the development and application of a phenotype prediction tool. The main differences in the procedures for developing a predictive model using the standard or alternative approach concern the selection of variables and the number of variables in the model. Consequently, the method of acquiring genetic data in the practical forensic applications of the next-generation predictive models may require whole-genome sequencing methods. Thus: (a) only phenotype-associated SNPs are included in prediction modelling, the models are not very extensive, and the methods of data acquisition can be less complex (SNaPshot, targeted MPS); (b) the selection of relevant variables (SNPs) is targeted towards improving the prediction accuracy of the model, and much more advanced variable selection methods are required. Some complex models may involve many thousands of SNPs, which, in biological traces, must be analysed using whole-genome sequencing methods that are effective for low DNA input samples.

2. ELUCIDATING THE HERITABILITY OF PHYSICAL CHARACTERISTICS

A large meta-analysis of twin studies has confirmed that all human traits are heritable and showed that most of the traits can be explained by an additive genetic variation [5]. The extreme similarity of physical appearance of monozygotic twins clearly indicates the role of genes, but their identification is not simple due to the complex nature of appearance traits. Linkage mapping, which relies on the co-segregation of causal DNA variants with marker variants (SNP or STR) within pedigrees, has been very successful at identifying the gene variants affecting simple mendelian traits [6], but mostly failed to identify the DNA variants involved in the determination of complex traits [7]. The breakthrough in explaining the heritability of complex phenotypes has come with the advent of genome-wide association studies (GWAS), which are effective at discovering common variants with small effect sizes on traits [7]. GWAS is used to identify associations between genotypes and phenotypes by testing for differences in the allele frequency of DNA variants between individuals who differ phenotypically. Technically, the analysis of hundreds of thousands of DNA variants in the genomes of these individuals enables finding those statistically associated with a specific phenotype [8].

2.1. Pigmentation Phenotype

GWAS data have shown highly successful in elucidating the heritability of physical appearance traits. The heritability of human pigmentation traits has been determined to be over 80%, indicating that 80% of the variation in pigmentation within a population is attributed to genetic differences between individuals, with a minimal contribution from environmental factors [9,10,11].Many candidate genes for human pigmentation were identified before the GWAS era through animal models and the linkage to diseases with mendelian inheritance modes, such as oculocutaneous albinism. Genome-wide association scans confirmed the importance of these genes and identified many of the novel gene variants influencing the variability of normal human pigmentation. The collected data confirmed a very promising perspective for the genetic prediction of pigmentation traits. The less complex nature of some pigmentation phenotypes, such as blue and brown eye colours and red hair colour, and the availability of DNA variants with relatively large effect sizes, similar to the genetic effects observed for mendelian traits, were particularly encouraging. The region on chromosome 15, including the OCA2 gene, was implicated in eye colour via linkage and subsequent fine-mapping analyses [12,13]. The evidence of a relationship between OCA2 genotypes and eye colour became stronger with additional reports [14,15,16]. This was an Icelandic GWAS that implicated the involvement of neighbouring HERC2 in the determination of eye colour and suggested that this genomic region was responsible for the regulation of OCA2 gene expression [17]. This speculation was soon confirmed by other studies that showed that the DNA variant rs12913832 was responsible for brown and blue eye colour in humans [18,19]. The postulated interaction between these two genes in determining eye colour was also confirmed [20]. Most of the

SNP heritability of red hair colour is explained by the single MC1R gene, which was also discovered long before the genome-wide association scans and confirmed in various population samples across the globe [**21,22**]. The effect of this gene was extended to skin colour and freckling [**23,24**]. These early genome-wide association scans for pigmentation also clearly demonstrated their agnostic power to detect novel, sometimes unexpected genotype–phenotype relationships, as in the case of the IRF4 gene, which is now an important predictor of pigmentation phenotypes [**17,25**]. The success of GWAS was clear, but a significant proportion of heritability remained missing, which could be attributed mainly to the insufficiently large sample sizes used in genome-wide association scans, insufficient phenotyping regimes generating heterogeneity, the insufficient density of the GWA arrays and the significance of non-additive variation [**26,27**]. Indeed, the improved statistical power to detect small effect-size variants more effectively in the next series of genome-wide association scans enabled the identification of multiple new DNA variants involved in the heritability of hair and eye colour. For example, a large study of 192,986 European individuals from 10 populations identified 50 new loci for eye colour [**28**]. The study revealed signals with genome-wide significance for 12,192 SNPs from 52 genomic regions in the discovery set of 157,485 individuals. By combining discovery and replication sets, the study finally identified 124 independent associations from 61 genomic regions and concluded that the known variants explain 53.2% of eye colour variation. Notably, the study also investigated Asian cohorts and found consistency in the genetic architecture of eye colour in populations from Europe and Asia [**28**].

Human skin colour is highly variable at continental and intercontinental levels, complicating research on the genetic architecture and heritability of this trait [**29**]. The rs1426654 in SLC24A5, discovered thanks to a Zebrafish study, plays an important role in skin colour differences at the continental level, explaining more than 30% of skin colour differences between African and European populations [**30**]. GWAS on skin colour conducted on various population samples discovered multiple genes and gene variants involved in skin colour variation at the intercontinental level [**25,31,32,33,34**]. Notably, the studies of African populations showed large differences in skin colour, revealing the high complexity of the genetic architecture of skin colour in Africa and the significance of genes unknown to European studies [**35,36**].

A meta-analysis that involved almost 300,000 genomes from individuals of European ancestry included in two different cohorts (23andMe, UK Biobank) discovered 124 loci relevant to human hair colour, mostly novel associations, including genes with strong effect, such as SLC45A1, DSTYK, FOSL2, LHX2, EDNRB, SHC4, KRT31, and BCAS1. The study was highly successful at explaining up to 34.6% (red hair) of the heritability of human hair colour, despite an imperfect phenotyping regime involving self-reported hair colour in adulthood [**37**]. Another study based on UK Biobank resources examined 343,234 genomes from participants reporting British descent and these were, thus, more homogeneous. This study assessed that all identified variants explain 90% of the SNP heritability of red hair colour but, surprisingly, it found that a DNA variant located 97 kb from the 5' end of the MC1R gene may be more important for explaining red hair colour than the polymorphism within the MC1R exon, and it identified an additional eight loci that contribute to the genetics of red hair colour. This research also revealed 213 variants important to the determination of blond hair colour, accounting for 73% of SNP heritability. In addition, a set of 56 DNA variants was found to be important for brown hair colour and was assessed to account for 47% of SNP heritability of this hair category [**38**].

2.2. Characteristics of Hair

Along with hair colour, other features describing the properties of human hair can be useful to define the physical appearance of an individual. Research shows that genetics plays a key role in the determination of hair features. However, the level of heritability may differ for various hair traits. Very high heritability (85–95%) was estimated for hair shape [**39**]. Heritability of around 70% was reported for monobrow and beard thickness [**40**]. Studies are contradictory in terms of the heritability level of hair loss (~40–80%) [**40,41,42,43**] and hair greying (~30–90%) [**40,44**], but the accuracy of the heritability measurement may be affected by the definition of heritability, the study design and the method of analysis used [**45**]. It is worth noting that heritability values calculated from the entire SNPs analysed in GWA studies tend to be underestimated compared to estimates of pedigree heritability, because the former do not include phenotypic variation due to rare variants that are not correctly determined by the SNPs genotyped on microarrays or common variants with small effect sizes that are not correctly identified if the sample size is not large enough. In turn, pedigree heritability may be biased by the common environmental factors to which families are typically exposed [**43,45**]. Notably, heritability estimates may vary due to changes in allele frequencies in populations caused by different evolutionary mechanisms and environmental contributions that change with the age of individuals [**46**]. The genetic basis of hair loss and hair shape are the most investigated so far. Androgenetic alopecia, known in men as male pattern baldness (MPB), is the most common type of progressive loss of hair from the scalp and is particularly frequent among men in Europe. Over the last >10 years, several GWA studies on hair loss have been carried out, with the vast majority of research conducted on Europeans [**43,47,48,49,50,51,52,53**]. These studies revealed multiple genes that are associated with the risk of MPB, with two loci showing the strongest effect of association, Xq12 (AR/EDA2R) and 20p11

(PAX1/FOXA2). Of these two loci, only 20p11 is known to act in Asians, indicating the significance of population heterogeneity [**54,55**]. A long list of additional loci, representing smaller effect sizes, identified through GWAS and/or candidate gene approaches, is available in the literature (e.g., HDAC9, WNT10, TARDBP, EBF1, SUCNR1, AUTS2, FGF5, IRF4, C1orf127, RUNX1, and TWIST2). Studies published in 2017–2018 led to significant advances in research on the genetics of hair loss. Four large GWA scans have been conducted on individuals of European descent. The first three of those studies, which investigated 20,000–50,000 genomes each, detected altogether more than 300 GWA signals, including 253 novel MPB associations [**42,52,53**]. The largest study, which investigated 200,000 genomes, allowed the identification of >600 genome-wide associations, explaining altogether 25% of the phenotypic variation observed in alopecia [**43**]. These large-scale studies not only discovered many new loci involved in alopecia, but also highlighted the implicated molecular pathways and discovered the genetic links of alopecia with different traits/conditions, including bone mineral density, puberty, metabolic traits, and Parkinson's disease. However, a significant part of MPB heritability remains missing. Recent studies showed that the use of advanced statistical methods and the incorporation of functional genomics data prior to association tests may improve the efficiency of SNP detection in GWAS and these approaches were proved to be successful in MPB research by increasing the number of SNP hits by an additional ~4% [**56,57**].

For hair morphology (shape), four GWA studies have been published so far, two of which were carried out on Europeans, with one study on Latin Americans and one on East Asians [**40,58,59,60**]. Hair shape, usually defined as straight vs. wavy vs. curly, is a highly distinctive feature of human appearance. As with hair loss, genetic heterogeneity between populations is observed with different mechanisms and genes underlying straight hair formation in Europeans and East Asians. The TCHH gene is known to act only in Europeans, while EDAR is the main contributor to straight hair in East Asians [**58,59,61**].

However, the proportion of known heritability attributed to both genes in respective populations was found to be small (<10%). The TCHH gene was discovered in the first GWA study published in 2009, which was conducted on three cohorts with a total of more than 4800 individuals of European descent [**58**]. TCHH was the only gene in this study that reached genome-wide significance, but suggestive associations were also disclosed for several additional loci, including the FRAS1 and WNT10 genes. The role of the EDAR gene in hair straightness and thickness in Asians was discovered through candidate gene analyses [**61,62**] and confirmed in a later GWA study conducted in 2016 on ~2900 Chinese people, with no additional genes reaching GWA significance in this study [**59**]. A GWA study conducted on >6000 Latin Americans discovered a novel association for PRSS53 [**40**]. The latest meta-analysis of European GWA studies, exploring a total of more than 16,000 samples, allowed the identification of 12 hair shape genes, including eight novel association signals (ERRFI1/SLC45A1, PEX14, PADI3, TGFA, LGR4, HOXC13, KRTAP, and PTK6) [**60**]. The study showed that a model consisting of 14 SNPs across novel and literature loci, together with sex, explains 10% of the total hair shape variability. Further research pointed to the role of gene–gene interactions in hair shape determination as one of the factors underlying missing heritability [**63**]. The RPTN gene has been implicated in straight hair formation in Europeans and East Asians, but throughout interactions with different previously known head hair shape genes.

Only a few studies have addressed the genetic basis of other hair traits. In recent years, the first genes responsible for the thickness of the eyebrows, e.g., EDAR, FOXL2, LIMS1, TMEM174, SOX2, and FOXD1 [**40,64,65**], monobrows, e.g., PAX3 and 5q13.2 [**40,51**], beard thickness, e.g., EDAR, LNX1, PREP, and FOXP2 [**40**], and hair greying, e.g., IRF4, and KIF1A [**40,66**], have been identified through whole-genome or whole-exome analyses.

2.3. Human Height

Approximately 80% of human height is determined by genetic inheritance. However, prior to the advent of Genome-Wide Association (GWA) investigations, only individual genes related to this feature were identified. The examination of human height genetics serves as a compelling illustration of the efficacy of elucidating the heritability of intricate characteristics via the GWAS methodology. A significant benefit of conducting height research is in the straightforwardness of assessing this particular characteristic, which ensures consistency in the collected phenotypic data. The genome-wide association scans for human stature have discovered gene variations that have a tiny impact size, providing unambiguous confirmation of the considerable polygenicity of this characteristic. The first three GWA studies of human height, which collectively included more than 50,000 samples, detected only 54 loci with a statistically significant association with stature [**67,68,69**].

Most of these loci have not been previously linked to human height and, in many cases, the known biological function did not make them candidates for the regulation of human stature. The genes discovered explained only about 5% of the variation in height, which was very discouraging, especially for predicting this distinctive feature. A huge meta-analysis that considered GWAS data for more than 180,000 genomes made only a small advance in explaining the heritability of human growth, enabling the discovery of 180 loci. The work demonstrated the importance of allelic heterogeneity in explaining the complex genetic architecture of human stature [**70**]. At the same time, it has been argued that testing each SNP individually for an association with a trait, which is typical for GWAS investigations, leads to missing many real associations, especially when the effect sizes of individual SNPs on a trait are small. By fitting all SNPs simultaneously, Yang et al. provided an unbiased estimate of the variance explained by the SNPs in total, and showed that common genetic variants are able to explain as much as 45% of the variance in human height [**71**]. However, consistently increasing the number of genomes analysed with high-density DNA microarrays has proven to be an effective method for elucidating the still-missing genetic variation responsible for human height. The large meta-analysis that included 700,000 European genomes (250,000 previously investigated [**72**] and 450,000 from the UK Biobank) identified 3290 near-independent SNPs associated with human stature which were found to explain 24.6% of variance of this trait [**73**]. Still, unpublished data suggest that the large proportion of missing heritability may be hiding in rare genetic variants (≤0.01) that can be detected via the whole genome sequencing of a sufficient number of genomes [**74**]. Notably, Zoledziewska et al. showed that human height can be under pressure from natural selection, presenting data showing that known height-decreasing alleles were found at higher frequency in Sardinians than would be expected to be caused by genetic drift [**75**]. Research on the genetic architecture of human stature, on a smaller scale, is also being conducted in populations in Asia and Africa. A meta-analysis of 93,926 individuals from East Asia identified 98 loci, including 17 novel for human height [**76**]. A GWA study based on 191,787 Japanese genomes disclosed 573 height-associated variants and assessed that 64 rare (<0.01) and low-frequency (<0.05) variants explain 1.7% of the height variance. The study revealed genes not previously associated with stature [**77**]. Eighty-three low-frequency variants affecting human height have also been reported in [**78**].

2.4. Facial Morphology

The human face encompasses a collection of interconnected and intricate physical characteristics that exhibit significant variation both between and within populations. These characteristics are considered to be the most distinguishing and distinctive human trait [79].The striking resemblance between the looks of monozygotic twins unequivocally suggests that the majority of this variation is genetically influenced.Despite this, research into the heritability of facial features has caused quite a few problems, probably due to the three-dimensional nature of human faces. Only a recent face heritability study performed on 952 British twins using an advanced phenotyping and landmarking system confirmed the high heritability (>65%) of many facial traits [**80**]. Indeed, contrary to some physical phenotype traits, collecting phenotypic data for faces can be challenging. A self-reported categorisation is less useful, and measurement ideally requires the involvement of methods that are able to capture the three-dimensionality of faces. The approaches used to collect facial appearance data for studying the genetics of craniofacial variation that can be found in the literature are standard 2D photographs, magnetic resonance imaging (MRI) and 3D scanning. The latter has quickly gained a dominant position in craniofacial genetics research. It should be noted that the phenotypic assessment of facial variability from 3D images is not an easy task and makes large-scale studies and comparisons between different studies difficult. Initially, the process relied on a labour-intensive process of the manual determination of landmarks, and later, several automated landmarking methods applicable to 3D images have facilitated research on the association of facial phenotype with genotype [**80,81,82,83**]. In one of the first works on the genetics of natural craniofacial variation, 11 DNA variants previously associated with cleft-lip phenotypes were tested in two European cohorts with the phenotypes captured using 2D photos or magnetic resonance images [**84**]. A DNA variant near the GREM1 gene was associated with nose width, and another near the CCDC26 gene was associated with bizygomatic distance. The first GWAS scan that was aimed at investigating normal facial variation identified only a single intronic DNA variant in the PAX3 gene, which showed association with nasion position. This first study was conducted on a relatively small group of 2185 adolescents. The study used a 3D laser scanning method to collect phenotypic data. The 22 identified landmarks were then used to generate 54 3D and 2D distances featuring different facial characteristics. Additionally, following a previous method, a principal component analysis enabled the identification of 14 independent groups of correlated coordinates [**85**]. These parameters were used in association testing, which identified four associations, but only PAX3 was replicated in an independent cohort of 1622 participants [**86**].

A larger GWAS analysis of almost 10,000 individuals of European origin from several cohorts used 3D MRI scans and 2D photos, and identified five genes involved in facial variation. PAX3, PRDM16, and TP63 have previously been linked to craniofacial development, while C5orf50 and COL17A1 were new findings [**87**]. The strongest signal was again obtained for PAX3, which soon gained further confirmation in an independent study of about 6000 Latin Americans investigated in the large CANDELA project [**40**]. It is worth noting that rare variants in PAX3, the most replicated gene for natural variation in facial appearance, cause Waardenburg syndrome, which involves some facial dysmorphism, including a broad nasal bridge. The phenotyping regime in Adhikari's study involved a simple approach based on standard 2D photographs, and the study also implicated DCHS2, RUNX2, GLI3, and PAX1 in nose morphology and EDAR in chin protrusion [**40**].

Another GWAS study, which included 3D images of 3118 individuals of European ancestry that were used to derive 20 facial distance measurements, identified several genomic regions and implicated MAFB, PAX9, MIPOL1, ALX3, HDAC8, and PAX1 in normal facial variation, including the measures of eye, nose, and facial breadth. The study also provided additional evidence for the association between

PRDM16 and C5orf50 and facial features [**88**]. Crouch et al. investigated the hypothesis that the DNA variants responsible for large effects on facial morphology exist in the human genome, and focused on individuals displaying extreme facial characteristics to find them. The study included 3D images of 1832 individuals from the general population as a discovery set and 1567 3D scans of twins from the TwinsUK databank, plus 33 of East Asians for replication. The original 3D scans were used to manually mark each face with 14 well-defined landmarks, allowing a mesh of 50,000–150,000 surface points in 3D space to be transformed into a set of 29,658 surface points for each face. This approach enabled the identification of three SNPs in PCDH15, MBTPS1, and TMEM163, genes that have previously been associated with various pathological phenotypes involving craniofacial dysmorphias [**89**]. The study by Claes et al. (2018) involved 2329 individuals at the discovery stage and an additional 1719 at the replication stage, and found associations for 15 loci with facial features, including four new genes, nine consistently confirmed, and two linked with pleiotropic facial phenotypic features. The study used an innovative, data-driven facial phenotyping approach based on structural correlations between about 10,000 3D quasi-landmarks, which enabled the hierarchical (global-to-local) clustering of the human face into segments [**90**]. This approach also yielded good results for a meta-analysis, which included 8246 European individuals and enabled the identification of 203 loci associated with normal facial variation [**91**] and for a study of facial features in East Africans, which investigated 2595 3D facial images collected on Tanzanian children [**92**]. The latter cohort was previously investigated, with two genes, SCHIP1 and PDE8A, identified that were associated with measures of human facial size [**83**]. GWA studies investigating human facial morphology in non-European cohorts are rare. Worth noting is a GWAS conducted on an exploratory panel of Uyghurs that identified six loci important for the genetic architecture of the human face, four of which were replicated in independent cohorts of Uyghur or southern Han Chinese [**93**].

3. DNA-BASED PREDICTIVE TOOLS FOR FORENSIC APPLICATIONS

Several factors determine the accuracy of DNA-based predictive methods, including high heritability of a trait, the identification of appropriate predictors, and the selection of the best mathematical approach to model development. The forensic community very early recognised the investigative potential of extracting phenotypes from DNA data. The practical importance of a simple amelogenin genetic sex test [**94**], and also of the inference of biogeographical ancestry [**95,96**], made it clear that a description of the phenotypic characteristics of a person of undetermined identity can provide important investigative leads. The variation of the MC1R gene was soon proposed as an indicator of red hair colour [**97**], while the predictive potential of the OCA2 variation was proposed for the inference of eye colour [**14**]. The availability of GWAS data has made it possible to develop tools for predicting human appearance traits more effectively. The research carried out has made it possible to develop predictive tools with varying performances and practicalities of application for different physical characteristics (**Table 1**).

Table 1. Examples of various approaches proposed for genetic prediction of physical traits.

Physical Trait	Statistical Model	Number of Predictors in the Model	Prediction Accuracy Parameters	Ref.
Eye colour	Multinomial logistic regression (IrisPlex) [1]	6 SNPs	$AUC_{brown} = 0.93$ [2] $AUC_{intermediate} = 0.72$ $AUC_{blue} = 0.91$	[**98**]
	Likelihood ratio	4 SNPs	$LR_{light\text{-}dark}$ depends on genotypes	[**99**]
	Multiple linear regression	3 SNPs	$R^2 = 0.764$	[**100**]
	No statistical model, classification based on genotypes	6 SNPs	Overall classification success rate (blue-green-brown): 98.94%	[**101**]
	Likelihood ratio	6 SNPs	$LR_{light\text{-}dark}$ depends on genotypes $AUC_{light\text{-}dark} = 0.925$	[**102**]
	Bayesian naïve classifier (Snipper)	23 SNPs	Classification success rate: blue = 98.27%, green-hazel = 97.81% brown = 96.67%.	[**103**]
	Multiple response classification tree	4 SNPs	Classification success rate: blue = 89% intermediate = 46% brown = 94%	[**104**]
	No statistical model, prediction based on genotypes	5 SNPs	Overall classification success rate (blue-green-brown): 97.64%	[**105**]

Physical Trait	Statistical Model	Number of Predictors in the Model	Prediction Accuracy Parameters	Ref.
Hair colour	Multinomial logistic regression + prediction guide (HIrisPlex) [1]	22 SNPs	Classification success rate: AUC_{blond} = 0.81 AUC_{brown} = 0.82 AUC_{black} = 0.87 AUC_{red} = 0.93	[106]
	Bayesian naïve classifier (Snipper)	12 SNPs	Classification success rate: blond = 92.3% brown = 76.7% black = 74.6% red = 85% Sex-related prediction accuracy differences noted	[107]
	Multinomial logistic regression	270 SNPs	AUC_{blond} = 0.74 AUC_{brown} = 0.68 AUC_{black} = 0.86 AUC_{red} = 0.86	[37]
Skin colour	Multiple linear regression, including interaction	3 SNPs	R^2 = 0.496	[100]
	No statistical model, classification based on genotypes	5 SNPs	Overall classification success rate (dark–medium–light): 62% 38% of results inconclusive	[105]
	Bayesian naïve classifier (Snipper)	10 SNPs	AUC_{white} = 0.999$AUC_{intermediate}$ = 0.803 AUC_{black} = 0.966	[108]
	Multinomial logistic regression (HIrisPlex-S) [1]	36 SNPs	AUC_{light} = 0.97 AUC_{dark} = 0.83 $AUC_{dark-black}$ = 0.96 or $AUC_{very-pale}$ = 0.74 AUC_{pale} = 0.72 $AUC_{intermediate}$ = 0.73 AUC_{dark} = 0.87 $AUC_{dark-black}$ = 0.97	[109]
	Multiple linear regression	9 SNPs	R^2 = 0.65	[110]

Physical Trait	Statistical Model	Number of Predictors in the Model	Prediction Accuracy Parameters	Ref.
Freckles	Binomial logistic regression	34 SNPs + sex	$AUC_{freckled}$ = 0.809	[111]
	Multinomial logistic regression	20 SNPs + sex	$AUC_{non\text{-}freckled}$ = 0.754 $AUC_{freckled}$ = 0.657 $AUC_{heavily\text{-}freckled}$ = 0.792	[112]
Hair loss	Binomial logistic regression	20 SNPs	AUC_{bald} = 0.66 AUC_{bald} = 0.76 in men ≥ 50 years old	[113]
	Binomial logistic regression	14 SNPs	$AUC_{early\text{-}onset\ baldness}$ = 0.74	[114]
	Polygenic scores (weighted allele sums)	261 autosomal SNPs; 70 X chromosomal SNPs	$AUC_{severe\ baldness}$ = 0.748 (autosomal SNPs)$AUC_{severe\ baldness}$ = 0.621 (X chromosome SNPs) With autosomal and X SNPs + age included in the model: $AUC_{severe\ baldness}$ = 0.79; $AUC_{moderate\ baldness}$ = 0.70; $AUC_{slight\ baldness}$ = 0.61	[52]
Hair shape	Binomial logistic regression	3 SNPs	$AUC_{straight}$ = 0.62	[115]
	Binomial and multinomial logistic regression	32 SNPs in binomial modelor33 SNPs in multinomial model	$AUC_{straight}$ = 0.66 in Europeans $AUC_{straight}$ = 0.79 in non-Europeans or $AUC_{straight}$ = 0.67 in Europeans AUC_{wavy} = 0.60 in Europeans AUC_{curly} = 0.60 in Europeans $AUC_{straight}$ = 0.80 in non-Europeans AUC_{wavy} = 0.61 in non-Europeans AUC_{curly} = 0.74 in non-Europeans	[116]
Hair greying	Binary and multi-class neural network	10 SNPs + age and sex in binary model or 12 SNPs + age and sex in multi-class model	$AUC_{greying}$ = 0.87 (mostly based on age)or $AUC_{no\ greying}$ = 0.86 $AUC_{mild\ greying}$ = 0.79 $AUC_{severe\ greying}$ = 0.86	[66]

Physical Trait	Statistical Model	Number of Predictors in the Model	Prediction Accuracy Parameters	Ref.
Height	Polygenic scores (weighted allele sums)	54 SNPs	$AUC_{tall\ stature} = 0.65$	[117]
	Polygenic scores (weighted allele sums)	180 SNPs	$AUC_{tall\ stature} = 0.75$	[118]
	Polygenic scores (weighted allele sums)	689 SNPs	$AUC_{tall\ stature} = 0.79$	[119]
	L_1-penalized regression (LASSO)	>20,000 SNPs	r = 0.64	[120]
Face	Partial least squares regression	Genomic ancestry (68 DNA variants) + sex + 24 SNPs	Genomic ancestry explains 9.6% of the total facial variation; sex independently from ancestry explains 12.9%; SNPs make a small contribution to improving facial distinctiveness	[82]
	Ridge regression	Genomic ancestry (1000 genomic Principal Components) + sex, BMI and age	Genomic ancestry and sex explain large proportion of the predictive accuracy of the model; age and BMI improve the accuracy of the model	[121]
	Simple quantitative method (principal component analysis and partial least square analysis used to extract new face traits)	277 SNPs	SSA statistic [3]: no difference between SNP-based prediction and random predictions in females; SNP-based predictions significantly better than random predictions in males	[93]

[1] SNaPshot and MPS forensically validated genetic tests for data collection available; [2] AUC—area under the ROC (receiver operating characteristic) curve, describes the general performance of the model, 1 means perfect prediction and 0.5 means random assignment; [3] SSA—a shape similarity statistic (shape space angle) developed to measure the angle between two shapes in the 3D face modelling data space.

3.1. Pigmentation Traits

Specifically, the identification of eye color markers with significant phenotypic impacts has facilitated the creation of very reliable genetic predictors for this characteristic. The IrisPlex prediction system is the most widely recognized tool utilized in the field of forensics. It consists of a genetic test for gathering data and a mathematical algorithm for accurately predicting the three distinct categories of eye color [98].The algorithm was developed based on the systematic selection of markers made by Liu et al., who reported 24 variants from eight genes, enabling the prediction of blue and brown eye colour with a prediction accuracy expressed by an AUC of 0.91 and 0.93, respectively [**122**]. AUC, which stands for area under the ROC (receiver operating characteristic) curve, describes the general performance of the model in such a way that 1 means perfect classification and 0.5 means random assignment to the phenotype categories. For forensic purposes, the number of markers from the originally identified 24 was restricted to the six with the largest effect [**98,122**]. The six crucial predictors included HERC2 rs12913832, OCA2 rs1800407, SLC24A4 rs12896399, SLC45A2 rs16891982, TYR rs1393350, and IRF4 rs12203592. The original IrisPlex method implements a multinomial logistic regression algorithm and a simple single base extension method based on SNaPshotminisequencing, which allows the PCR amplification and genotyping of several SNPs in a multiplex reaction. Importantly, the products of primer extension are analysed using capillary electrophoresis platforms, which are commonly used in human identification testing laboratories. Other tools based on other mathematical solutions were soon developed but, essentially, each of these algorithms relied on exploiting information in the HERC2-OCA2 gene complex. In general, these works were limited to the development of predictive algorithms using various sets of samples and mathematical approaches, but did not present specific tools for the collection of genetic data [**99,100,101,102,103,104**]. Notably, IrisPlex and other forensic methods of eye colour prediction can accurately predict blue and brown iris colours, but have difficulty with the prediction of intermediate eye colours [**3**]. Moreover, in some populations, the effect of sex was noted on prediction results [**123,124,125**].

The IrisPlex tool for the genotyping and prediction of eye colour evolved to HIrisPlex [**106**] and finally to the HIrisPlex-S tool [**109**], which were developed based on the same strategy as IrisPlex. The algorithm for hair colour prediction implemented in HIrisPlex was developed based on the investigation of a Polish population sample, which enabled the selection of 22 crucial SNPs from 11 genes for hair colour. The study showed a high level of accuracy for red and black hair colour prediction (AUC ~ 0.9) and a lower prediction accuracy for blond and brown hair colour (AUC ~ 0.8) [**126**]. The skin colour predictor was proposed by Walsh et al. after a systematic study of skin colour candidate variants in a sample of 2025 individuals from 31 worldwide populations. The algorithm predicted skin colour with very high accuracy, with an AUC = 0.97 for light skin colour, 0.83 dark, and 0.96 for dark-black skin colour [**127**]. Notably, it has been demonstrated that the original SNaPshot protocol can be replaced by the targeted massive parallel sequencing (MPS) method [**128**], and the HIrisPlex-S method was also adopted in a tool combining pigmentation prediction capability with ancestry inference developed by the VISAGE consortium [**129**]. Other studies also investigated the possibility of hair and skin colour prediction in the forensic field [**100,105,107,108,110**]. The Snipper Application suite deserves more attention because it provides an online tool that allows the performance of predictive calculations based on data generated by any genotyping method. The tool was originally developed for the statistical interpretation of data in ancestry inference studies, but a number of new functionalities have subsequently been added to enable the prediction of pigmentation and even age [**130**]. A more complete prediction of pigmentation will be provided by the developed algorithms for freckle prediction [**111,112**]. It is worth noting that the use of extended DNA variant sets for prediction has begun to be explored, which may lead to the development of next-generation prediction tools. For example, the previously described association work of Hysi et al. was extended to predictive modelling. Hair colour prediction was compared in two independent cohorts using prediction models based on the 258 associated SNPs and the original HIrisPlex method, and these new models outperformed the previous HIrisPlex model [**37**]. Further development of pigmentation predictors may also require the use of sex information, and age will naturally be needed for the final interpretation of the data [**37,123**]. This issue is also addressed later in the article, as sex in particular can be important for predicting other appearance traits.

3.2. Hair Loss

Numerous association studies conducted for MPB raised questions about the predictive ability of the discovered genetic variants. In 2015, a compact regression model was developed based on analysis of five SNPs from five genomic regions (Xq12, 20p11, EBF1, TARDBP, and HDAC9), trained and validated on >600 samples from six European populations [**113**]. The model was shown to enable the prediction of hair loss in Europeans at an acceptable level, but only in two extreme phenotype categories, i.e., young men with significant alopecia vs. older men without symptoms of alopecia with AUC of 0.76. In the same study, Marcińska et al. also pointed to the potential role of allelic heterogeneity in determining scalp hair loss. Expanding the number of DNA variants in both crucial regions, i.e., Xq12 and 20p11, improved the accuracy of prediction, suggesting that there might be more functional variants in these loci. The extended 20-SNP regression model predicted hair loss with an AUC of 0.66 in all samples of all age categories and had the highest AUC value for the age category of ≥50 years old (AUC = 0.76; sensitivity = 67.7%; specificity = 90%), where the sensitivity refers to the ability of the model to correctly classify individuals with the particular phenotype (here baldness), while the specificity refers to the ability of the model to correctly classify individuals without this phenotype [**113**].

Liu et al. conducted a parallel study on the prediction of MPB in >2700 Europeans and developed a 14-SNP model that was found to predict early-onset MPB cases with a cross-validated AUC of 0.74 [**114**]. The accuracy of hair loss prediction status in elderly and middle-aged individuals was lower, with an AUC of 0.69–0.71. In 2017, Hagenaars and colleagues developed a polygenic predictor based on the genome-wide data generated for a large cohort of 40,000 individuals and showed that it can discriminate individuals with no signs of hair loss from those with severe baldness, with an AUC = 0.78, sensitivity = 0.74, and specificity = 0.69 [**52**].

3.3. Hair Shape and Other Hair *Characteristics*

The first preliminary model for head hair shape was developed as a follow-up to the first GWA study conducted on hair characteristics [**58**], and included an analysis of three SNPs in three genes (TCHH, WNT10A, FRAS1), and was trained on data generated for 528 samples from Polish individuals [**115**]. The model was reported to predict straight hair with high accuracy but low specificity (cross-validated AUC = 0.622, sensitivity = 93.2%, specificity = 15.4%). The application of the model on an independent test set consisting of samples from six European populations and using a 65% probability threshold allowed for higher sensitivity (81.4%) and improved specificity (50.0%) of prediction, but at the same time with a very high rate of inconclusive results (66.9%). In 2018, a large-scale prediction study for hair shape prediction was conducted with more than 9600 samples used for predictor selection and model development and more than 2400 samples used for prediction model validation, collected from both European and non-European populations [**116**]. The binomial logistic regression model was developed to predict hair shape, defined as straight vs. non-straight, based on 32 informative SNPs from 26 loci.

The model was reported to explain ~12% of hair shape variation and can predict straight vs. non-straight hair in European populations with an accuracy of AUC of 0.66, a sensitivity of 84.1% and a specificity of 34.2%. It was shown that the same set of SNP markers can predict hair shape with significantly different accuracies in Europeans and non-Europeans. For non-European samples, the AUC value was 0.79, sensitivity = 82.9%, and specificity = 49.8%. The higher prediction accuracy obtained for non-European populations compared to Europeans is due to the effect of the EDAR gene, which has a significant effect on the determination of straight hair in non-European populations, primarily East Asian. In addition to the binomial model, a multinomial logistic regression model was developed to allow for a higher resolution of hair shape prediction, considering three categories—straight, wavy and curly—based on an analysis of 33 SNP positions.

There are few or no prediction studies of the remaining hair features. In 2016, Adhikari et al. predicted different hair traits using the GWAS data generated for Latin Americans and reported the highest accuracy of prediction for beard thickness and the lowest for hair greying, with ~18% and ~7% of the phenotypic variation explained by the associated SNPs, respectively [**40**]. Interestingly, for both of these traits, a large effect of age and sex on prediction was observed, explaining the additional ~11% and ~20% of the phenotypic variation, respectively, for beard thickness and greying. Age was found to be a main predictor of hair greying in a study conducted in 2020, explaining around 48% of the variation observed in hair greying in a cohort of 849 people from Poland [**66**]. A binary neural network model for greying vs. no greying prediction was developed in this study based on information relating to age, sex, and 10 SNPs selected using whole-exome sequencing data analysis (e.g., KIF1A rs59733750, SEMA4D rs45483393) and literature resources (IRF4 rs12203592, FGF5 rs7680591). The model achieved a high accuracy of prediction with a cross-validated AUC = 0.87 (sensitivity = 0.73; specificity = 0.85) but most of the prediction information was driven by age itself, while SNPs were found to explain merely ~7% of the variation in hair greying. As mentioned earlier, age is a very important factor in predicting hair loss. Sex and age were also shown to slightly improve the accuracy of prediction of hair shape [**116**].

This implies that there is a need to determine the sex and age of an individual from the analysed biological sample. Information on a person's sex is usually available in criminal investigations due to the inclusion of marker for the amelogenin gene located on the X and Y chromosome in standard STR DNA profiling, as previously mentioned, whereas age can be estimated via epigenetic analysis [**131**].

3.4. Human Stature

Efforts to predict human height using forensic methods have been few and have focused on creating algorithms that lack data collection capabilities. The causes derive from the constraints of DNA analysis technology and arise from the necessity to examine a multitude of DNA variations. Although the original GWAS scans for human height discovered 54 DNA variations that accounted for only 5% of the heritability, Aulchenko et al. conducted a test to determine if these variants could accurately predict extreme height. However, this turned out to be possible with only limited accuracy. Tall stature prediction was possible at AUC of 0.65, thus only moderately improving the accuracy resulting from a random hit (AUC = 0.5) [**117**]. Using the 180 height markers identified in the Lango Allen et al. paper improved the prediction of tall stature to AUC of 0.75 [**118**]. The study suggested the importance of allelic heterogeneity for the prediction of human stature. Further increasing the number of predictors to 697 reported in the paper by [**72**] enabled the prediction of tall stature with an AUC of 0.79 [**119**]. The possibilities of human height prediction have also been explored outside the forensic mainstream using a non-standard approach that has nevertheless yielded very promising results, enabling the prediction of the full range of human height at a good level of accuracy [**120**]. Based on the results obtained, the authors suggested changing the approach to phenotype prediction, pointing out the benefits of also including as predictors polymorphisms that do not show an association with a given trait, but only on the basis of the improved prediction accuracy obtained after their inclusion in the prediction model [**132**].

3.5. The Human Face

Creating a forensic drawing by following the directions provided by a witness in a criminal investigation is a longstanding method employed to ascertain the identity of the offender. Individuals identify one another by discerning the considerable diversity of face characteristics. Hence, possessing a comprehensive comprehension of the genetic aspects of human facial diversity and the ability to anticipate this intricate phenotypic is an exceptionally thrilling potential for forensic DNA intelligence. The limited extent of heritability elucidated for craniofacial variables does not bode well for the anticipation of human facial phenotypes. Nevertheless, attempts have been made to develop models that would allow the prediction of facial appearance. The proposed methods are based on the indirect prediction of facial phenotypes, with ancestry and sex prediction DNA data playing a key role in this regard. The method by Claes et al. implements a bootstrapped response-based imputation modelling that makes use of information on genomic ancestry and sex first to create a sketch called a base-face. At the second stage, the information in 24 SNPs associated with facial variation is used to improve the prediction outcome [**82**]. A similar strategy was proposed by Lippert et al., who used the whole genome sequencing data to gain information about the sex and ancestry proportions of the individual [**121**]. The data on genetic face predictors did not improve facial appearance predictions, but the study showed a positive effect on the prediction of age and body mass index. The genetic prediction of facial features was also explored by Qiao at el., who developed a quantitative model based on multiple SNP loci and tried to simulate 3D face models. The study suggests that epistasis is part of the genetic architecture of facial features and concludes that the model developed should be treated as an exploratory basis for future, more advanced predictive models [**93**].

4. APPEARANCE PREDICTION IN THE ERA OF BIG DATA

4.1. Appearance Trait Predicition as a Supervised Learning Task

The use of DNA markers to predict human externally visible characteristics can be viewed as a supervised learning problem. In this problem, the appearance trait being considered is the response variable, while the genetic markers serve as explanatory variables, also known as features or predictors. Supervised learning models are trained using a dataset that contains observations with known values for the target variable. Three distinct tasks can be identified based on the type of the target variable: regression (for a quantitative characteristic, such as human height), binary classification (for a binary trait, such as the presence of freckles), and multi-class classification (for a categorical trait, such as eye color).The specificity of the problem and the greatest challenge lies in the large number of potential features (genetic markers), which may significantly exceed the number of observations in the training data. Due to this, the use of traditional models and estimation methods (such as the maximum likelihood method in logistic regression) is not feasible. The simplest solution is to use some initial filtering method to reduce the total number of markers. However, simple filters only assess the marginal dependence between the variable and the trait; they may exclude variables that are potentially useful for the model, for example, variables that contribute by interacting with already selected ones. Therefore, there is a need to apply the estimation methods as well as feature selection approaches specially tailored to high-dimensional settings. This is one of the greatest challenges in designing learning models for appearance trait prediction.

Finally, it is important to note that traditional genome-wide association studies focus on detecting the genetic variants associated with the trait with high statistical confidence, which, in particular, includes controlling the probability of at least one rejection via multiple-testing procedures. When the prediction is the main task, the paradigm shift is needed, because focusing on the accuracy of the model becomes the main objective [**133**]. This approach requires the careful selection of variables. On one hand, unlike in GWAS, it is allowed to include a certain number of non-significant variables in the model, since the excessive pruning of SNPs, which may result in the discarding of some significant variables, can negatively affect prediction accuracy [**132**]. On the other hand, including too many spurious variables may cause the overfitting of the model and decrease its accuracy [**134**].

4.2. Linear Easily Interpretable Models

The linear model and its generalizations are highly effective methods for predicting appearance traits, despite their simplicity. The theory [135] and empirical results [136,137] indicate that in several instances, the relationship between the trait and genetic markers can be effectively represented using linear models. Multiple studies suggest that simpler models, such as ensemble approaches or neural networks, often perform equally well or even better than more sophisticated models [120,132,135,136,137], as they are less prone to overfitting. A distinct advantage of the linear models is their interpretability; the parameter value indicates how the given variable influences the dependent variable for fixed values of the remaining variables. Within the linear models, there are many methods of parameter estimation, among which the regularised (also known as penalised) maximum likelihood methods play the most prominent role in modern genetic data analysis. First, for the regularisation methods, there are theoretical guarantees that the solution of the related optimisation problem exists and is unique, even for a high-dimensional setting. Second, some forms of the regularisation, such as lasso, ensure the sparsity of the vector of estimated coefficients, meaning that a majority of coefficients will be zero. Under some unfortunately stringent conditions, this majority will correspond to non-significant variables in the model. Thus, the selected regularisation techniques can be seen as methods of simultaneous parameter estimation and feature selection. Below, we discuss the three most important generalised linear models (linear regression, logistic regression, and multinomial regression) and the methods of parameter estimation within them.

In the case of the quantitative trait, it is natural to consider the linear regression model, which assumes that for an i-th observation, we have $yi=\beta 0+xTi\beta+\epsilon i$,where yi is the value of the target variable, $\beta 0$ is an intercept, β=($\beta 1$,...,βp)T,..., is the coefficients vector, ϵi is noise, and xi=(xi,1,...,xi,p)T is a vector of features. Coordinates xi,1,...,xi,p,1,..., denote the genetic markers for the i-th observation. They can be coded numerically as 0, 1, or 2, where 0 indicates the homozygosity of the major allele, 1 the heterozygosity and 2 the homozygosity of the minor allele. In the penalised least squares method, we solve:

$$\hat{\beta}_0, \hat{\beta} = \arg \min_{b_0 \in R, b \in R^p} \sum_{i=1}^{n} (y_i - b_0 - x_i^T b)^2 + \lambda \mathrm{pen}(b),$$

where λ>00 is the regularisation parameter that controls the penalty strength and pen(b)pen is the penalty. For example, in the lasso method, pen(b)=||b||1=Σpj=1|bj|pen, we discuss other choices below. In the case of a binary trait, the logistic regression model is usually used in which the posterior probability is modelled as:

$$P(y_i = 1 | x_i) = \frac{\exp(\beta_0 + x_i^T \beta)}{1 + \exp(\beta_0 + x_i^T \beta)}$$

and parameters are estimated using the penalised maximum likelihood method:

$$\hat{\beta}_0, \hat{\beta} = \arg \max_{b_0 \in R, b \in R^p} \sum_{i=1}^{n} [y_i \log(\sigma(b_0 + x_i^T b)) + (1 - y_i) \log(1 - \sigma(b_0 + x_i^T b))] + \lambda \mathrm{pen}(b),$$

where $\sigma(s)$=exp(s)/(1+exp(s)) is the sigmoid logistic function. The multinomial logistic regression (MLR) extends the logistic model when the number of categories of the dependent variable K>2. This is the most commonly used model, as usually the considered trait has multiple categories (eye colour, skin colour, hair type, etc.). The posterior probability for the *k*-th category is:

$$P(y_i = k|x_i) = \frac{\exp(\beta_{0k} + x_i^T \beta_k)}{1 + \sum_{k=1}^{K-1} \exp(\beta_{0k} + x_i^T \beta_k)},$$

for *k*=1,...,*K*−1,=1,..., where *βk* is a coefficients vector corresponding to the *k*-th category and *P*(*yi*=*K*|*xi*)=1-$\sum_{k=1}^{K-1} P(y_i = k|x_i)$ In this model, we have *K*×*p* parameters, which are estimated using the penalised maximum likelihood method. The interaction terms *xi*,×*xi*,*k* can be included in the above models, at the cost of a significant increase in the number of parameters. In addition to linear models, additive models are an important class of models in which, instead of the linear combination $\beta_0 + x_i^T \beta$, the combination of *M* non-linear base functions $\beta_0 + \sum_{m=1}^{M} \beta_m h_m(x_i)$is used. In this group, the notable approach is the MARS method (multivariate adaptive regression splines; see Section 9 in [**134**]) in which the functions *hmh* are constructed as products of so-called hinge functions in a forward stage-wise manner. Importantly, the functions *hmh* in MARS can capture non-linear dependencies as well as interactions between variables. Note that the considered model is linear in predictors *hm*(*xi*)*h* and is an important example of the transformation of predictors method.

Regarding regularisation in the above models, the lasso penalty pen(*b*)=||*b*||1pen is the most popular choice, which was successfully used in appearance trait prediction, e.g., in prediction of human height [**120**] or eye colour [**137**]. The lasso method selects features with non-zero estimated coefficients, and the number selected depends on parameter *λ*>0. A small value of *λ* will result in a larger number of features included in the model, whereas for a larger *λ*, we obtain a more parsimonious model. The optimal value of *λ* is chosen using cross-validation or by minimising the prediction error with a validation set. An alternative to the lasso is ridge penalty pen(*b*)=||*b*||2pen which, instead of performing feature selection, only shrinks the estimated parameters towards zero. The ridge penalty facilitates a reduction in the variance of the estimators, especially when the variables are highly correlated, and thus may yield an even higher accuracy for the prediction than the lasso method.

Although the lasso method has many excellent properties and high predictive power, in recent years, several modifications have been proposed in statistical and machine learning literature. For example, it has been noticed that the lasso method produces biased estimators for truly significant variables with large coefficients, and this bias does not necessarily disappear for a large sample size. To overcome this drawback, non-convex penalties, such as SCAD (smoothly clipped absolute deviation) [**138**] or MCP (minimax concave penalty) [**139**] have been proposed and effective algorithms for solving the related optimisation problems have been developed [**140**]. Another important line of research is focused on controlling the false discovery rate (FDR) (the expected fraction of non-significant variables that are selected for the model) instead of the much stronger control of probability that at least one non-significant variable is selected (familywise error rate). Unfortunately, the standard lasso does not control the FDR, which means that, among the selected variables, we can expect a significant portion of spurious variables. The problem is exacerbated by the fact that there is no known way of testing the significance of a specific feature based on its estimated lasso coefficient that would allow the application of one of multiple testing approaches, such as the Benjamini-Hochberg procedure [**141**], to control the FDR.

A notable alternative approach is the knockoff filter method [**142**]. It can be seen as a refinement of randomisation methods [**143,144**] that, by permuting the values of a studied predictor (which renders the resulting artificial predictor non-significant), creates a benchmark situation in which its usefulness can be checked. The basic idea in [**142**] is to construct extra variables called 'knockoff' variables, which are noisy copies of original ones but which have a certain similar correlation structure, as they allow for FDR control when standard variable selection methods (such as lasso) are applied. Namely, the lasso method is run using both the original variables and knockoff variables (thus there are $2 \times p 2 \times$ variables in total). The original variable is deemed useful when its pertaining estimated coefficient is significantly larger than that of the corresponding knockoff.

The nonconvex penalties, as well as the randomisation methods, seem to be worthwhile alternatives to the lasso method for predicting human traits. The above methods are implemented, e.g., in R software, see packages glmnet (lasso and ridge), ncvreg (MCP, SCAD), knockoff (knockoff filter), and earth (MARS method).

4.3. Complex Black-Box Models

Black-box models are a type of predictive models that may capture intricate relationships between explanatory variables and the dependent variable, including interaction terms. They have the potential to attain higher accuracy compared to linear models. The primary constraints include the significant computational intricacy, the challenge in comprehending the model, and the requirement for parameter adjustment. Ensemble methods and neural networks are the dominant techniques in this group. The former are usually based on decision trees [**145**] and overcome two limitations of single trees: their instability and tendency to overfitting. The simplest approach is bagging (bootstrap aggregating) [**146**] in which each tree in the ensemble is trained using a bootstrap sample, i.e., a sample drawn with replacements from the original training data. In order to classify a new instance, each decision tree provides the classification for the input data. The majority vote classification is then chosen as the final prediction. In the case of regression, the predictions from individual tress are averaged. Another important class of models are random subspace methods (RSM), in which each base classifier is learnt using the randomly selected subset of variables [**147,148**]. One of the most successful and commonly used methods is random forest (RF), which can be seen as a combination of bagging and RSM. The RF uses a modified tree learning algorithm that selects, at each candidate split in the learning process, a random subset of the features of size m, where m is a hyper-parameter. Making m smaller helps to avoid the danger of overfitting. Nowadays, the most powerful class of ensemble methods are gradient boosting (GB) algorithms (Section 10 in [**134**]). In GB, the subsequent models $F1(x)$,...,$FM(x)$ are learned sequentially, and the last model $FM(x)$ serves as a final model. The main advantage of GB algorithms is that they are able to optimise different loss functions, depending on the considered task. The classifier in step m+1 (usually a decision tree) is learnt using current training data, in which the residuals from the previous model are treated as the current target variable (where the squared loss is considered, and the residuals are yi-$Fm(xi)$. The residuals are related to the so-called functional gradient of the loss function and, therefore, GB methods can be seen as gradient descent algorithms, which take steps in the direction of the steepest descent and converge to the minimum of the loss function. The common property of all boosting algorithms is that the current model zooms in on samples where its predecessor failed. Usually, some regularisation techniques are used in boosting algorithms to prevent overfitting. There are many versions of gradient boosting algorithms, among which XGB (extreme gradient boosting) is considered to be one of the most powerful variants [**149**]. The ensemble methods are controlled by different parameters, whose optimal choice may significantly improve the performance: the number of trees, the size of the random subspace (in RF and RSM), as well as the regularisation and pruning parameters.

The ensemble methods described above (RF and XGB) are often used to assess the importance of the features. The simplest approach is based on a permutation scheme and is very similar to the randomisation feature selection described above. The first method (called mean decrease accuracy) involves fitting two ensemble models (e.g., RF or XGB): the first is based on the original training data and the second is based on training data in which the values of the j-th variable are randomly permuted. The variable importance measure for the j-th variable is defined as the difference in accuracies corresponding to these two models. A large value of the difference indicates the significance of the variable. The second measure (called mean decrease impurity) is based on observing how well the given variable separates the classes. The Boruta algorithm [**150**], based on the above two measures, contains a testing procedure that allows the rejecting of the noisy variables. Other more sophisticated variable importance measures are also advocated for, e.g., the MCFS method [**151**], in which one of its major advantages is that the predictive power of each tree in the ensemble is taken into account in the measure definition.

The second important group of black-box models is artificial neural networks (ANN) [**152**]. The latest advances in computational and optimisation methods have made it possible to train networks with very complex architectures corresponding to large families of functions, such as convolution networks (in image recognition) and recurrent networks (in text analysis). The deep networks used today may consist of hundreds of hidden layers and can model very complex dependencies [**153**]. In appearance trait prediction, the feed-forward neural network is usually used. In such networks, the input signal (the vector of features for the *i*-th observation) is transmitted from the input layer to the output layer, which yields the prediction of the response. The hidden layers consist of artificial neurons in which the linear combination of the signals from the previous layers is computed and the signal is passed through the activation function as the input for the following layers. The models are trained using gradient algorithms (the ADAM algorithm [**154**] is now the state-of-the-art method) and the back-propagation algorithm is used to effectively compute the gradient of the considered risk function [**153**]. A number of parameters need to be tuned in ANN, such as the number of layers, the number of neurons in each layer, and the value of the learning rate. Other spectacular advances with ANN, such as variational autoencoders (VAE), which enable latent feature analysis (see [**155**]), are of potential interest in appearance trait prediction. For the methods described here, see R packages randomForest, xgboost, rmcfs, Boruta, and tensorflow.

4.4. Feature Selection

Feature selection is a crucial aspect in constructing predictive models, as it minimizes overfitting and enables the identification of the relationship between variables. Specifically, it helps to identify the qualities that have an impact on the target variable. In the aforementioned models, the process of selecting features is typically incorporated inside the learning algorithms. In linear models and neural networks, selection is accomplished through regularization, while in tree-based approaches, the appropriate characteristics are chosen during the construction of the tree. Nevertheless, incorporating an excessive number of potential characteristics can substantially escalate the computational expense of fitting the model. Therefore, it is frequently necessary in practical situations to employ a rapid initial filtering technique. Methods rooted in information theory have become increasingly prominent in the machine learning field in recent years [156]. These models are characterized by their speed, lack of reliance on pre-defined structures, and their ability to identify non-linear relationships and interactions among variables, while also considering redundancies. The fundamental measure employed in these strategies is mutual information (MI):

$$I(Y, X_k) = \sum_{x,y} P(X_k = x, Y = y) \log \frac{P(X_k = x, Y = y)}{P(X_k = x)P(Y = y)}$$

which is a non-parametric measure of dependence between some feature Xk and target variable Y. Moreover, analogously defined, the conditional mutual information $(Y,Xk|Z)$ quantifies the dependence strength between Xk and Y given the possibly multivariate variable Z. It is commonly used in feature selection of a new predictor Xk when Z consists of predictors already chosen. Another important quantity used in genome-wise interaction studies (GWIS) is interaction information (II):

$$II(Y, X_j, X_k) = I((X_k, X_j), Y) - I(Y, X_k) - I(Y, X_j)$$

which measures the interaction strength between Xk and Xj for the prediction of Y. The positive value of II indicates a synergistic interaction, whereas a negative value indicates redundancy. II has been successfully used in many genetic studies to detect epistasis [**157,158**], and also in the context of appearance trait prediction, such as human pigmentation [**159**]. It has been shown that the methods based on II are able to detect interactions that remain undetected by the logistic regression model [**160**].

The existing filters based on MI are forward sequential procedures that, in each step, add a candidate feature Xk to the set of already selected features S. The quality of a candidate feature can be assessed using various criteria, and the representative one is CIFE (conditional infomax feature extraction) [**156,161**]. It adds candidate Xk, being the maximizer of the CIFE takes into account the marginal dependence between a candidate feature and the target variable, as well as interactions between the candidate feature and the previously selected features. Methods taking into account higher order interactions are also considered [**162**]. In practice, it is important to decide at which step to stop the procedure of adding new candidate variables, with the possible solution based on the approximate distribution of the criterion function when a candidate feature is not significant, as proposed in [**163**].

5. THE NEED FOR A HIGH-THROUGHPUT, LOW-INPUT DNA SEQUENCING METHOD IN FORENSIC SCIENCE

The limitations of DNA sequencing technologies used in the forensic field are increasingly problematic because they are hindering the implementation of new methods that can improve law enforcement and justice, and which are therefore important for the safety of society. The lack of a suitable method for generating large amounts of SNP data from degraded DNA, validated for use in forensics, was considered to be a barrier to the forensic implementation of investigative genetic genealogy, an approach that was very successful at solving a number of criminal cases [**1,164**]. Such a method also seems to be essential for developing next-generation tools for the DNA-based prediction of appearance traits, which requires information derived from hundreds or even thousands of SNPs. It may be argued that the optimal method for all the applications developed for forensic DNA intelligence would be whole-genome sequencing (WGS). Notably, WGS that uses high-throughput methods (massively parallel sequencing) has revolutionised the studies of ancient DNA and enabled a better understanding of human evolutionary history. Similarities between forensic genetics and palaeogenetics, especially in terms of the specificity of research material with a high content of inhibitors and small amounts of highly fragmented DNA, and the enormous success of palaeogenetics in the analysis of such samples, prompts a closer look at the methods developed in this field. Several technological advancements were crucial for the effective analysis of ancient DNA, including the very efficient extraction of short ancient DNA fragments, the implementation of the uracil-DNA glycosylase (UDG) protocol for the selective removal of damaged sections of ancient DNA, improved protocols for library preparation, and, finally, progress has also been made in high-throughput DNA sequencing [**165,166**]. The major advantage for ancient DNA research brought about by high-throughput sequencing technology is the ability to sequence very short DNA fragments. Research material analysed in forensic DNA laboratories is not as degraded as ancient samples, and current DNA extraction methods are efficient and effective at removing inhibitors. Therefore, the transfer of DNA analysis protocols from palaeogenomics to forensic genomics should perhaps primarily focus on library preparation methods that work well with low-input DNA. Standard library preparation protocols are optimised for large amounts of DNA and perform poorly in the case of samples containing degraded DNA. However, a number of modified protocols have been proposed to reduce the requirement for DNA inputs to be at subnanogram quantities.

One category of protocols involves library construction based on double-stranded DNA. A first protocol was described by Meyer and Kircher in 2010, and this was laborious and had limitations that resulted in the losses of ancient DNA sequences due to incompatible adapter combinations and three purification steps prior to amplification [**167**]. Double-stranded library preparation protocols involve the blunt-end repair of the degraded DNA fragments, the non-directional blunt-end ligation of two adapters and the fill-in of the nicks formatted between adapters and the DNA fragment [**168**]. A more advanced alternative of double stranded library preparation method is the protocol proposed by Carøe et al., named blunt-end-single-tube. As the name suggests, the protocol is carried out in a single tube and relies on heat denaturation instead of purification between the subsequent steps of end-repair, the ligation of double-stranded adapters to the 5′ ends, and adapter fill-in [**169**].

The second approach for library preparation from samples containing low amounts of degraded DNA is particularly interesting, as it implies a process of library construction based on single-stranded DNA, allowing the use of DNA that was preserved in a single-stranded state and which is considered to be more efficient compared to double-stranded approaches. The original protocol for single-stranded library preparation, although it recovered more endogenous DNA, was very expensive and laborious [**170**]. However, the protocol evolved to a simplified version proposed in Gansauge et al., 2017 [**171**]. This is a method that involves the dephosphorylation of the template DNA, the splinted ligation of a biotinylated adapter to the 3′ end, bonding to streptavidin beads, annealing an extension primer to allow the synthesis of a second strand, and the ligation of the 5′ end of a double-stranded adapter to the 3′ end of the newly synthesized strand. The authors also proposed an automated version of this protocol [**172**]. An interesting modification of the single-strand library preparation method was recently proposed by Kapp et al. (2021). The advantage of the method, named the Santa Cruz Reaction, relies on simplicity and cost effectiveness. The method converts single-stranded DNA into sequencing libraries using a single enzymatic reaction, enabling the simultaneous directional splinted ligation of Illumina's P5 and P7 adapters [**173**]. Technological improvements in ancient DNA analysis have resulted in significant progress in sequencing efficiency. Whole-genome data from ancient hominin material were generated with an average sequence coverage of only 1.3-fold in 2010 [**174**] and 30-fold in 2012 [**175**]. The usefulness of these protocols was also confirmed in clinical research of problematic biological material, including formalin-fixed paraffin embedded tissues [**176**]. The future will show whether the protocols developed in palaeogenomics can be easily transferred to forensic genomics. This would undoubtedly be extremely helpful for the further development of forensic DNA intelligence methods.

6. AT A GLANCE

Studies on the genetic structure of natural variation in the physical characteristics of humans are expanding in scope and encompassing many human populations. Forensic research places significant emphasis on the genetic prediction of physical appearance attributes, however the current technologies are primarily focused on less intricate traits, particularly pigmentation. Significantly, the forensic community has successfully applied predictive methods in ancient DNA research. These methods have been utilized in the field of molecular anthropology [177,178,179] and in the identification of historical figures [180,181,182]. This serves as additional proof that molecular anthropology and forensic genetics share many similarities.

Commercial kits have incorporated several DNA-based prognostic capabilities that were created by the forensic community. The renowned ForenSeq kit enables the examination of HIrisPlex SNPs, therefore facilitating the estimation of eye and hair color [183]. The HIrisPlex-S variations can be found in the Ion AmpliSeq™ PhenoTrivium Panel [184]. Accurately anticipating dependable outlines in forensic science is greatly sought after during the investigative phase. Consequently, there have been accounts of law enforcement agencies employing private firms that specialize in this field, specifically for the purpose of forecasting face appearances. ParabonNanoLabs offers the Snapshot Forensic DNA Phenotyping System, which promises to accurately predict genetic ancestry, eye color, hair color, skin color, freckling, and face shape [185]. Additional research provides the chance to gain a deeper comprehension of the evolutionary and genetic foundation of human physical characteristics. The potential for future research on the heritability of complex traits and the investigation of the significance of uncommon DNA variants, as well as the interactions between genes of the second and higher orders, appears intriguing. Understanding heredity will enhance the accuracy of predicting physical traits. Without a doubt, the advancement of next-generation prediction techniques necessitates enhancements in the technology of DNA polymorphism analysis employed in forensic investigations. These changes must involve the utilization of larger sets of predictors and more advanced statistical and machine learning algorithms. To accurately interpret the results, it is essential to possess knowledge about the individual's age, which can be most effectively ascertained by the examination of DNA methylation. Nevertheless, the analysis of DNA methylation necessitates substantial quantities of DNA. Consequently, in the pursuit of investigating biological traces for intelligence-related objectives, it would be advantageous to cultivate more discerning techniques for predicting age. The adoption of novel predictive algorithms will also demand answers to key ethical problems emerging from the use of high-throughput DNA sequencing tools.

7. CONCISE SUMMARY

The concept of forensic DNA intelligence involves extracting any pertinent information from genomic data to assist in directing the inquiry. The indications of the phenotype that can be observed externally are very significant in practical terms. The substantial heritability of the physical phenotype implies that genetic information can be readily anticipated, however this has only been achievable with qualities that include fewer polygenes. Forensic experts have created predictive tools using DNA analysis techniques that focus on a small set of crucial indicators and utilize targeted large parallel sequencing. To accurately forecast the genetics of various appearance traits, it is necessary to utilize large datasets and advanced machine learning techniques. An important obstacle in the development of universal genomic prediction algorithms will be the acquisition of adequately extensive data sets. These should be generated utilizing whole-genome sequencing technologies in order to facilitate the detection of uncommon DNA variants associated with the determination of physical traits. The accuracy of the forensic sketch produced from the DNA data is contingent upon the incorporation of an age variable. However, the prediction of this can be achieved by analyzing epigenetic data. A significant constraint that hinders the widespread adoption of whole-genome techniques in forensics is the sluggish advancement in the creation and application of high-throughput, low DNA input sequencing technology. The case of palaeoanthropology indicates that similar techniques may potentially be applied in the field of forensics.

REFERENCES

1. Kling, D.; Phillips, C.; Kennett, D.; Tillmar, A. Investigative genetic genealogy: Current methods, knowledge and practice. Forensic Sci. Int. Genet. **2021**, 52, 102474. **[Google Scholar] [CrossRef]**
2. Phillips, C. Forensic genetic analysis of bio-geographical ancestry. Forensic Sci. Int. Genet. **2015**, 18, 49–65. **[Google Scholar] [CrossRef] [PubMed]**
3. Kayser, M. Forensic DNA Phenotyping: Predicting human appearance from crime scene material for investigative purposes. Forensic Sci. Int. Genet. **2015**, 18, 33–48. **[Google Scholar] [CrossRef]**
4. Lee, H.Y.; Lee, S.D.; Shin, K.J. Forensic DNA methylation profiling from evidence material for investigative leads. BMB Rep. **2016**, 49, 359–369. **[Google Scholar] [CrossRef] [PubMed] [Green Version]**
5. Polderman, T.J.; Benyamin, B.; de Leeuw, C.A.; Sullivan, P.F.; van Bochoven, A.; Visscher, P.M.; Posthuma, D. Meta-analysis of the heritability of human traits based on fifty years of twin studies. Nat. Genet. **2015**, 47, 702–709. **[Google Scholar] [CrossRef] [Green Version]**
6. Botstein, D.; Risch, N. Discovering genotypes underlying human phenotypes: Past successes for mendelian disease, future approaches for complex disease. Nat. Genet. **2003**, 33, 228–237. **[Google Scholar] [CrossRef]**
7. Visscher, P.M.; Brown, M.A.; McCarthy, M.I.; Yang, J. Five years of GWAS discovery. Am. J. Hum. Genet. **2012**, 90, 7–24. **[Google Scholar] [CrossRef] [PubMed] [Green Version]**
8. Uffelmann, E.; Huang, Q.Q.; Munung, N.S.; DeVries, J.; Okada, Y.; Martin, A.R.; Martin, H.C.; Lappalainen, T.; Posthuma, D. Genome-wide association studies. Nat. Rev. Methods Primers **2021**, 1, 59. **[Google Scholar] [CrossRef]**
9. Clark, P.; Stark, A.E.; Walsh, R.J.; Jardine, R.; Martin, N.G. A twin study of skin reflectance. Ann. Hum. Biol. **1981**, 8, 529–541. **[Google Scholar] [CrossRef] [PubMed] [Green Version]**

10. Lin, B.D.; Mbarek, H.; Willemsen, G.; Dolan, C.V.; Fedko, I.O.; Abdellaoui, A.; De Geus, E.J.; Boomsma, D.I.; Hottenga, J.-J. Heritability and Genome-Wide Association Studies for Hair Color in a Dutch Twin Family Based Sample. Genes **2015**, 6, 559–576. **[Google Scholar] [CrossRef] [Green Version]**
11. Bito, L.Z.; Matheny, A.; Cruickshanks, K.J.; Nondahl, D.M.; Carino, O.B. Eye Color Changes Past Early Childhood: The Louisville Twin Study. Arch. Ophthalmol. **1997**, 115, 659–663. **[Google Scholar] [CrossRef]**
12. Eiberg, H.; Mohr, J. Assignment of genes coding for brown eye colour (BEY2) and brown hair colour (HCL3) on chromosome 15q. Eur. J. Hum. Genet. **1996**, 4, 237–241. **[Google Scholar] [CrossRef] [PubMed]**
13. Rebbeck, T.R.; Kanetsky, P.A.; Walker, A.H.; Holmes, R.; Halpern, A.C.; Schuchter, L.M.; Elder, D.E.; Guerry, D. P gene as an inherited biomarker of human eye color. Cancer Epidemiol. Biomark. Prev. **2002**, 11, 782–784. **[Google Scholar]**
14. Frudakis, T.; Thomas, M.; Gaskin, Z.; Venkateswarlu, K.; Chandra, K.S.; Ginjupalli, S.; Gunturi, S.; Natrajan, S.; Ponnuswamy, V.K.; Ponnuswamy, K.N. Sequences associated with human iris pigmentation. Genetics **2003**, 165, 2071–2083. **[Google Scholar] [CrossRef] [PubMed]**
15. Duffy, D.L.; Montgomery, G.W.; Chen, W.; Zhao, Z.Z.; Le, L.; James, M.R.; Hayward, N.K.; Martin, N.G.; Sturm, R.A. A three-single-nucleotide polymorphism haplotype in intron 1 of OCA2 explains most human eye-color variation. Am. J. Hum. Genet. **2007**, 80, 241–252. **[Google Scholar] [CrossRef] [PubMed] [Green Version]**
16. Branicki, W.; Brudnik, U.; Kupiec, T.; Wolańska-Nowak, P.; Szczerbińska, A.; Wojas-Pelc, A. Association of polymorphic sites in the OCA2 gene with eye colour using the tree scanning method. Ann. Hum. Genet. **2008**, 72, 184–192. **[Google Scholar] [CrossRef]**
17. Sulem, P.; Gudbjartsson, D.F.; Stacey, S.N.; Helgason, A.; Rafnar, T.; Magnusson, K.P.; Manolescu, A.; Karason, A.; Palsson, A.; Thorleifsson, G.; et al. Genetic determinants of hair, eye and skin pigmentation in Europeans. Nat. Genet. **2007**, 39, 1443–1452. **[Google Scholar] [CrossRef]**
18. Sturm, R.A.; Duffy, D.L.; Zhao, Z.Z.; Leite, F.P.; Stark, M.S.; Hayward, N.K.; Martin, N.G.; Montgomery, G.W. A single SNP in an evolutionary conserved region within intron 86 of the HERC2 gene determines human blue-brown eye color. Am. J. Hum. Genet. **2008**, 82, 424–431. **[Google Scholar] [CrossRef] [Green Version]**
19. Eiberg, H.; Troelsen, J.; Nielsen, M.; Mikkelsen, A.; Mengel-From, J.; Kjaer, K.W.; Hansen, L. Blue eye color in humans may be caused by a perfectly

associated founder mutation in a regulatory element located within the HERC2 gene inhibiting OCA2 expression. Hum. Genet. **2008**, 123, 177–187. **[Google Scholar] [CrossRef]**

20. Visser, M.; Kayser, M.; Grosveld, F.; Palstra, R.J. Genetic variation in regulatory DNA elements: The case of OCA2 transcriptional regulation. Pigment Cell Melanoma Res. **2014**, 27, 169–177. **[Google Scholar] [CrossRef] [PubMed]**
21. Valverde, P.; Healy, E.; Jackson, I.; Rees, J.L.; Thody, A.J. Variants of the melanocyte-stimulating hormone receptor gene are associated with red hair and fair skin in humans. Nat. Genet. **1995**, 11, 328–330. **[Google Scholar] [CrossRef] [PubMed]**
22. Rees, J.L. Genetics of hair and skin color. Annu. Rev. Genet. **2003**, 37, 67–90. **[Google Scholar] [CrossRef] [PubMed]**
23. Flanagan, N.; Healy, E.; Ray, A.; Philips, S.; Todd, C.; Jackson, I.J.; Birch-Machin, M.A.; Rees, J.L. Pleiotropic effects of the melanocortin 1 receptor (MC1R) gene on human pigmentation. Hum. Mol. Genet. **2000**, 9, 2531–2537. **[Google Scholar] [CrossRef] [PubMed] [Green Version]**
24. Bastiaens, M.; terHuurne, J.; Gruis, N.; Bergman, W.; Westendorp, R.; Vermeer, B.J.; Bouwes Bavinck, J.N. The melanocortin-1-receptor gene is the major freckle gene. Hum. Mol. Genet. **2001**, 10, 1701–1708. **[Google Scholar] [CrossRef] [Green Version]**
25. Han, J.; Kraft, P.; Nan, H.; Guo, Q.; Chen, C.; Qureshi, A.; Hankinson, S.E.; Hu, F.B.; Duffy, D.L.; Zhao, Z.Z.; et al. A genome-wide association study identifies novel alleles associated with hair color and skin pigmentation. PLoS Genet. **2008**, 4, e1000074. **[Google Scholar] [CrossRef]**
26. Manolio, T.A.; Collins, F.S.; Cox, N.J.; Goldstein, D.B.; Hindorff, L.A.; Hunter, D.J.; McCarthy, M.I.; Ramos, E.M.; Cardon, L.R.; Chakravarti, A.; et al. Finding the missing heritability of complex diseases. Nature **2009**, 461, 747–753. **[Google Scholar] [CrossRef] [PubMed] [Green Version]**
27. Nelson, R.M.; Pettersson, M.E.; Carlborg, Ö. A century after Fisher: Time for a new paradigm in quantitative genetics. Trends Genet. **2013**, 29, 669–676. **[Google Scholar] [CrossRef]**
28. Simcoe, M.; Valdes, A.; Liu, F.; Furlotte, N.A.; Evans, D.M.; Hemani, G.; Ring, S.M.; Smith, G.D.; Duffy, D.L.; Zhu, G.; et al. Genome-wide association study in almost 195,000 individuals identifies 50 previously unidentified genetic loci for eye color. Sci. Adv. **2021**, 7, eabd1239. **[Google Scholar] [CrossRef] [PubMed]**
29. Norton, H.L. The color of normal: How a Eurocentric focus erases pigmentation complexity. Am. J. Hum. Biol. **2021**, 33, e23554. **[Google Scholar] [CrossRef]**

30. Lamason, R.L.; Mohideen, M.A.; Mest, J.R.; Wong, A.C.; Norton, H.L.; Aros, M.C.; Jurynec, M.J.; Mao, X.; Humphreville, V.R.; Humbert, J.E.; et al. SLC24A5, a putative cation exchanger, affects pigmentation in zebrafish and humans. Science **2005**, 310, 1782–1786. **[Google Scholar] [CrossRef] [Green Version]**

31. Liu, F.; Visser, M.; Duffy, D.L.; Hysi, P.G.; Jacobs, L.C.; Lao, O.; Zhong, K.; Walsh, S.; Chaitanya, L.; Wollstein, A.; et al. Genetics of skin color variation in Europeans: Genome-wide association studies with functional follow-up. Hum. Genet. **2015**, 134, 823–835. **[Google Scholar] [CrossRef] [Green Version]**

32. Sulem, P.; Gudbjartsson, D.F.; Stacey, S.N.; Helgason, A.; Rafnar, T.; Jakobsdottir, M.; Steinberg, S.; Gudjonsson, S.A.; Palsson, A.; Thorleifsson, G.; et al. Two newly identified genetic determinants of pigmentation in Europeans. Nat. Genet. **2008**, 40, 835–837. **[Google Scholar] [CrossRef] [PubMed]**

33. Edwards, M.; Bigham, A.; Tan, J.; Li, S.; Gozdzik, A.; Ross, K.; Jin, L.; Parra, E.J. Association of the OCA2 polymorphism His615Arg with melanin content in east Asian populations: Further evidence of convergent evolution of skin pigmentation. PLoS Genet. **2010**, 6, e1000867. **[Google Scholar] [CrossRef] [Green Version]**

34. Stokowski, R.P.; Pant, P.V.; Dadd, T.; Fereday, A.; Hinds, D.A.; Jarman, C.; Filsell, W.; Ginger, R.S.; Green, M.R.; van der Ouderaa, F.J.; et al. A genomewide association study of skin pigmentation in a South Asian population. Am. J. Hum. Genet. **2007**, 81, 1119–1132. **[Google Scholar] [CrossRef] [Green Version]**

35. Crawford, N.G.; Kelly, D.E.; Hansen, M.E.B.; Beltrame, M.H.; Fan, S.; Bowman, S.L.; Jewett, E.; Ranciaro, A.; Thompson, S.; Lo, Y.; et al. Loci associated with skin pigmentation identified in African populations. Science **2017**, 358, eaan8433. **[Google Scholar] [CrossRef] [PubMed] [Green Version]**

36. Martin, A.R.; Lin, M.; Granka, J.M.; Myrick, J.W.; Liu, X.; Sockell, A.; Atkinson, E.G.; Werely, C.J.; Möller, M.; Sandhu, M.S.; et al. An Unexpectedly Complex Architecture for Skin Pigmentation in Africans. Cell **2017**, 171, 1340–1353. **[Google Scholar] [CrossRef] [Green Version]**

37. Hysi, P.G.; Valdes, A.M.; Liu, F.; Furlotte, N.A.; Evans, D.M.; Bataille, V.; Visconti, A.; Hemani, G.; McMahon, G.; Ring, S.M.; et al. Genome-wide association meta-analysis of individuals of European ancestry identifies new loci explaining a substantial fraction of hair color variation and heritability. Nat. Genet. **2018**, 50, 652–656. **[Google Scholar] [CrossRef] [Green Version]**

38. Morgan, M.D.; Pairo-Castineira, E.; Rawlik, K.; Canela-Xandri, O.; Rees, J.; Sims, D.; Tenesa, A.; Jackson, I.J. Genome-wide study of hair colour in UK Biobank explains most of the SNP heritability. Nat. Commun. **2018**, 9, 5271. **[Google Scholar] [CrossRef] [PubMed] [Green Version]**

39. Medland, S.E.; Zhu, G.; Martin, N.G. Estimating the heritability of hair curliness in twins of European ancestry. Twin Res. Hum. Genet. **2009**, 12, 514–518. **[Google Scholar] [CrossRef] [PubMed]**

40. Adhikari, K.; Fontanil, T.; Cal, S.; Mendoza-Revilla, J.; Fuentes-Guajardo, M.; Chacón-Duque, J.C.; Al-Saadi, F.; Johansson, J.A.; Quinto-Sanchez, M.; Acuña-Alonzo, V.; et al. A genome-wide association scan in admixed Latin Americans identifies loci influencing facial and scalp hair features. Nat. Commun. **2016,** 7, 10815. **[Google Scholar] [CrossRef] [Green Version]**

41. Nyholt, D.R.; Gillespie, N.A.; Heath, A.C.; Martin, N.G. Genetic basis of male pattern baldness. J. Investig. Dermatol. **2003**, 121, 1561–1564. **[Google Scholar] [CrossRef] [PubMed]**

42. Pirastu, N.; Joshi, P.K.; de Vries, P.S.; Cornelis, M.C.; McKeigue, P.M.; Keum, N.; Franceschini, N.; Colombo, M.; Giovannucci, E.L.; Spiliopoulou, A.; et al. GWAS for male-pattern baldness identifies 71 susceptibility loci explaining 38% of the risk. Nat. Commun. **2017**, 8, 1584, Erratum in: Nat Commun. **2018**, 9, 2536. **[Google Scholar] [CrossRef] [PubMed]**

43. Yap, C.X.; Sidorenko, J.; Wu, Y.; Kemper, K.E.; Yang, J.; Wray, N.R.; Robinson, M.R.; Visscher, P.M. Dissection of genetic variation and evidence for pleiotropy in male pattern baldness. Nat. Commun. **2018**, 9, 5407. **[Google Scholar] [CrossRef] [PubMed]**

44. Gunn, D.A.; Rexbye, H.; Griffiths, C.E.; Murray, P.G.; Fereday, A.; Catt, S.D.; Tomlin, C.C.; Strongitharm, B.H.; Perrett, D.I.; Catt, M. Why some women look young for their age. PLoS ONE **2009**, 4, e8021. **[Google Scholar] [CrossRef] [Green Version]**

45. Weissbrod, O.; Flint, J.; Rosset, S. Estimating SNP-Based Heritability and Genetic Correlation in Case-Control Studies Directly and with Summary Statistics. Am. J. Hum. Genet. **2018**, 103, 89–99. **[Google Scholar] [CrossRef] [PubMed] [Green Version]**

46. Visscher, P.M.; Hill, W.G.; Wray, N.R. Heritability in the genomics era—concepts and misconceptions. Nat. Rev. Genet. **2008**, 9, 255–266. **[Google Scholar] [CrossRef] [PubMed]**

47. Richards, J.B.; Yuan, X.; Geller, F.; Waterworth, D.; Bataille, V.; Glass, D.; Song, K.; Waeber, G.; Vollenweider, P.; Aben, K.K.; et al. Male-pattern baldness susceptibility locus at 20p11. Nat. Genet. **2008**, 40, 1282–1284. **[Google Scholar] [CrossRef]**

48. Hillmer, A.M.; Brockschmidt, F.F.; Hanneken, S.; Eigelshoven, S.; Steffens, M.; Flaquer, A.; Herms, S.; Becker, T.; Kortüm, A.K.; Nyholt, D.R.; et al.

Susceptibility variants for male-pattern baldness on chromosome 20p11. Nat. Genet. **2008**, 40, 1279–1281. **[Google Scholar] [CrossRef] [PubMed]**

49. Brockschmidt, F.F.; Heilmann, S.; Ellis, J.A.; Eigelshoven, S.; Hanneken, S.; Herold, C.; Moebus, S.; Alblas, M.A.; Lippke, B.; Kluck, N.; et al. Susceptibility variants on chromosome 7p21.1 suggest HDAC9 as a new candidate gene for male-pattern baldness. Br. J. Dermatol. **2011**, 165, 1293–1302. **[Google Scholar] [CrossRef]**
50. Li, R.; Brockschmidt, F.F.; Kiefer, A.K.; Stefansson, H.; Nyholt, D.R.; Song, K.; Vermeulen, S.H.; Kanoni, S.; Glass, D.; Medland, S.E.; et al. Six novel susceptibility Loci for early-onset androgenetic alopecia and their unexpected association with common diseases. PLoS Genet. **2012**, 8, e1002746. **[Google Scholar] [CrossRef] [Green Version]**
51. Pickrell, J.K.; Berisa, T.; Liu, J.Z.; Ségurel, L.; Tung, J.Y.; Hinds, D.A. Detection and interpretation of shared genetic influences on 42 human traits. Nat. Genet. **2016**, 48, 709–717. **[Google Scholar] [CrossRef] [Green Version]**
52. Hagenaars, S.P.; Hill, W.D.; Harris, S.E.; Ritchie, S.J.; Davies, G.; Liewald, D.C.; Gale, C.R.; Porteous, D.J.; Deary, I.J.; Marioni, R.E. Genetic prediction of male pattern baldness. PLoS Genet. **2017**, 13, e1006594. **[Google Scholar] [CrossRef] [PubMed]**
53. Heilmann-Heimbach, S.; Herold, C.; Hochfeld, L.M.; Hillmer, A.M.; Nyholt, D.R.; Hecker, J.; Javed, A.; Chew, E.G.; Pechlivanis, S.; Drichel, D.; et al. Meta-analysis identifies novel risk loci and yields systematic insights into the biology of male-pattern baldness. Nat. Commun. **2017**, 8, 14694. **[Google Scholar] [CrossRef]**
54. Liang, B.; Yang, C.; Zuo, X.; Li, Y.; Ding, Y.; Sheng, Y.; Zhou, F.; Cheng, H.; Zheng, X.; Chen, G.; et al. Genetic variants at 20p11 confer risk to androgenetic alopecia in the Chinese Han population. PLoS ONE **2013**, 8, e71771. **[Google Scholar] [CrossRef]**
55. Zhuo, F.L.; Xu, W.; Wang, L.; Wu, Y.; Xu, Z.L.; Zhao, J.Y. Androgen receptor gene polymorphisms and risk for androgenetic alopecia: A meta-analysis. Clin. Exp. Dermatol. **2012**, 37, 104–111. **[Google Scholar] [CrossRef]**
56. Loh, P.R.; Kichaev, G.; Gazal, S.; Schoech, A.P.; Price, A.L. Mixed-model association for biobank-scale datasets. Nat. Genet. **2018**, 50, 906–908. **[Google Scholar] [CrossRef]**
57. Kichaev, G.; Bhatia, G.; Loh, P.R.; Gazal, S.; Burch, K.; Freund, M.K.; Schoech, A.; Pasaniuc, B.; Price, A.L. Leveraging Polygenic Functional Enrichment to Improve GWAS Power. Am. J. Hum. Genet. **2019**, 104, 65–75. **[Google Scholar] [CrossRef] [PubMed] [Green Version]**

58. Medland, S.E.; Nyholt, D.R.; Painter, J.N.; McEvoy, B.P.; McRae, A.F.; Zhu, G.; Gordon, S.D.; Ferreira, M.A.; Wright, M.J.; Henders, A.K.; et al. Common variants in the trichohyalin gene are associated with straight hair in Europeans. Am. J. Hum. Genet. **2009**, 85, 750–755. **[Google Scholar] [CrossRef] [PubMed] [Green Version]**

59. Wu, S.; Tan, J.; Yang, Y.; Peng, Q.; Zhang, M.; Li, J.; Lu, D.; Liu, Y.; Lou, H.; Feng, Q.; et al. Genome-wide scans reveal variants at EDAR predominantly affecting hair straightness in Han Chinese and Uyghur populations. Hum. Genet. **2016**, 135, 1279–1286. **[Google Scholar] [CrossRef]**

60. Liu, F.; Chen, Y.; Zhu, G.; Hysi, P.G.; Wu, S.; Adhikari, K.; Breslin, K.; Pospiech, E.; Hamer, M.A.; Peng, F.; et al. Meta-analysis of genome-wide association studies identifies 8 novel loci involved in shape variation of human head hair. Hum. Mol. Genet. **2018**, 27, 559–575. **[Google Scholar] [CrossRef]**

61. Fujimoto, A.; Kimura, R.; Ohashi, J.; Omi, K.; Yuliwulandari, R.; Batubara, L.; Mustofa, M.S.; Samakkarn, U.; Settheetham-Ishida, W.; Ishida, T.; et al. A scan for genetic determinants of human hair morphology: EDAR is associated with Asian hair thickness. Hum. Mol. Genet. **2008**, 17, 835–843. **[Google Scholar] [CrossRef]**

62. Tan, J.; Yang, Y.; Tang, K.; Sabeti, P.C.; Jin, L.; Wang, S. The adaptive variant EDARV370A is associated with straight hair in East Asians. Hum. Genet. **2013**, 132, 1187–1191. **[Google Scholar] [CrossRef]**

63. Pośpiech, E.; Lee, S.D.; Kukla-Bartoszek, M.; Karłowska-Pik, J.; Woźniak, A.; Boroń, M.; Zubańska, M.; Bronikowska, A.; Hong, S.R.; Lee, J.H.; et al. Variation in the RPTN gene may facilitate straight hair formation in Europeans and East Asians. J. Dermatol. Sci. **2018**, 91, 331–334. **[Google Scholar] [CrossRef]**

64. Endo, C.; Johnson, T.A.; Morino, R.; Nakazono, K.; Kamitsuji, S.; Akita, M.; Kawajiri, M.; Yamasaki, T.; Kami, A.; Hoshi, Y.; et al. Genome-wide association study in Japanese females identifies fifteen novel skin-related trait associations. Sci. Rep. **2018**, 8, 8974. **[Google Scholar] [CrossRef] [PubMed] [Green Version]**

65. Wu, S.; Zhang, M.; Yang, X.; Peng, F.; Zhang, J.; Tan, J.; Yang, Y.; Wang, L.; Hu, Y.; Peng, Q.; et al. Genome-wide association studies and CRISPR/Cas9-mediated gene editing identify regulatory variants influencing eyebrow thickness in humans. PLoS Genet. **2018**, 14, e1007640. **[Google Scholar] [CrossRef] [PubMed]**

66. Pośpiech, E.; Kukla-Bartoszek, M.; Karłowska-Pik, J.; Zieliński, P.; Woźniak, A.; Boroń, M.; Dąbrowski, M.; Zubańska, M.; Jarosz, A.; Grzybowski, T.; et al. Exploring the possibility of predicting human head hair greying from DNA using whole-exome and targeted NGS data. BMC Genom. **2020**, 21, 538. **[Google Scholar] [CrossRef]**

67. Gudbjartsson, D.F.; Walters, G.B.; Thorleifsson, G.; Stefansson, H.; Halldorsson, B.V.; Zusmanovich, P.; Sulem, P.; Thorlacius, S.; Gylfason, A.; Steinberg, S.; et al. Many sequence variants affecting diversity of adult human height. Nat. Genet. **2008**, 40, 609–615. **[Google Scholar] [CrossRef]**

68. Lettre, G.; Jackson, A.U.; Gieger, C.; Schumacher, F.R.; Berndt, S.I.; Sanna, S.; Eyheramendy, S.; Voight, B.F.; Butler, J.L.; Guiducci, C.; et al. Identification of ten loci associated with height highlights new biological pathways in human growth. Nat. Genet. **2008**, 40, 584–591. **[Google Scholar] [CrossRef] [PubMed]**

69. Weedon, M.N.; Lango, H.; Lindgren, C.M.; Wallace, C.; Evans, D.M.; Mangino, M.; Freathy, R.M.; Perry, J.R.; Stevens, S.; Hall, A.S.; et al. Genome-wide association analysis identifies 20 loci that influence adult height. Nat. Genet. **2008**, 40, 575–583. **[Google Scholar] [CrossRef] [Green Version]**

70. Lango Allen, H.; Estrada, K.; Lettre, G.; Berndt, S.I.; Weedon, M.N.; Rivadeneira, F.; Willer, C.J.; Jackson, A.U.; Vedantam, S.; Raychaudhuri, S.; et al. Hundreds of variants clustered in genomic loci and biological pathways affect human height. Nature **2010**, 467, 832–838. **[Google Scholar] [CrossRef] [Green Version]**

71. Yang, J.; Benyamin, B.; McEvoy, B.P.; Gordon, S.; Henders, A.K.; Nyholt, D.R.; Madden, P.A.; Heath, A.C.; Martin, N.G.; Montgomery, G.W.; et al. Common SNPs explain a large proportion of the heritability for human height. Nat. Genet. **2010**, 42, 565–569. **[Google Scholar] [CrossRef] [Green Version]**

72. Wood, A.R.; Esko, T.; Yang, J.; Vedantam, S.; Pers, T.H.; Gustafsson, S.; Chu, A.Y.; Estrada, K.; Luan, J.; Kutalik, Z.; et al. Defining the role of common variation in the genomic and biological architecture of adult human height. Nat. Genet. **2014**, 46, 1173–1186. **[Google Scholar] [CrossRef] [Green Version]**

73. Yengo, L.; Sidorenko, J.; Kemper, K.E.; Zheng, Z.; Wood, A.R.; Weedon, M.N.; Frayling, T.M.; Hirschhorn, J.; Yang, J.; Visscher, P.M. Meta-analysis of genome-wide association studies for height and body mass index in ~700,000 individuals of European ancestry. Hum. Mol. Genet. **2018**, 27, 3641–3649. **[Google Scholar] [CrossRef] [PubMed]**

74. Kaiser, J. Growth spurt for height genetics. Science **2020**, 370, 645. **[Google Scholar] [CrossRef] [PubMed]**

75. Zoledziewska, M.; Sidore, C.; Chiang, C.W.K.; Sanna, S.; Mulas, A.; Steri, M.; Busonero, F.; Marcus, J.H.; Marongiu, M.; Maschio, A.; et al. Height-reducing variants and selection for short stature in Sardinia. Nat. Genet. **2015**, 47, 1352–1356. **[Google Scholar] [CrossRef] [PubMed]**

76. He, M.; Xu, M.; Zhang, B.; Liang, J.; Chen, P.; Lee, J.Y.; Johnson, T.A.; Li, H.; Yang, X.; Dai, J.; et al. Meta-analysis of genome-wide association studies of

adult height in East Asians identifies 17 novel loci. Hum. Mol. Genet. **2015**, 24, 1791–1800. **[Google Scholar] [CrossRef]**

77. Akiyama, M.; Ishigaki, K.; Sakaue, S.; Momozawa, Y.; Horikoshi, M.; Hirata, M.; Matsuda, K.; Ikegawa, S.; Takahashi, A.; Kanai, M.; et al. Characterizing rare and low-frequency height-associated variants in the Japanese population. Nat. Commun. **2019**, 10, 4393. **[Google Scholar] [CrossRef] [Green Version]**
78. Marouli, E.; Graff, M.; Medina-Gomez, C.; Lo, K.S.; Wood, A.R.; Kjaer, T.R.; Fine, R.S.; Lu, Y.; Schurmann, C.; Highland, H.M.; et al. Rare and low-frequency coding variants alter human adult height. Nature **2017**, 542, 186–190. **[Google Scholar] [CrossRef] [Green Version]**
79. Roosenboom, J.; Hens, G.; Mattern, B.C.; Shriver, M.D.; Claes, P. Exploring the Underlying Genetics of Craniofacial Morphology through Various Sources of Knowledge. Biomed. Res. Int. **2016**, 2016, 3054578. **[Google Scholar] [CrossRef] [PubMed]**
80. Tsagkrasoulis, D.; Hysi, P.; Spector, T.; Montana, G. Heritability maps of human face morphology through large-scale automated three-dimensional phenotyping. Sci. Rep. **2017**, 7, 45885. **[Google Scholar] [CrossRef] [Green Version]**
81. Guo, J.; Mei, X.; Tang, K. Automatic landmark annotation and dense correspondence registration for 3D human facial images. BMC Bioinform. **2013**, 14, 232. **[Google Scholar] [CrossRef] [Green Version]**
82. Claes, P.; Liberton, D.K.; Daniels, K.; Rosana, K.M.; Quillen, E.E.; Pearson, L.N.; McEvoy, B.; Bauchet, M.; Zaidi, A.A.; Yao, W.; et al. Modeling 3D facial shape from DNA. PLoS Genet. **2014**, 10, e1004224. **[Google Scholar] [CrossRef] [PubMed] [Green Version]**
83. Cole, J.B.; Manyama, M.; Kimwaga, E.; Mathayo, J.; Larson, J.R.; Liberton, D.K.; Lukowiak, K.; Ferrara, T.M.; Riccardi, S.L.; Li, M.; et al. Genomewide Association Study of African Children Identifies Association of SCHIP1 and PDE8A with Facial Size and Shape. PLoS Genet. **2016**, 12, e1006174. **[Google Scholar] [CrossRef]**
84. Boehringer, S.; van der Lijn, F.; Liu, F.; Günther, M.; Sinigerova, S.; Nowak, S.; Ludwig, K.U.; Herberz, R.; Klein, S.; Hofman, A.; et al. Genetic determination of human facial morphology: Links between cleft-lips and normal variation. Eur. J. Hum. Genet. **2011**, 19, 1192–1197. **[Google Scholar] [CrossRef] [PubMed]**
85. Toma, A.M.; Zhurov, A.I.; Playle, R.; Marshall, D.; Rosin, P.L.; Richmond, S. The assessment of facial variation in 4747 British school children. Eur. J. Orthod. **2012**, 34, 655–664. **[Google Scholar] [CrossRef] [PubMed]**

86. Paternoster, L.; Zhurov, A.I.; Toma, A.M.; Kemp, J.P.; St Pourcain, B.; Timpson, N.J.; McMahon, G.; McArdle, W.; Ring, S.M.; Smith, G.D.; et al. Genome-wide association study of three-dimensional facial morphology identifies a variant in PAX3 associated with nasion position. Am. J. Hum. Genet. **2012**, 90, 478–485. **[Google Scholar] [CrossRef] [Green Version]**

87. Liu, F.; van der Lijn, F.; Schurmann, C.; Zhu, G.; Chakravarty, M.M.; Hysi, P.G.; Wollstein, A.; Lao, O.; de Bruijne, M.; Ikram, M.A.; et al. A genome-wide association study identifies five loci influencing facial morphology in Europeans. PLoS Genet. **2012**, 8, e1002932. **[Google Scholar] [CrossRef] [PubMed] [Green Version]**

88. Shaffer, J.R.; Orlova, E.; Lee, M.K.; Leslie, E.J.; Raffensperger, Z.D.; Heike, C.L.; Cunningham, M.L.; Hecht, J.T.; Kau, C.H.; Nidey, N.L.; et al. Genome-Wide Association Study Reveals Multiple Loci Influencing Normal Human Facial Morphology. PLoS Genet. **2016**, 12, e1006149. **[Google Scholar] [CrossRef] [PubMed]**

89. Crouch, D.J.M.; Winney, B.; Koppen, W.P.; Christmas, W.J.; Hutnik, K.; Day, T.; Meena, D.; Boumertit, A.; Hysi, P.; Nessa, A.; et al. Genetics of the human face: Identification of large-effect single gene variants. Proc. Natl. Acad. Sci. USA **2018**, 115, E676–E685. **[Google Scholar] [CrossRef] [Green Version]**

90. Claes, P.; Roosenboom, J.; White, J.D.; Swigut, T.; Sero, D.; Li, J.; Lee, M.K.; Zaidi, A.; Mattern, B.C.; Liebowitz, C.; et al. Genome-wide mapping of global-to-local genetic effects on human facial shape. Nat. Genet. **2018**, 50, 414–423. **[Google Scholar] [CrossRef] [PubMed]**

91. White, J.D.; Indencleef, K.; Naqvi, S.; Eller, R.J.; Hoskens, H.; Roosenboom, J.; Lee, M.K.; Li, J.; Mohammed, J.; Richmond, S.; et al. Insights into the genetic architecture of the human face. Nat. Genet. **2021**, 53, 45–53. **[Google Scholar] [CrossRef] [PubMed]**

92. Liu, C.; Lee, M.K.; Naqvi, S.; Hoskens, H.; Liu, D.; White, J.D.; Indencleef, K.; Matthews, H.; Eller, R.J.; Li, J.; et al. Genome scans of facial features in East Africans and cross-population comparisons reveal novel associations. PLoS Genet. **2021**, 17, e1009695. **[Google Scholar] [CrossRef]**

93. Qiao, L.; Yang, Y.; Fu, P.; Hu, S.; Zhou, H.; Peng, S.; Tan, J.; Lu, Y.; Lou, H.; Lu, D.; et al. Genome-wide variants of Eurasian facial shape differentiation and a prospective model of DNA based face prediction. J. Genet. Genom. **2018**, 45, 419–432. **[Google Scholar] [CrossRef]**

94. Sullivan, K.M.; Mannucci, A.; Kimpton, C.P.; Gill, P. A rapid and quantitative DNA sex test: Fluorescence-based PCR analysis of X-Y homologous gene amelogenin. Biotechniques **1993**, 15, 636–638, 640–641. **[Google Scholar] [PubMed]**

95. Evett, I.W.; Pinchin, R.; Buffery, C. An investigation of the feasibility of inferring ethnic origin from DNA profiles. J. Forensic Sci. Soc. **1992**, 32, 301–306. **[Google Scholar] [CrossRef]**

96. Shriver, M.D.; Smith, M.W.; Jin, L.; Marcini, A.; Akey, J.M.; Deka, R.; Ferrell, R.E. Ethnic-affiliation estimation by use of population-specific DNA markers. Am. J. Hum. Genet. **1997**, 60, 957–964. **[Google Scholar]**

97. Grimes, E.A.; Noake, P.J.; Dixon, L.; Urquhart, A. Sequence polymorphism in the human melanocortin 1 receptor gene as an indicator of the red hair phenotype. Forensic Sci. Int. **2001**, 122, 124–129. **[Google Scholar] [CrossRef]**

98. Walsh, S.; Liu, F.; Ballantyne, K.N.; van Oven, M.; Lao, O.; Kayser, M. IrisPlex: A sensitive DNA tool for accurate prediction of blue and brown eye colour in the absence of ancestry information. Forensic Sci. Int. Genet. **2011**, 5, 170–180. **[Google Scholar] [CrossRef]**

99. Mengel-From, J.; Børsting, C.; Sanchez, J.J.; Eiberg, H.; Morling, N. Human eye colour and HERC2, OCA2 and MATP. Forensic Sci. Int. Genet. **2010**, 4, 323–328. **[Google Scholar] [CrossRef]**

100. Valenzuela, R.K.; Henderson, M.S.; Walsh, M.H.; Garrison, N.A.; Kelch, J.T.; Cohen-Barak, O.; Erickson, D.T.; John Meaney, F.; Bruce Walsh, J.; Cheng, K.C.; et al. Predicting phenotype from genotype: Normal pigmentation. J. Forensic Sci. **2010**, 55, 315–322. **[Google Scholar] [CrossRef] [PubMed] [Green Version]**

101. Spichenok, O.; Budimlija, Z.M.; Mitchell, A.A.; Jenny, A.; Kovacevic, L.; Marjanovic, D.; Caragine, T.; Prinz, M.; Wurmbach, E. Prediction of eye and skin color in diverse populations using seven SNPs. Forensic Sci. Int. Genet. **2011**, 5, 472–478. **[Google Scholar] [CrossRef] [PubMed]**

102. Pośpiech, E.; Draus-Barini, J.; Kupiec, T.; Wojas-Pelc, A.; Branicki, W. Prediction of eye color from genetic data using Bayesian approach. J. Forensic Sci. **2012**, 57, 880–886. **[Google Scholar] [CrossRef]**

103. Ruiz, Y.; Phillips, C.; Gomez-Tato, A.; Alvarez-Dios, J.; de Cal, M.C.; Cruz, R.; Maroñas, O.; Söchtig, J.; Fondevila, M.; Rodriguez-Cid, M.J.; et al. Further development of forensic eye color predictive tests. Forensic Sci. Int. Genet. **2013**, 7, 28–40. **[Google Scholar] [CrossRef]**

104. Allwood, J.S.; Harbison, S. SNP model development for the prediction of eye colour in New Zealand. Forensic Sci. Int. Genet. **2013**, 7, 444–452. **[Google Scholar] [CrossRef] [PubMed]**

105. Hart, K.L.; Kimura, S.L.; Mushailov, V.; Budimlija, Z.M.; Prinz, M.; Wurmbach, E. Improved eye- and skin-color prediction based on 8 SNPs. Croat. Med. J. **2013**, 54, 248–256. **[Google Scholar] [CrossRef] [Green Version]**

106. Walsh, S.; Liu, F.; Wollstein, A.; Kovatsi, L.; Ralf, A.; Kosiniak-Kamysz, A.; Branicki, W.; Kayser, M. The HIrisPlex system for simultaneous prediction of hair and eye colour from DNA. Forensic Sci. Int. Genet. **2013**, 7, 98–115. **[Google Scholar] [CrossRef] [Green Version]**

107. Söchtig, J.; Phillips, C.; Maroñas, O.; Gómez-Tato, A.; Cruz, R.; Alvarez-Dios, J.; de Cal, M.Á.; Ruiz, Y.; Reich, K.; Fondevila, M.; et al. Exploration of SNP variants affecting hair colour prediction in Europeans. Int. J. Legal Med. **2015**, 129, 963–975. **[Google Scholar] [CrossRef] [PubMed]**

108. Maroñas, O.; Phillips, C.; Söchtig, J.; Gomez-Tato, A.; Cruz, R.; Alvarez-Dios, J.; de Cal, M.C.; Ruiz, Y.; Fondevila, M.; Carracedo, Á.; et al. Development of a forensic skin colour predictive test. Forensic Sci. Int. Genet. **2014**, 13, 34–44. **[Google Scholar] [CrossRef]**

109. Chaitanya, L.; Breslin, K.; Zuñiga, S.; Wirken, L.; Pośpiech, E.; Kukla-Bartoszek, M.; Sijen, T.; Knijff, P.; Liu, F.; Branicki, W.; et al. The HIrisPlex-S system for eye, hair and skin colour prediction from DNA: Introduction and forensic developmental validation. Forensic Sci. Int. Genet. **2018**, 35, 123–135. **[Google Scholar] [CrossRef] [Green Version]**

110. Andersen, J.D.; Meyer, O.S.; Simão, F.; Jannuzzi, J.; Carvalho, E.; Andersen, M.M.; Pereira, V.; Børsting, C.; Morling, N.; Gusmão, L. Skin pigmentation and genetic variants in an admixed Brazilian population of primarily European ancestry. Int. J. Legal Med. **2020**, 134, 1569–1579. **[Google Scholar] [CrossRef]**

111. Hernando, B.; Ibañez, M.V.; Deserio-Cuesta, J.A.; Soria-Navarro, R.; Vilar-Sastre, I.; Martinez-Cadenas, C. Genetic determinants of freckle occurrence in the Spanish population: Towards ephelides prediction from human DNA samples. Forensic Sci. Int. Genet. **2018**, 33, 38–47. **[Google Scholar] [CrossRef]**

112. Kukla-Bartoszek, M.; Pośpiech, E.; Woźniak, A.; Boroń, M.; Karłowska-Pik, J.; Teisseyre, P.; Zubańska, M.; Bronikowska, A.; Grzybowski, T.; Płoski, R.; et al. DNA-based predictive models for the presence of freckles. Forensic Sci. Int. Genet. **2019**, 42, 252–259. **[Google Scholar] [CrossRef] [Green Version]**

113. Marcińska, M.; Pośpiech, E.; Abidi, S.; Andersen, J.D.; van den Berge, M.; Carracedo, Á.; Eduardoff, M.; Marczakiewicz-Lustig, A.; Morling, N.; Sijen, T.; et al. Evaluation of DNA variants associated with androgenetic alopecia and their potential to predict male pattern baldness. PLoS ONE **2015**, 10, e0127852. **[Google Scholar] [CrossRef] [PubMed]**

114. Liu, F.; Hamer, M.A.; Heilmann, S.; Herold, C.; Moebus, S.; Hofman, A.; Uitterlinden, A.G.; Nöthen, M.M.; van Duijn, C.M.; Nijsten, T.E.; et al. Prediction of male-pattern baldness from genotypes. Eur. J. Hum. Genet. **2016**, 24, 895–902. **[Google Scholar] [CrossRef] [PubMed] [Green Version]**

115. Pośpiech, E.; Karłowska-Pik, J.; Marcińska, M.; Abidi, S.; Andersen, J.D.; Berge, M.V.D.; Carracedo, Á.; Eduardoff, M.; Freire-Aradas, A.; Morling, N.; et al. Evaluation of the predictive capacity of DNA variants associated with straight hair in Europeans. Forensic Sci. Int. Genet. **2015**, 19, 280–288. **[Google Scholar] [CrossRef] [PubMed] [Green Version]**

116. Pośpiech, E.; Chen, Y.; Kukla-Bartoszek, M.; Breslin, K.; Aliferi, A.; Andersen, J.D.; Ballard, D.; Chaitanya, L.; Freire-Aradas, A.; van der Gaag, K.J.; et al. Towards broadening Forensic DNA Phenotyping beyond pigmentation: Improving the prediction of head hair shape from DNA. Forensic Sci. Int. Genet. **2018**, 37, 241–251. **[Google Scholar] [CrossRef] [Green Version]**

117. Aulchenko, Y.S.; Struchalin, M.V.; Belonogova, N.M.; Axenovich, T.I.; Weedon, M.N.; Hofman, A.; Uitterlinden, A.G.; Kayser, M.; Oostra, B.A.; van Duijn, C.M.; et al. Predicting human height by Victorian and genomic methods. Eur. J. Hum. Genet. **2009**, 17, 1070–1075. **[Google Scholar] [CrossRef] [PubMed] [Green Version]**

118. Liu, F.; Hendriks, A.E.; Ralf, A.; Boot, A.M.; Benyi, E.; Sävendahl, L.; Oostra, B.A.; van Duijn, C.; Hofman, A.; Rivadeneira, F.; et al. Common DNA variants predict tall stature in Europeans. Hum. Genet. **2014**, 133, 587–597. **[Google Scholar] [CrossRef]**

119. Liu, F.; Zhong, K.; Jing, X.; Uitterlinden, A.G.; Hendriks, A.E.J.; Drop, S.L.S.; Kayser, M. Update on the predictability of tall stature from DNA markers in Europeans. Forensic Sci. Int. Genet. **2019**, 42, 8–13. **[Google Scholar] [CrossRef] [Green Version]**

120. Lello, L.; Avery, S.G.; Tellier, L.; Vazquez, A.I.; de Los Campos, G.; Hsu, S.D.H. Accurate Genomic Prediction of Human Height. Genetics **2018**, 210, 477–497. **[Google Scholar] [CrossRef] [Green Version]**

121. Lippert, C.; Sabatini, R.; Maher, M.C.; Kang, E.Y.; Lee, S.; Arikan, O.; Harley, A.; Bernal, A.; Garst, P.; Lavrenko, V.; et al. Identification of individuals by trait prediction using whole-genome sequencing data. Proc. Natl. Acad. Sci. USA **2017**, 114, 10166–10171. **[Google Scholar] [CrossRef] [Green Version]**

122. Liu, F.; van Duijn, K.; Vingerling, J.R.; Hofman, A.; Uitterlinden, A.G.; Janssens, A.C.; Kayser, M. Eye color and the prediction of complex phenotypes from genotypes. Curr. Biol. **2009**, 19, R192–R193. **[Google Scholar] [CrossRef] [PubMed] [Green Version]**

123. Martinez-Cadenas, C.; Peña-Chilet, M.; Ibarrola-Villava, M.; Ribas, G. Gender is a major factor explaining discrepancies in eye colour prediction based on HERC2/OCA2 genotype and the IrisPlex model. Forensic Sci. Int. Genet. **2013**, 7, 453–460. **[Google Scholar] [CrossRef] [Green Version]**

124. Pietroni, C.; Andersen, J.D.; Johansen, P.; Andersen, M.M.; Harder, S.; Paulsen, R.; Børsting, C.; Morling, N. The effect of gender on eye colour variation in European populations and an evaluation of the IrisPlex prediction model. Forensic Sci. Int. Genet. **2014**, 1, 1–6. **[Google Scholar] [CrossRef] [PubMed] [Green Version]**

125. Pośpiech, E.; Karłowska-Pik, J.; Ziemkiewicz, B.; Kukla, M.; Skowron, M.; Wojas-Pelc, A.; Branicki, W. Further evidence for population specific differences in the effect of DNA markers and gender on eye colour prediction in forensics. Int. J. Legal. Med. **2016**, 130, 923–934. **[Google Scholar] [CrossRef] [Green Version]**

126. Branicki, W.; Liu, F.; van Duijn, K.; Draus-Barini, J.; Pośpiech, E.; Walsh, S.; Kupiec, T.; Wojas-Pelc, A.; Kayser, M. Model-based prediction of human hair color using DNA variants. Hum. Genet. **2011**, 129, 443–454. **[Google Scholar] [CrossRef] [PubMed] [Green Version]**

127. Walsh, S.; Chaitanya, L.; Breslin, K.; Muralidharan, C.; Bronikowska, A.; Pospiech, E.; Koller, J.; Kovatsi, L.; Wollstein, A.; Branicki, W.; et al. Global skin colour prediction from DNA. Hum. Genet. **2017**, 136, 847–863. **[Google Scholar] [CrossRef] [Green Version]**

128. Breslin, K.; Wills, B.; Ralf, A.; Ventayol Garcia, M.; Kukla-Bartoszek, M.; Pospiech, E.; Freire-Aradas, A.; Xavier, C.; Ingold, S.; de La Puente, M.; et al. HIrisPlex-S system for eye, hair, and skin color prediction from DNA: Massively parallel sequencing solutions for two common forensically used platforms. Forensic Sci. Int. Genet. **2019**, 43, 102152. **[Google Scholar] [CrossRef] [PubMed]**

129. Xavier, C.; de la Puente, M.; Mosquera-Miguel, A.; Freire-Aradas, A.; Kalamara, V.; Vidaki, A.; Gross, T.; Revoir, A.; Pośpiech, E.; Kartasińska, E.; et al. Development and validation of the VISAGE AmpliSeq basic tool to predict appearance and ancestry from DNA. Forensic Sci. Int. Genet. **2020**, 48, 102336. **[Google Scholar] [CrossRef]**

130. Phillips, C.; Salas, A.; Sánchez, J.J.; Fondevila, M.; Gómez-Tato, A.; Alvarez-Dios, J.; Calaza, M.; de Cal, M.C.; Ballard, D.; Lareu, M.V.; et al. Inferring ancestral origin using a single multiplex assay of ancestry-informative marker SNPs. Forensic Sci. Int. Genet. **2007**, 1, 273–280. **[Google Scholar] [CrossRef] [PubMed]**

131. Noroozi, R.; Ghafouri-Fard, S.; Pisarek, A.; Rudnicka, J.; Spólnicka, M.; Branicki, W.; Taheri, M.; Pośpiech, E. DNA methylation-based age clocks: From age prediction to age reversion. Ageing Res. Rev. **2021**, 68, 101314. **[Google Scholar] [CrossRef]**

132. De Los Campos, G.; Vazquez, A.I.; Hsu, S.; Lello, L. Complex-Trait Prediction in the Era of Big Data. Trends Genet. **2018**, 34, 746–754. **[Google Scholar]** **[CrossRef]**

133. Shmueli, G. To Explain or to Predict? Stat. Sci. **2010**, 25, 289–310. **[Google Scholar]** **[CrossRef]**

134. Hastie, T.; Tibshirani, R.; Friedman, J. The Elements of Statistical Learning, 2nd ed.; Springer: New York, NY, USA, 2009. **[Google Scholar]**

135. Hill, G.H.; Goddard, M.E.; Vissher, P.M. Data and Theory Point to Mainly Additive Genetic Variance for Complex Traits. PLoS Genet. **2008**, 4, 1–10. **[Google Scholar]** **[CrossRef]** **[Green Version]**

136. Katsara, M.A.; Branicki, W.; Walsh, S.; Kayser, M.; Nothnagel, M. Evaluation of supervised machine-learning methods for predicting appearance traits from DNA. Forensic Sci. Int. Genet. **2021**, 53, 1–9. **[Google Scholar]** **[CrossRef]** **[PubMed]**

137. Kukla-Bartoszek, M.; Teisseyre, P.; Pośpiech, E.; Karłowska-Pik, J.; Zieliński, P.; Woźniak, A.; Boroń, M.; Dąbrowski, M.; Zubańska, M.; Jarosz, A.; et al. Searching for improvements in predicting human eye colour from DNA. Int. J. Legal Med. **2021**, 135, 2175–2187. **[Google Scholar]** **[CrossRef]** **[PubMed]**

138. Fan, J.; Li, R. Variable selection via nonconcave penalized likelihood and its oracle properties. J. Amer. Stat. Assoc. **2001**, 96, 1348–1361. **[Google Scholar]** **[CrossRef]**

139. Zhang, C.H. Nearly unbiased variable selection under minimax concave penalty. Ann. Stat. **2001**, 38, 894–942. **[Google Scholar]** **[CrossRef]** **[Green Version]**

140. Breheny, P.; Huang, J. Coordinate descent algorithms for nonconvex penalized regression, with applications to biological feature selection. Ann. Appl. Stat. **2011**, 5, 232–253. **[Google Scholar]** **[CrossRef]** **[Green Version]**

141. Benjamini, Y.; Hochberg, Y. Controlling the false discovery rate: A practical and multiple approach to multiple testing. J. R. Stat. Soc. Ser. B **1995**, 57, 289–300. **[Google Scholar]**

142. Barber, R.F.; Candes, E.J. Controlling the False Discovery Rate by knockoffs. Ann. Stat. **2015**, 43, 2055–2085. **[Google Scholar]** **[CrossRef]** **[Green Version]**

143. Tsamardinos, I.; Borboudakis, G. Permutation testing improves Bayesian Network learning. In Proceedings of the Joint European Conference on Machine Learning and Knowledge Discovery in Databases, Barcelona, Spain, 19–23 September 2010; pp. 322–337. **[Google Scholar]**

144. Tansey, W.; Veitch, V.; Zhang, H.; Rabadan, R.; Blei, D. The Holdout Randomisation Test for Feature Selection in Black Box Models. J. Comput. Graph. Stat. **2021**, 1–37. Available online: **https://arxiv.org/abs/1811.00645** (accessed on 8 December 2021).
145. Bishop, C. Pattern Recognition and Machine Learning, 1st ed.; Springer: New York, NY, USA, 2006. **[Google Scholar]**
146. Breiman, L. Bagging Predictors. Mach. Learn. **1996**, 24, 123–140. **[Google Scholar] [CrossRef] [Green Version]**
147. Ho, T.K. The Random Subspace Method for Constructing Decision Forests. IEEE Trans. Pattern Anal. Mach. Intell. **1998**, 20, 832–844. **[Google Scholar]**
148. Mielniczuk, J.; Teisseyre, P. Using Random Subspace Method for Prediction and Variable Importance Assessment in Regression. Comput. Stat. Data Anal. **2014**, 71, 725–742. **[Google Scholar] [CrossRef]**
149. Chen, T.; Guestrin, C. XGBoost: A Scalable Tree Boosting System. In Proceedings of the 22nd ACM SIGKDD International Conference on Knowledge Discovery and Data Mining, San Francisco, CA, USA, 13–17 August 2016; pp. 785–794. **[Google Scholar]**
150. Kursa, M.; Rudnicki, W. Feature Selection with the Boruta Package. J. Stat. Softw. **2010**, 36, 1–13. **[Google Scholar] [CrossRef] [Green Version]**
151. Dramiński, M.; Rada-Iglesias, A.; Enroth, S.; Wadelius, C.; Koronacki, J.; Komorowski, J. Monte Carlo feature selection for supervised classification. Bioinformatics **2008**, 24, 110–117. **[Google Scholar] [CrossRef] [PubMed] [Green Version]**
152. Rosenblatt, F. The Perceptron—A Perceiving and Recognizing Automaton, Report. 1957. Available online: **https://blogs.umass.edu/brain-wars/files/2016/03/rosenblatt-1957.pdf** (accessed on 8 December 2021).
153. Goodfellow, J.; Bengio, Y.; Courville, A. Deep Learning, 1st ed.; MIT Press: Cambridge, MA, USA, 2016. **[Google Scholar]**
154. Kingma, D.; Ba, J. Adam: A Method for Stochastic Optimization. In Proceedings of the International Conference on Learning Representations, San Diego, CA, USA, 7–9 May 2015; pp. 1–13. **[Google Scholar]**
155. Kingsma, D.; Welling, M. Autoencoding variational Bayes. In Proceedings of the 2nd Conference on Learning Representations, Banff, AB, Canada, 14–16 April 2014; pp. 1–14. **[Google Scholar]**
156. Brown, G.; Pocock, A.; Zhao, M.-J.; Luján, M. Conditional Likelihood Maximisation: A Unifying Framework for Information Theoretic Feature Selection. J. Mach. Learn. Res. **2012**, 13, 27–66. **[Google Scholar]**

157. Moore, J.H.; Hu, T. Epistatic analysis using information theory. Methods Mol. Biol. **2015**, 1253, 257–268. **[Google Scholar] [PubMed]**

158. Cordell, H.J. Epistasis: What it means, what it doesn't mean, and statistical methods to detect it in humans. Hum. Mol. Genet. **2002**, 11, 2463–2468. **[Google Scholar] [CrossRef] [Green Version]**

159. Pośpiech, E.; Wojas-Pelc, A.; Walsh, S.; Liu, F.; Maeda, H.; Ishikawa, T.; Skowron, M.; Kayser, M.; Branicki, W. The common occurrence of epistasis in the determination of human pigmentation and its impact on DNA-based pigmentation phenotype prediction. Forensic Sci. Int. Genet. **2014**, 11, 64–72. **[Google Scholar] [CrossRef] [PubMed]**

160. Mielniczuk, J.; Teisseyre, P. Deeper Look at Two Concepts of Measuring Gene-Gene Interactions: Logistic Regression and Interaction Information Revisited. Genet. Epidemiol. **2018**, 42, 187–200. **[Google Scholar] [CrossRef] [PubMed]**

161. Lin, D.; Tang, X. Conditional infomax learning: An integrated framework for feature extraction and fusion. In Proceedings of the European Conference on Computer Vision, Graz, Austria, 7–13 May 2006; pp. 68–82. **[Google Scholar]**

162. Vinh, N.X.; Zhou, S.; Chan, J.; Bailey, J. Can high-order dependencies improve mutual information based feature selection? Pattern Recognit. **2016**, 53, 46–58. **[Google Scholar] [CrossRef] [Green Version]**

163. Mielniczuk, J.; Teisseyre, P. Stopping rules for mutual information-based feature selection. Neurocomputing **2019**, 358, 255–274. **[Google Scholar] [CrossRef]**

164. Tillmar, A.; Sjölund, P.; Lundqvist, B.; Klippmark, T.; Älgenäs, C.; Green, H. Whole-genome sequencing of human remains to enable genealogy DNA database searches—A case report. Forensic Sci. Int. Genet. **2020**, 46, 102233. **[Google Scholar] [CrossRef] [PubMed]**

165. Hofman, C.A.; Warinner, C. Ancient DNA 101: An introductory guide in the era of high-throughput sequencing. SAA Rec. **2019**, 19, 18–25. **[Google Scholar]**

166. Hofreiter, M.; Sneberger, J.; Pospisek, M.; Vanek, D. Progress in forensic bone DNA analysis: Lessons learned from ancient DNA. Forensic Sci. Int. Genet. **2021**, 54, 102538. **[Google Scholar] [CrossRef]**

167. Meyer, M.; Kircher, M. Illumina sequencing library preparation for highly multiplexed target capture and sequencing. Cold Spring Harb. Protoc. **2010**, 2010, pdb.prot5448. **[Google Scholar] [CrossRef]**

168. Psonis, N.; Vassou, D.; Kafetzopoulos, D. Testing a series of modifications on genomic library preparation methods for ancient or degraded DNA. Anal. Biochem. **2021**, 623, 114193. **[Google Scholar] [CrossRef]**

169. Carøe, C.; Gopalakrishnan, S.; Vinner, L.; Mak, S.S.T.; Sinding, M.-H.S.; Samaniego, J.A.; Wales, N.; Sicheritz-Pontén, T.; Gilbert, M.T.P. Single-tube library preparation for degraded DNA. Methods Ecol. Evol. **2018**, 9, 410–419. **[Google Scholar] [CrossRef]**

170. Gansauge, M.T.; Meyer, M. Single-stranded DNA library preparation for the sequencing of ancient or damaged DNA. Nat. Protoc. **2013**, 8, 737–748. **[Google Scholar] [CrossRef]**

171. Gansauge, M.T.; Gerber, T.; Glocke, I.; Korlevic, P.; Lippik, L.; Nagel, S.; Riehl, L.M.; Schmidt, A.; Meyer, M. Single-stranded DNA library preparation from highly degraded DNA using T4 DNA ligase. Nucleic Acids Res. **2017**, 45, e79. **[Google Scholar] [CrossRef] [Green Version]**

172. Gansauge, M.T.; Aximu-Petri, A.; Nagel, S.; Meyer, M. Manual and automated preparation of single-stranded DNA libraries for the sequencing of DNA from ancient biological remains and other sources of highly degraded DNA. Nat. Protoc. **2020**, 15, 2279–2300. **[Google Scholar] [CrossRef] [PubMed]**

173. Kapp, J.D.; Green, R.E.; Shapiro, B. A Fast and Efficient Single-stranded Genomic Library Preparation Method Optimized for Ancient DNA. J. Hered. **2021**, 112, 241–249. **[Google Scholar] [CrossRef] [PubMed]**

174. Green, R.E.; Krause, J.; Briggs, A.W.; Maricic, T.; Stenzel, U.; Kircher, M.; Patterson, N.; Li, H.; Zhai, W.; Fritz, M.H.; et al. A draft sequence of the Neandertal genome. Science **2010**, 328, 710–722. **[Google Scholar] [CrossRef] [PubMed] [Green Version]**

175. Meyer, M.; Kircher, M.; Gansauge, M.T.; Li, H.; Racimo, F.; Mallick, S.; Schraiber, J.G.; Jay, F.; Prüfer, K.; de Filippo, C.; et al. A high-coverage genome sequence from an archaic Denisovan individual. Science **2012**, 338, 222–226. **[Google Scholar] [CrossRef] [PubMed] [Green Version]**

176. Stiller, M.; Sucker, A.; Griewank, K.; Aust, D.; Baretton, G.B.; Schadendorf, D.; Horn, S. Single-strand DNA library preparation improves sequencing of formalin-fixed and paraffin-embedded (FFPE) cancer DNA. Oncotarget **2016**, 7, 59115–59128. **[Google Scholar] [CrossRef] [Green Version]**

177. Rasmussen, M.; Li, Y.; Lindgreen, S.; Pedersen, J.S.; Albrechtsen, A.; Moltke, I.; Metspalu, M.; Metspalu, E.; Kivisild, T.; Gupta, R.; et al. Ancient human genome sequence of an extinct Palaeo-Eskimo. Nature **2010**, 463, 757–762. **[Google Scholar] [CrossRef]**

178. Keller, A.; Graefen, A.; Ball, M.; Matzas, M.; Boisguerin, V.; Maixner, F.; Leidinger, P.; Backes, C.; Khairat, R.; Forster, M.; et al. New insights into the Tyrolean Iceman's origin and phenotype as inferred by whole-genome sequencing. Nat. Commun. **2012**, 3, 698. **[Google Scholar] [CrossRef] [PubMed] [Green Version]**

179. Olalde, I.; Allentoft, M.E.; Sánchez-Quinto, F.; Santpere, G.; Chiang, C.W.; DeGiorgio, M.; Prado-Martinez, J.; Rodríguez, J.A.; Rasmussen, S.; Quilez, J.; et al. Derived immune and ancestral pigmentation alleles in a 7000-year-old Mesolithic European. Nature **2014**, 507, 225–228. **[Google Scholar] [CrossRef] [Green Version]**

180. Bogdanowicz, W.; Allen, M.; Branicki, W.; Lembring, M.; Gajewska, M.; Kupiec, T. Genetic identification of putative remains of the famous astronomer Nicolaus Copernicus. Proc. Natl. Acad. Sci. USA **2009**, 106, 12279–12282. **[Google Scholar] [CrossRef] [Green Version]**

181. Kupiec, T.; Branicki, W. Genetic examination of the putative skull of Jan Kochanowski reveals its female sex. Croat. Med. J. **2011**, 52, 403–409. **[Google Scholar] [CrossRef] [PubMed]**

182. King, T.E.; Fortes, G.G.; Balaresque, P.; Thomas, M.G.; Balding, D.; Maisano Delser, P.; Neumann, R.; Parson, W.; Knapp, M.; Walsh, S.; et al. Identification of the remains of King Richard III. Nat. Commun. **2014**, 5, 5631. **[Google Scholar] [CrossRef] [PubMed]**

183. Salvo, N.M.; Janssen, K.; Kirsebom, M.K.; Meyer, O.S.; Berg, T.; Olsen, G.H. Predicting eye and hair colour in a Norwegian population using Verogen'sForenSeq™ DNA signature prep kit. Forensic Sci. Int. Genet. **2021**, 56, 102620. **[Google Scholar] [CrossRef]**

184. Diepenbroek, M.; Bayer, B.; Schwender, K.; Schiller, R.; Lim, J.; Lagacé, R.; Anslinger, K. Evaluation of the Ion AmpliSeq™ PhenoTrivium Panel: MPS-Based Assay for Ancestry and Phenotype Predictions Challenged by Casework Samples. Genes **2020**, 11, 1398. **[Google Scholar] [CrossRef] [PubMed]**

185. ParabonNanoLabs. Available online: **https://snapshot.parabon-nanolabs.com** (accessed on 8 December 2021).

09

CREATION AND ASSESSMENT OF THE ANCESTRY INFORMATIVE MARKER PANEL FOR THE VISAGE BASIC TOOL

1. INTRODUCTION

In the last ten years, forensic DNA analysis has been extended beyond identification tests that link a suspect to crime-scene evidence using STR profiling, into areas of genetic analysis designed to predict a range of physical characteristics of unidentified trace donors, mainly defined by single nucleotide polymorphisms (SNPs). Such SNP tests, applicable when no suspect has been identified by investigators, have been termed forensic DNA phenotyping (FDP), and until recently, consisted of tests to infer bio-geographical ancestry (BGA) [**1**], or to predict certain externally visible characteristics (EVCs) [**2**]. These SNP-based tests have now been supplemented with DNA analyses that measure the methylation status of carefully chosen CpG sites showing age-correlated methylation patterns in order to estimate a donor's chronological age from the same DNA samples used for BGA and EVC tests [**3**]. The array of FDP tests now being adopted can serve to progress a major criminal investigation lacking strong leads, resurrect cold cases by providing new genetic data about old crime-scene DNA samples, and aid in the identification of the missing or historical remains [**4**]. While FDP tests have been gaining traction as supplementary analysis regimes available to forensic laboratories, the emergence of massively parallel sequencing (MPS) now provides major enhancements for forensic DNA analysis, including improved sensitivity to analyse minimal amounts of evidential material, larger multiplexes that can combine conventional identification STRs with SNPs for FDP analysis, and greater detail about the detectable variation within a sequence. The VISible Attributes through GEnomics (VISAGE) Consortium was initiated in 2017 to develop new MPS-based tools for predicting the BGA, appearance based on common EVCs, and age of an unidentified crime-scene DNA donor.

VISAGE adopted a two-step program to create MPS tools for FDP: developing a Basic Tool as a pilot assay, followed by the development of an Enhanced Tool with more markers and extended capabilities. The VISAGE Basic Tool (herein BT) is the first forensic MPS test combining markers for predicting eye, hair, and skin colour with those for BGA inference in a single assay, along with a saliva-blood focused age estimation assay requiring a parallel assay and workflow due to the bisulphite conversion steps needed to measure methylation. The VISAGE BT was founded on marker panels which have been shown to be informative for the three pigmentation traits [**5,6,7**] and for continental-scale population differentiation [**8,9,10,11,12**]. The level of multiplexing necessary to accommodate sufficient SNPs to yield optimum predictions of both EVCs and continental BGA was in part dictated by experience of building multiplexes for forensic MPS analysis [**8,12,13**]. Therefore, for the BT assay, which acts as a pilot test, we decided to design a moderate PCR scale of 150 to 160 SNPs by combining the 41 well-established HIrisPlex-S markers, which have been successfully applied in previous SNaPshot and MPS assays [**5,6,7,13**], with up to 120 ancestry-informative marker (AIM) SNPs. A panel of 120 AIM SNPs represents a reduced multiplex size compared to the one commercially available forensic ancestry panel for MPS, i.e., the Thermo Fisher Precision ID Ancestry Panel, comprising 165 AIMs [**14**], although similar in scale to another panel of 127 AIMs [**8**]. For this reason, we selected markers with the maximum possible ancestry informativeness for any given population, and then balanced these to ensure the major population groups had broadly comparable levels of differentiation. In contrast to the previous development of the 127-SNP Global AIMs panel (gAIMs [**8**]), South Asians, i.e., individuals from the Indian subcontinent, were treated as a separate population group.

This paper describes the compilation of component SNPs into the ancestry informative marker set forming the major portion of the VISAGE Basic Tool for appearance-ancestry. The development of the AIMs set and its evaluation involved four stages: i. Selection of markers and balancing of their relative population informativeness proportions in the multiplex to ensure comparable levels of continental population group differentiation; ii. Generation of a large-scale reference dataset built on open-access, genome-wide variant datasets, plus our own MPS genotyping of in-house population samples from which to apply the statistical analysis pipelines accompanying the BT assay; iii. Genotype concordance studies and an audit of existing genome-wide variant datasets for the selected AIM SNPs by analysing whole-genome sequence data released by the 1000 Genomes Project in 2020 [**15,16,17**]; and iv. Evaluation of the panel's capacity to make efficient population differentiations using existing likelihood-based ancestry inference tests.

2. MATERIALS AND METHODS

2.1. Selection and Balancing of Component Ancestry Informative SNPs

The BT assay design targeted an AIMs panel of approximately 120 SNPs, based on the fact that ~25% of the full multiplex would be occupied with the 41 markers of HIrisPlex-S, and shared use of key SNPs rs16891982 (in SLC45A2 gene), rs1426654 (SLC24A5), rs12913832 (HERC2) for both ancestry and appearance predictive purposes. Because tri-allelic SNPs have been found to be useful for the detection of mixed DNA [**18**], but when carefully selected have also been informative for ancestry to comparable levels as binary SNPs [**19**], we expanded their number in the multiplex above those of the previous gAIMs panel (which had six tri-allelic SNPs of a total 127 loci [**8**]). Twenty tri-allelic SNPs showing the highest levels of population divergence were selected from a very large candidate pool created from a genome-wide compilation of this type of human variation [**20**].

Careful consideration was made to balance the differentiation of the five main continental population groups of sub-Saharan Africa, Europe, East Asia, Oceania and America (herein, AFR, EUR, EAS, OCE and AMR) with differentiation of the South Asian sub-group (SAS). We decided to target 60–70 SNPs for continental differentiation, plus 20 SNPs to distinguish South Asia from the neighbouring population groups of Europe and East Asia.

SNPs for continental differentiation were compiled from four well-established AIM sets: i. the 127-SNP gAIMs ancestry panel; ii. the 446-SNP LACE (Latin American Cancer Epidemiology) ancestry panel [**21**]; iii–iv. the 165-SNP Thermo Fisher Precision ID Ancestry Panel (PIAP) [**14**], which includes the widely used 56-SNP Kiddlab ancestry panel [**22**]. SNPs differentiating South Asian and European populations were compiled from the above panels and three dedicated AIM sets for such geographic distinctions: v. the best European differentiating SNPs from the EUROFORGEN NAME panel [**23**]; vi. the Shriver group's US admixture mapping panel, with many highly European-informative loci [**24**]; and vii. the Eurasiaplex South Asian informative panel [**9**].

The continental SNPs in BT were balanced in terms of their individual population differentiation power to equilibrate as far as possible the five continental groups, ensuring that no one population group had excessive numbers of indicative SNPs, which could potentially bias calculations of co-ancestry proportions in persons with admixed backgrounds (e.g., excessive numbers of African-informative SNPs in such a small panel could overestimate this co-ancestry compared to the others). For each SNP, this process records the population specific divergence (In_{AFR}; In_{EUR}; $In_{E\ ASN}$; etc., the metric divergence is capitalised and measures the degree of differentiation per marker) to guide the removal or addition of SNPs for a specific population comparison in order to improve overall In balance. To reach this balance, the Snipper online ancestry analysis portal [**25**] was used to estimate cumulative In values, as previously described for the development of the gAIMs panel [**8**]. As BT had a smaller number of SNPs than gAIMs, we did not expect to reach a comparably narrow range of finely balanced In values.

2.2. Compilation of a 4132-Sample Population Dataset

A comprehensive population dataset for the BT ancestry SNPs was generated by compiling online whole-genome-sequencing variant data from 3965 samples and adding in-house genotyping of 167 samples from six populations, chosen to cover geographic gaps in data for several under-represented regions, i.e., 30 from Eritrea, 16 from Somalia, 32 from Morocco, 32 from Central Iraq, 28 from the Kurdistan region of Iraq and 29 from Turkey (Turkish resident in Germany). An additional 277 DNA samples from the HGDP-CEPH human diversity panel were genotyped with the BT assay with the goal of further extending the geographic coverage of Oceanian, Native American and Middle East (herein ME) population variation, i.e., regions not covered by 1000 Genomes Phase 3 populations. However, the 1000 Genomes Consortium completed whole-genome-sequencing of the full HGDP-CEPH panel in 2019 soon after our in-house genotyping had been completed, so we compiled the complete dataset from 1000 Genomes and used the overlapping sample data to measure the MPS genotyping concordance of BT. This was accomplished for the whole marker set of BT (i.e., including the 41 appearance markers) to gauge sequencing performance across the complete multiplex.

Of the total 4132 SNP genotype profiles compiled, 520 were used as a standardised six population group reference dataset for uploading as training sets to the Snipper ancestry analysis portal, with the aim of providing the closest possible equivalence of sample sizes amongst the continental and South Asian regions. The standardised reference dataset consisted of: sub-Saharan Africans represented by 108 1000 Genomes 30X sequence coverage (1KG-30) Yoruba from Nigeria (YRI); Europeans by 99 1KG-30 CEPH Europeans from Utah (CEU); East Asians by 103 1KG-30 Han Chinese from Beijing (CHB); South Asians by 103 1KG-30 Gujarati from Houston (GIH); Oceanians by 28 HGDP-CEPH Papuans from Bougainvillea and Papua New Guinea; Native Americans by 79 samples, comprising 61 HGDP-CEPH samples from Maya, Pima populations, Colombians and Amazonian Surui and Karitiana populations, supplemented by 18 1KG-30 Peruvians from Lima, Peru (PEL) which we had previously analysed and showed no detectable non-American co-ancestry (in-silico analysis of 572,743 Affymetrix Human Origins SNPs.

Although we established the above standardised reference dataset, the additional populations compiled can be flexibly included in Snipper or can replace those in the reference set at the user's discretion by adjusting the Excel-based training set file uploaded to the 'multiple profiles' classifier portal (**http://mathgene.usc.es/snipper/analysismultipleprofiles.html**, accessed on 20 August 2021), which generates a Bayes likelihood ratio statistical test for ancestry and a matched 2D principal component analysis (PCA) plot. For maximum flexibility, the other population data was arranged into a series of worksheets in the same core Excel reference file, allowing the end-user to select alternative reference populations from 1000 Genomes or HGDP-CEPH (e.g., HGDP-CEPH Pakistani South Asian samples rather than 1KG-30 Gujarati, or other populations from the Indian sub-continent). The same user-driven options apply to the VISAGE in-house population samples provided in a separate worksheet. The admixed populations in 1000 Genomes, comprising 96 African Caribbean individuals in Barbados (ACB), 61 Americans of African Ancestry in SW USA (ASW), 64 individuals with Mexican Ancestry from Los Angeles USA (MXL,) 94 Colombians from Medellin, Colombia (CLM), 104 Puerto Ricans from Puerto Rico (PUR), 67 of 85 PEL (i.e., with detected co-ancestry) were also compiled in a separate worksheet but would not be expected to be useful as training set data from which representative allele frequency estimates could be obtained, given their high levels of individual admixture.

Genome-wide variant data from Simons Foundation human genome diversity project (herein SGDP) has been available for several years [**27**], and offers additional information on geographic areas outside of those covered by 1000 Genomes or the HGDP-CEPH sampling regimes, in particular, Northeast Asia (broadly, Eastern Siberia east towards the Bering Straits); Southeast Island Asia; and Central South Asia (broadly, the Caucasus' east towards the central Asian Steppe immediately north of South Asia). There are 278 genome-wide SNP datasets, of which 22 overlap with 1000 Genomes and 126 overlap with the HGDP-CEPH panel samples, leaving 130 unique samples, from 67 populations. The small sample size of SGDP highlights the very limited number of 1, 2 or 3 samples per region. Nevertheless, we compiled the 130 SGDP-unique BT AIM profiles into a dedicated worksheet and completed population analyses using the standardised reference set.

Genome-wide variant data from the Estonian Biocentre genome diversity project (herein, EGDP) largely mirrors the sampling regimes of SGDP [**28**], with a maximum of 16 samples per region, but mainly 1, 2 or 3 per region. EGDP has 402 whole-genome datasets from the sampling of 126 populations that almost all complement those of SGDP and provides extensive coverage of regions in Siberia, Northeast Asia, Eastern Europe, and Central South Asia. As with SGDP, the 402 EGDP BT AIM profiles were compiled into a dedicated worksheet and population analyses made with the standardised reference set. Note that the tri-allelic SNPs forming part of the BT AIMs panel are not reported by EGDP and an additional four ancestry SNPs do not have genotypes, so data completeness is ~83.5% (96/115 SNPs).

2.3. Genotyping Concordance amongst MPS Sequence Data and Online Databases

Genotyping concordance for the BT SNPs was assessed in two ways. First, a direct comparison was made between the MPS genotypes generated during developmental runs genotyping 277 HGDP-CEPH DNA samples for all 153 SNPs in BT, and the SNP genotypes reported by 1000 Genomes for the same DNA samples [**16**], providing 42,381 comparisons. Second, the genotypes listed by 1000 Genomes Phase 3 database for 2504 worldwide population samples (and available in the Ensembl browser at: **http://www.ensembl.org/Homo_sapiens/Info/Index**, accessed on 20 August 2021) were compared to the high coverage re-sequencing dataset for the same samples, released in early 2020 by the New York Genome Centre [**17**]. The high sequence coverage genotypes correspond to an average 30X coverage, while the current Phase 3 genotypes were produced from an average 2-3X coverage. We considered the high coverage data to represent more reliable genotype calls for the SNPs of BT, so these were compiled as the major part of the reference population data we used for statistical analysis of ancestry, as described above.

The Coriell control DNA samples originally used as the genotyping concordance standards in the inter-laboratory evaluations of the BT assay [**29**] were also run as positive controls on each sequencing run performed for the in-house population studies.

2.4. Evaluation of Ancestry and Co-Ancestry Inference Efficiency of the BT AIMs

The efficiency of the BT AIMs to infer ancestry was assessed for a six-group differentiation of African, European, East Asian, South Asian, American and Oceanian ancestries. To measure classification error, one-out cross-validation of the standardised reference dataset of 520 samples was performed using the verbose cross validation option in Snipper (**http://mathgene.usc.es/Snipper/analysispopfile2_new.html**, accessed on 20 August 2021). For all other samples, STRUCTURE, PCA and neighbour joining tree (NJT) analyses were performed on each of the separate population sets, comprising admixed and unadmixed 1000 Genomes samples not used as reference data; HGDP-CEPH samples not used as reference data (i.e., no Oceanian, American population data); SGDP samples, with the six in-house populations included in the same analysis run; and EGDP samples (for 100 binary SNPs of 115 ancestry SNPs in BT). STRUCTURE v.2.3.4 [**30**] was used for runs consisting of five iterations per K (genetic cluster values K:2 to K:8 evaluated) consisting of 100,000 burnin steps and 100,000 MCMC steps, using correlated allele frequencies under the Admixture model. The optimum 'K' cluster number was inferred by plotting log probability of K and magnitude of ΔK, following the analyses of Evanno et al. [**31**]. Allele frequencies were updated only using individuals marked POPFLAG = 1 at the optimum genetic cluster number of K:6. Cluster membership proportion plots were constructed with CLUMPAK v.1.1 [**32**]. Multi-dimensional scaling (MDS) analysis and construction of neighbour-joining trees was implemented using R software v.3.5.0 [**33**] over an allele-distance matrix computed with the pegas R package [**34**].

The reliable identification of co-ancestry in DNA donors with admixed backgrounds can be considered important information that can be reported to investigators. Although there is likely to be some imprecision in the estimation of co-ancestry ratios when using relatively small-scale AIMs panels like BT, if the markers have been carefully balanced, they are more likely to be free of bias towards one particular co-ancestral population group and therefore match more closely the actual co-ancestry proportions in such individuals. To measure the reliability of co-ancestry estimation from identifying genetic clusters using the BT AIMs, we ran all 504 admixed 1000 Genomes samples described above (including all 85 PEL), together with the unadmixed populations from AFR, EUR, AMR and EAS, to keep the identified genetic clusters simple (K:4). The ACB and ASW samples represent typical African Caribbean and African American co-ancestry patterns of majority African co-ancestry and 0–30% European co-ancestry. The MXL, CLB, PUR and PEL samples represent more complex three-way co-ancestry patterns of major European co-ancestry, with Native American and African co-ancestries at varied ratios, with a few PEL individuals showing detectable East Asian co-ancestry [**15**]. We compared the BT data to the co-ancestry ratio estimates from the detailed genetic cluster analysis of the same 1000 Genomes-CEPH populations using 572,743 Affymetrix Human Origins SNPs (see **Section 2.2**. Although the parallel analyses with the Human Origins SNPs used the ADMIXTURE algorithm [**35**] to identify clusters, because data input for this algorithm uses only binary variant data, we applied STRUCTURE to ensure the tri-allelic SNP genotypes were assessed. Co-ancestry ratios were grouped into 10-percentiles (i.e., bins of one tenth of the samples from any one population) and the mean ratios of each of these 10-percentile groups in both analyses were assessed for goodness-of-fit using linear regression. Finally, we included a comparison with the genetic distance algorithm (GDA) co-ancestry estimator available in Snipper, developed from the work of Cheung et al. 2017 [**36**].

2.5. Evaluation of Ancestry and Co-Ancestry Inference Efficiency of the BT AIMs

The current gnomAD version 3.1 genome database compiles variation in almost 100,000 individuals from ten populations, so it provides a very efficient system for the detection of rare variation which could be potentially population informative. We screened the gnomAD 3.1 database to make a genomic audit of rare variations associated with the selected BT ancestry SNPs, comprising two types: i. rare, but potentially informative 'flanking' SNPs present on the same amplified fragment as the target SNP; and ii. additional polymorphic alleles in the binary ancestry SNPs, in the form of a third nucleotide substitution—creating a tri-allelic SNP where the allele-3 is either very rare or linked to a specific population group and hitherto undetected. Cataloguing rare third nucleotide substitutions is an important MPS quality control step, as it forewarns the user that the detected nucleotide at the target site is not a spurious sequencing result, but has been detected as a low frequency allele. We confined out searches for flanking SNPs within an arbitrary +/- 25 nucleotides of the target SNP position.

3. RESULTS AND DISCUSSION

3.1. Ancestry Informative SNPs in BT

The final BT ancestry panel consists of 100 binary SNPs, with 7 SNPs providing information about sub-Saharan African populations, 15 about European populations, 16 about East Asian populations, 20 about South Asian populations, 13 about Oceanian populations, and 17 about American people.The additional 12 ancestry single nucleotide polymorphisms (SNPs) out of the total 100 genetic locations were chosen due to their significant divergence between European and other Eurasian population clusters, specifically East and South Asian as well as Middle Eastern populations. Table 1 presents the origin of each binary SNPs mentioned in the earlier forensic AIMs panel studies discussed in Section 2.1 [8,9,21,22,23,24]. Additionally, it includes one OCE-informative SNP from a separate study that generated the Pacifiplex panel [11].Out of 100 single nucleotide polymorphisms (SNPs), 28 have been chosen as forensic ancestry informative markers (AIMs) in several panels.

Table 1. Commonality between SNPs selected for the BT ancestry panel and established forensic ancestry panels: Kiddlab 56; Thermo Fisher Precision ID Ancestry Panel (PIAP); Euroforgen Global AIMs (gAIMs); the LACE panel; the NAME panel; Eurasiaplex; and Shriver et al. US admixture mapping panel [24]. The two markers lower right are BT appearance SNPs previously selected as AIMs.

No.	Pop.	SNP	KK/PIAP	gAIMs	LACE	Other	No.	Pop.	SNP	KK/PIAP	gAIMs	LACE	Other	No.	Pop.	SNP	KK/PIAP	gAIMs	LACE	Other
1	AFR	rs10497191	Kiddlab	-	LACE		1	AME	rs10012227	-	gAIMs	-		1	Eurasia	rs1495085	-	-	-	NAME
2	AFR	rs1197062	-	gAIMs	LACE		2	AME	rs10483251	-	gAIMs	LACE		2	Eurasia	rs1757928	-	-	-	NAME
3	AFR	rs1369290	-	gAIMs	-		3	AME	rs12130799	PIAP	-	-		3	Eurasia	rs2337024	-	-	-	NAME
4	AFR	rs2789823	-	gAIMs	-		4	AME	rs12498138	Kiddlab	gAIMs	-		4	Eurasia	rs6989963	-	-	-	NAME
5	AFR	rs2814778	Kiddlab	gAIMs	-		5	AME	rs12629908	PIAP	-	-		5	Eurasia	rs6990312	Kiddlab	-	-	
6	AFR	rs310644	Kiddlab	gAIMs	-		6	AME	rs1452501	-	gAIMs	LACE		6	Eurasia	rs7148809	-	-	-	NAME
7	AFR	rs4737753	-	-	-	NAME	7	AME	rs1557553	-	gAIMs	LACE		7	Eurasia	rs12203115	-	-	-	NAME
1	EUR	rs11778591	-	gAIMs	LACE		8	AME	rs17130385	-	gAIMs	LACE		8	Eurasia	rs2227203	-	-	-	NAME
2	EUR	rs12142199	-	gAIMs	-		9	AME	rs17359176	-	gAIMs	LACE		9	Eurasia	rs39897	-	-	-	Eurasiaplex
3	EUR	rs12913832	Kiddlab	gAIMs	-		10	AME	rs174570	Kiddlab	gAIMs	LACE		10	Eurasia	rs4308478	-	-	-	NAME
4	EUR	rs1426654	Kiddlab	gAIMs	-		11	AME	rs2302013	-	gAIMs	-		11	Eurasia	rs7570971	-	-	-	NAME
5	EUR	rs16891982	Kiddlab	gAIMs	-		12	AME	rs2471552	-	gAIMs	-		12	Eurasia	rs984038	-	-	-	NAME
6	EUR	rs2715883	-	gAIMs	-		13	AME	rs3737576	Kiddlab	-	-		1	SAS	rs1040934	-	-	-	Shriver
7	EUR	rs3759171	-	gAIMs	LACE		14	AME	rs4792928	-	gAIMs	-		2	SAS	rs1063677	-	-	-	Shriver
8	EUR	rs705308	PIAP	-	-		15	AME	rs5757362	-	-	LACE		3	SAS	rs10764919	-	-	LACE	
9	EUR	rs7084970	-	gAIMs	-		16	AME	rs8137373	-	gAIMs	-		4	SAS	rs10962599	-	-	-	Eurasiaplex
10	EUR	rs7531501	-	gAIMs	-		17	AME	rs870347	Kiddlab	-	-		5	SAS	rs13267318	-	-	-	Shriver
11	EUR	rs8072587	-	gAIMs	-		1	EAS	rs10079352	-	gAIMs	LACE		6	SAS	rs13280988	-	-	LACE	
12	EUR	rs820371	-	gAIMs	LACE		2	EAS	rs1229984	Kiddlab	gAIMs	-		7	SAS	rs17625895	-	-	-	Eurasiaplex
13	EUR	rs862500	-	gAIMs	LACE		3	EAS	rs12594144	-	gAIMs	-		8	SAS	rs1796048	-	-	-	Shriver
14	EUR	rs917115	Kiddlab	gAIMs	-		4	EAS	rs1371048	-	gAIMs	-		9	SAS	rs1924381	-	gAIMs	LACE	
15	EUR	rs9522149	Kiddlab	gAIMs	-		5	EAS	rs17822931	-	gAIMs	-		10	SAS	rs2026999	-	-	-	Shriver
1	OCE	rs10149275	-	gAIMs	-		6	EAS	rs1834619	Kiddlab	gAIMs	-		11	SAS	rs2196051	Kiddlab	-	-	Eurasiaplex
2	OCE	rs16830500	-	gAIMs	-		7	EAS	rs2180052	-	gAIMs	-		12	SAS	rs2238151	Kiddlab	-	-	
3	OCE	rs2139931	-	gAIMs	-		8	EAS	rs3827760	Kiddlab	gAIMs	-		13	SAS	rs2269793	PIAP	-	-	
4	OCE	rs2274636	-	gAIMs	-		9	EAS	rs434504[illegible]	-	gAIMs	-		14	SAS	rs2472304	-	-	-	Eurasiaplex

No.	Pop.	SNP	KK/PIAP	gAIMs	LACE	Other	No.	Pop.	SNP	KK/PIAP	gAIMs	LACE	Other	No.	Pop.	SNP	KK/PIAP	gAIMs	LACE	Other
5	OCE	rs26951	-	gAIMs	-		10	EAS	rs459920	Kiddlab	-	-		15	SAS	rs2503770	-	gAIMs	LACE	
6	OCE	rs3751050	-	gAIMs	-		11	EAS	rs4657449	-	gAIMs	-		16	SAS	rs26247	-	-	-	Shriver
7	OCE	rs3804030	-	gAIMs	-		12	EAS	rs4781011	PIAP	-	-		17	SAS	rs3844336	-	-	-	Shriver
8	OCE	rs4391951	-	gAIMs	-		13	EAS	rs4918664	Kiddlab	gAIMs	-		18	SAS	rs7080350	-	-	LACE	
9	OCE	rs4959270	-	x	-	Pacifiplex *	14	EAS	rs4935501	-	gAIMs	-		19	SAS	rs7568054	-	-	LACE	
10	OCE	rs6054465	-	gAIMs	-		15	EAS	rs7226659	Kiddlab	-	-		20	SAS	rs756913	-	-	-	Eurasiaplex
11	OCE	rs715605	-	gAIMs	-		16	EAS	rs8104441	-	gAIMs	-								
12	OCE	rs9908046	-	gAIMs	-									MYH15 °	EAS	rs6437783	-	gAIMs	-	-
13	OCE	rs9934011	-	gAIMs	-									OCA2 °	EAS	rs1800414	Kiddlab	-	-	-

* A single SNP developed for the Pacifiplex panel was not incorporated into gAIMs. ° Gene locations of the two BT appearance SNPs previously selected for other ancestry panels.

Balancing population specific divergence (PSD) values (excluding the 12 Eurasian divergent SNPs) was successful to a large extent and the cumulative PSD values for each of the six population groups are shown in **Figure 1**. AFR, EUR, OCE and AMR were well balanced with cumulative PSD values of 13.54, 13.30, 11.99 and 11.8, respectively. EAS with a cumulative value of 9.43 did not have enough informative SNPs to reach these levels of divergence, while SAS, with much less differentiation from EUR and EAS, only reached a cumulative value of 2.7. It is noteworthy that two BT appearance SNPs, rs6437783 (in MYH15 gene) and rs1800414 (OCA2), shown in **Table 1**, had been selected for previous forensic ancestry panels as an EAS-informative SNP in gAIMs and Kiddlab AIM sets, respectively. Given the lower cumulative PSD value for EAS compared to other population groups, these two markers would be worth considering as joint ancestry-appearance SNPs along with the three already used in this way.

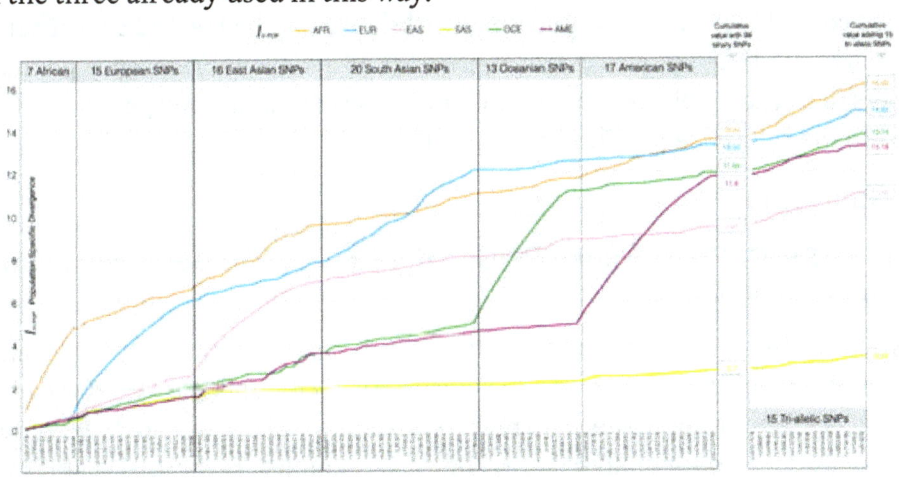

Figure 1. Accumulating population specific divergence values for each of the main population groups and the six sets of SNPs informative for their differentiation. The cumulative values are shown obtained from 88 binary SNPs (i.e., excluding 12 Eurasian-informative SNPs) and from the addition of the 15 tri-allelic SNPs in BT (VISAGE Basic Tool).

From a candidate list of 20 tri-allelic SNPs, rs11238577, rs11990024, rs9845503, rs7853487 and rs809540 were rejected from the assay design, bringing the total number of AIMs in BT to 115, including the three shared appearance SNPs. When the 15 tri-allelic SNPs were added to the cumulative PSD plot of **Figure 1** the balance was marginally improved for EAS with a cumulative PSD value of 11.01 closer to the average value for the other population groups.

Allele frequency estimates of the 115 BT AIMs based on the standardised reference grid outlined in **Section 2.2** (YRI, CEU, CHB, GIH, plus HGDP-CEPH Americans and Oceanians). Middle East allele frequency estimates are included based on 134 HGDP-CEPH samples from the Israeli Bedouin, Druze and Palestinian populations. The allele frequencies of 12 Eurasian-informative SNPs in the relevant population groups. For comparison purposes we included North African (NAF) allele frequency estimates based on HGDP-CEPH Mozabite from Algeria, and delta values were estimated for EUR compared to a NAF-ME-SAS average).

3.2. *Aggregation of Reference and Test Population Datasets*

The Excel worksheets necessary for generating Bayes likelihood calculations and linked PCA analyses by uploading the BT ancestry SNP genotype data to Snipper. The active worksheet of reference and query SNP profiles uploaded to Snipper is in position 1 in Excel and has the label '1' applied to all reference population profiles in the rightmost column, and '0' to unknown profiles such as those compiled from a forensic sample. The values in cells A1, B1, C1 provide numbers of reference/query profiles, markers, and populations in the worksheet, respectively. All other SNP profiles compiled in the six supporting worksheets can be treated as test samples (i.e., marked with a '0'), or used as alternative or additional reference population datasets (e.g., the HGDP-CEPH or VISAGE in-house ME population genotypes can be added to the reference profiles as a seventh population group).

3.3. Genotyping Concordance

3.3.1. *HGDP-CEPH in-House BT Genotypes vs. 1000 Genomes Whole-Genome-Sequence Data*

The pairwise genotype comparisons between in-house data for HGDP-CEPH samples and the data from 1000 Genomes published in 2020 [**16**]. This file examines all SNPs in BT except for one appearance marker, rs796296176, which did not have genotype data from the in-house analyses of HGDP-CEPH samples. Five HGDP-CEPH Middle East samples had excessive numbers of data gaps from in-house sequencing and were not included in genotype comparisons. Of the 153 total markers in BT, two ancestry SNPs had higher than average discordancy rates, indicating a problem with genotyping either from 1000 Genomes sequence analysis, or the BT MPS assay. First, tri-allelic SNP rs2737126 had 15/277 (5.4%) genotype discordancy, seemingly arising from failure to detect a G allele, when present as a GT or CG heterozygote, but not for all such genotypes. This phenomenon was not explained by detailed scrutiny of sequence data at this variant site. Second, the binary SNP rs3804030 had a disproportionately high genotype discordancy rate of 29/277 (10.47%), which appeared to be due to a failure to detect the rare, OCE-indicative C allele outside of Oceanian populations examined by 1000 Genomes. Interestingly, no discordances were seen for this SNP amongst pairwise comparisons of 27 HGDP-CEPH Oceanians.

The 151 SNPs of BT without apparent problems, the genotyping concordance was very high, reaching 99.96% concordance with 17 discordances largely appearing at random across the data grid, rather than systematically as detected in the above two SNPs. This high level of genotype concordance between the BT assay developed vs. 1000 Genomes whole genome sequence-based variant detection indicates the robustness of the MPS method and the BT multiplex developed by VISAGE. The no-call rate (unreported genotypes) was also low at 0.2% for 1000 Genomes, and 0.6% for our MPS genotyping.

3.3.2. 1000 Genomes Phase 3 Genotypes vs. 1000 Genomes High Sequence Coverage Genotypes

File S3B gives the pairwise comparisons for all BT SNPs between the current 1000 Genomes Phase 3 genotypes listed online by Ensembl, and the genotypes published following high coverage sequence analysis of the same samples by the New York Genome Centre [**17**]. As we have relied extensively on the online genotype data produced by 1000 Genomes Phase 3 for several years, the cross-checks of genotype calls comparing 30X and 2-3X sequence coverage that this concordance analysis provides are important. Amongst all 153 BT SNPs, 73 had zero genotype discordances and 66 showed largely inconsequential discordances numbering 1–5 genotype differences between each sequencing dataset (a locus-specific concordance of 99.96–99.8%). However, 14 SNPs had higher levels of six or more discordances, comprising 11 ancestry SNPs. Three ancestry SNPs: rs2789823, rs9522149 and rs2196051 had concordance rates ≤ 98.2% due to 25, 27 and 46 discordances, respectively. The BT ancestry SNPs genotype discordances of two or more in number are summarised in **Figure 2.** It can be assumed that higher sequence coverage provides more secure genotyping for a small, but significant proportion of SNPs in the 1000 Genomes variant database, of which 14 with higher-than-average levels of discordancy are part of BT. For this reason, all reference population data compiled from 1000 Genomes for VISAGE ancestry analyses with BT are based on the high coverage (30X) genotype datasets, which have yet to be made available in the Ensemble variant browser for 1000 Genomes.

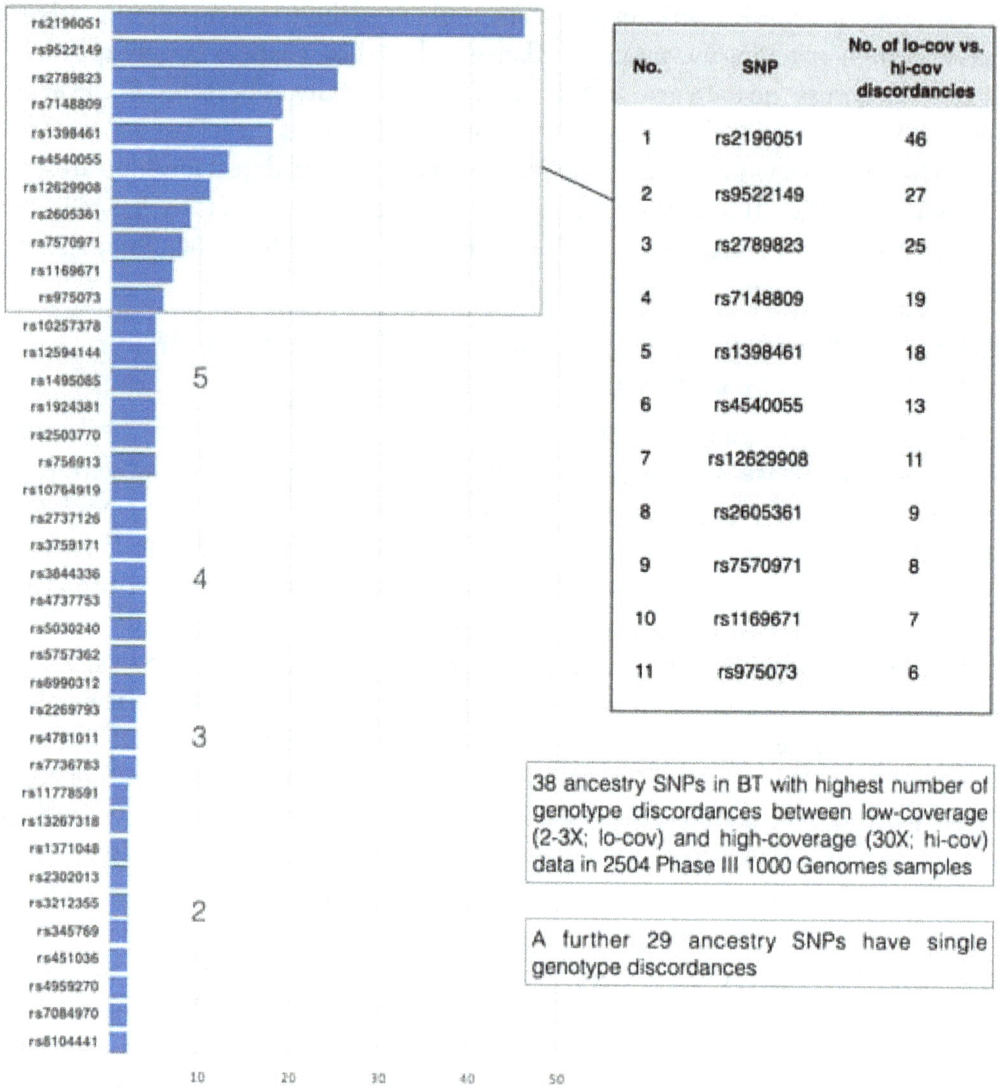

Figure 2. The 38 BT ancestry SNPs with the highest numbers of discordant genotypes between 1000 Genomes low coverage vs. high coverage sequence data. An additional 29 had only one discordant genotype. The full set of genotype comparisons for all BT SNPs and all 1000 Genomes samples are given in File S3B.

3.4. Ancestry Inference Efficiency of the BT Ancestry SNPs

One-out cross validation of the reference dataset gave 100% correct classification in all cases, i.e., all 520 reference profiles were successfully assigned to their true population of origin. The likelihood ratio values produced by cross validation were consistently high and most samples gave likelihoods greater than 'The profile is more than 1 billion times more likely to be from the true population of origin than another population' (data not shown).

Figure 3A shows the STRUCTURE analysis K:6 cluster plots for the reference populations (1–6) in worksheet 1. **Figure** 3B shows the accompanying probability of data and Delta K statistical analyses indicating an optimum cluster number of 6 for these analyses. **Figure** 3C shows colour-matched MDS plots for the same samples for coordinate 1 vs. 2 (left plot), 1 vs. 3 (mid) and 2 vs. 3. Only a small degree of overlap between the OCE and EAS MDS clusters-of-points remains when comparing all three coordinate plots. **Figure** 3D shows the Neighbour Joining Tree (NJT) distance matrix results, which indicate a clear arrangement of branch lengths and spatial separation, apart from two SAS outliers close to the OCE set. The summary of cross-validation classification results in **Figure** 3E completes the ancestry analysis of these sample sets.

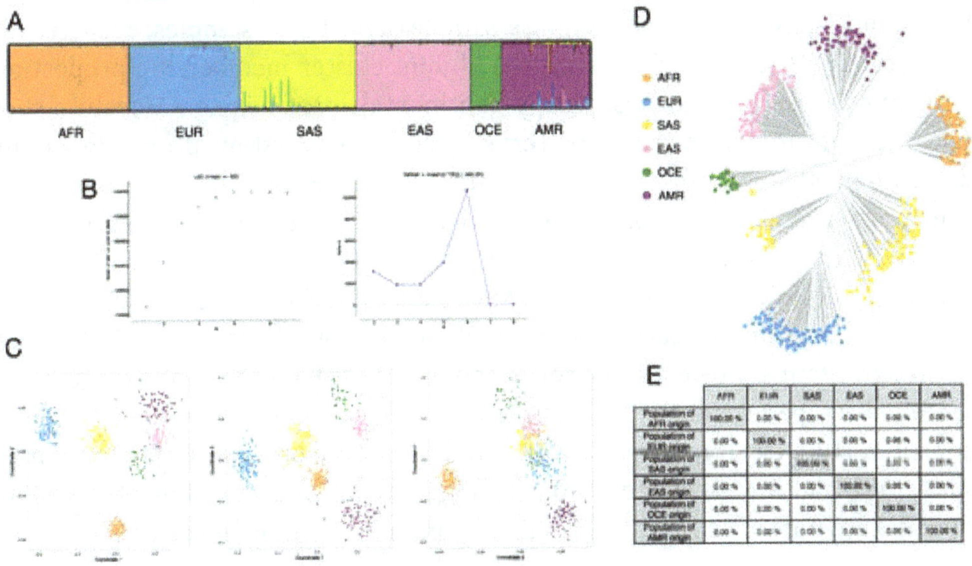

Figure 3. Ancestry analysis with 115 BT ancestry SNPs of the six populations of the standardised reference dataset (AFR: brown; EUR: blue; SAS: yellow; EAS: pink; OCE: green; AMR: purple), with consistent colours across three statistical analyses of A, C and D. (A) STRUCTURE cluster membership proportions at K = 6, indicated to be the optimum K number of genetic clusters by: (B) the mean L(K) (log probability of data) and ΔK plots from STRUCTURE runs, following the analyses of Evanno et al. [31]. (C) Multi-dimensional scaling (MDS) analysis showing principal component (PC) 1 vs. PC2 coordinates, PC1 vs. PC3 and PC2 vs. PC3 two-dimensional plots. (D) Neighbour joining tree (NJT) analysis. (E) Summary classification success table of cross validation of the standardised reference set.

Summarises the same type of population analyses as **Figure 3** applied to unadmixed (8–11, 14–25) and admixed (12–13, 26–29) 1000 Genomes samples (30X coverage genotypes) analysed against the reference population set. In nearly all cases, unadmixed samples show low levels of joint cluster membership. The admixed African populations give similar patterns to those found in other studies (but see **Section 3.5**) with European co-ancestry ranging from 5–30% K2 cluster membership. The admixed American samples from 1000 Genomes also show the expected proportions from K:2 and K:6 in the STRUCTURE analysis, with K:1 cluster membership forming the third African co-ancestry component, most evident in Puerto Ricans. The carefully curated Peruvian reference Native American samples are clearly discernible on the left of the columns of the K6 cluster. Equally consistently, admixed samples occupy the middle ground between the MDS clusters-of-points formed by the unadmixed samples, depending on the degree of their separation in coordinates 1 vs. 3 or 1 vs. 2 MDS plots, particularly the admixed Africans in 1 vs. 2.

Identical analysis output and using the same reference populations for HGDP-CEPH samples, SGDP-VISAGE in-house samples and EGDP samples, respectively. The HGDP-CEPH samples show a degree of joint cluster membership proportions in regions whose populations occupy continental margins, e.g., Mozabite show African-European co-ancestry patterns (joint membership proportions) and Pakistani populations show some European co-ancestry. The SGDP and EGDP sample analyses are the most varied, reflecting the more widespread sampling locations and emphasis on continental margin regions such as Central South Asia. The SGDP-EGDP Oceanian and American samples give clear, unequivocal cluster memberships, underlining the careful choice of informative SNPs for these population groups. However, it should be noted that BT and all other equivalent MPS ancestry panels show Oceanian ancestry to be only a small proportion of the STRUCTURE cluster patterns in the single SGDP Maori and Hawaiian samples, indicating that AIMs selected from analysis of Melanesians (i.e., HGDP-CEPH Papuans) are not sufficiently informative to infer Polynesian ancestry.

3.5. Co-Ancestry Analysis of Known Admixed Individuals in 1000 Genomes with BT Ancestry SNPs

3.5.1. Comparison of Co-Ancestry Patterns Obtained with the Human Origins Panel and BT

Figure 4 shows a direct pairwise comparison of the co-ancestry patterns (cluster membership proportions) of 504 admixed samples from 1000 Genomes, analysed in combination with the standardised reference set with the >572,000 Human Origins array SNPs (using ADMIXTURE due to SNP data density) and the 115 ancestry SNPs of BT (using STRUCTURE). The genetic cluster proportions from both analyses on which the **Figure 4** cluster plots are based. These plots show a very good match of co-ancestry patterns in the two African admixed ACB and ASW populations. The correlation analysis and r^2 values aligned below the cluster plots in **Figure 4** indicate high levels of correlation between Origins and BT co-ancestry proportion estimates for ACB and ASW, notably for the AFR proportions (although they are combined with AMR co-ancestry in these assessments). The EUR co-ancestry proportions tend to be slightly underestimated by BT SNPs or go undetected when very small.

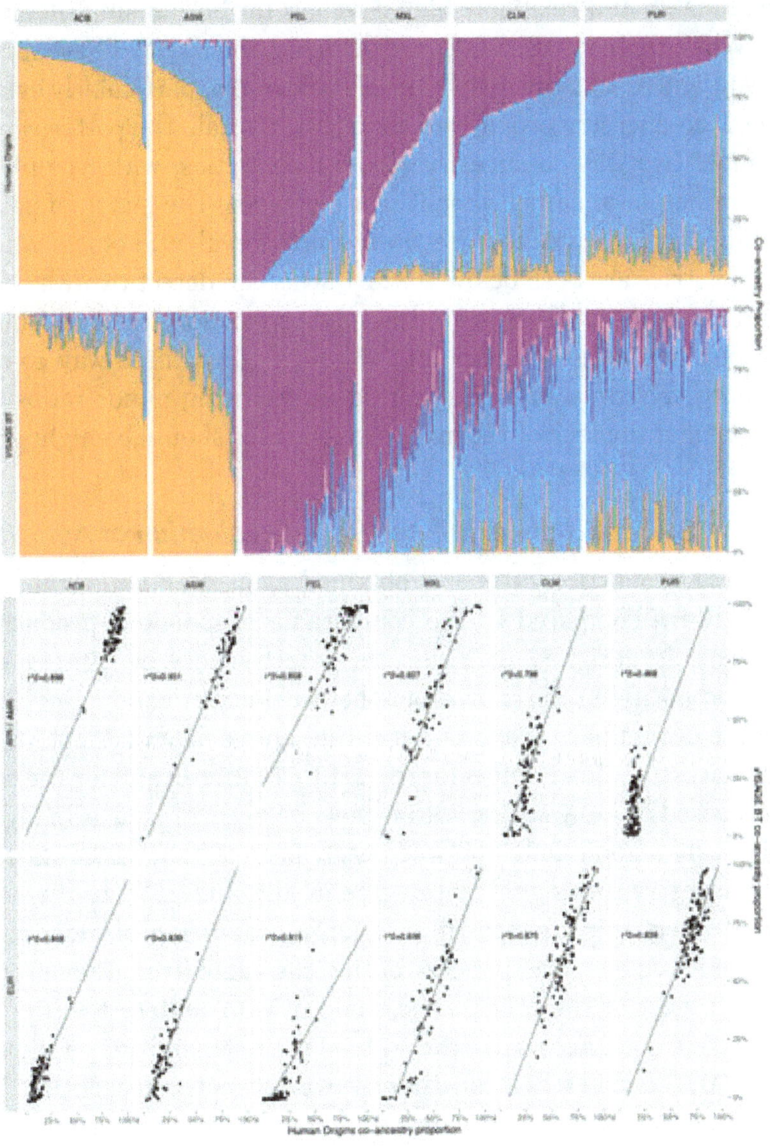

Figure 4. Pairwise comparison of individual co-ancestry proportions (cluster membership proportions) in 504 admixed samples from 1000 Genomes, analysed using the standardised reference set with Human Origins array, comprising >572,000 SNPs (using ADMIXTURE) and 115 VISAGE BT ancestry SNPs (using STRUCTURE). Co-ancestry proportions in four genetic clusters representing, African, European, Native American and East Asian, ancestries are given in File S4. The r^2 correlation analysis plots of each admixed population group are shown below the corresponding cluster patterns.

The four admixed populations with AMR co-ancestry are arranged in descending overall proportions of this co-ancestry and all show the same tendency for BT SNPs to underestimate the EUR proportions, but the PEL, MXL and CLM patterns still show a good match and relatively high r^2 values for both main EUR and AMR co-ancestries. When three co-ancestries are detected, the BT SNPs have less precision to detect AMR and AFR co-ancestry at levels below 25%, particularly evident in the PUR non-EUR co-ancestry proportion estimates. Overall, the patterns match very well for simple two-way co-ancestry across most ratios, with BT only failing to detect very minor co-ancestry when it falls below 5%. The match of patterns only tends to reduce when 3-way co-ancestry is more prevalent, notably when the two minor co-ancestries are both below 10%. BT SNPs can detect two-way co-ancestry using STRUCTURE with sufficient accuracy for proportions to be reliably reported down to about 10% minor co-ancestry, although when three-way co-ancestry is detected, more caution would be required in reporting minor ratios below this 10% threshold and the lack of accuracy in such cases should be highlighted in the report.

3.5.2. Using GDA as a Simple Snipper-Based Evaluation of Admixture

The coancestry proportion estimates obtained from the STRUCTURE analysis of the BT SNPs were compared to the comparable proportions produced by GDA in Snipper.This is designed to assess the effectiveness of GDA in identifying admixture and notifying the user about the necessity of conducting STRUCTURE analysis, if the preliminary examination of the sample data does not indicate clear unadmixed ancestry. Cluster plots for the STRUCTURE run and for the co-ancestry proportions based on GDA values, with r^2 plots below arranged as in **Figure 4**. The r^2 values indicate a good match between each approach, but GDA underestimates the EUR co-ancestry to a significant degree in ACB and ASW, to the point where GDA did not detect this co-ancestry in a large proportion of individuals, and it was underestimated by more than 50% of the true value (from Human Origins SNP array data) in most of the others. The trend of GDA underestimating European co-ancestry continues across all the PEL, MXL, CLM and PUR samples, where additionally, AFR co-ancestry is consistently overestimated in each population. The EUR underestimation is partly explained by detection of significant proportions of EAS co-ancestry by GDA, likely to be falsely created by a close relationship between AMR and EAS population groups, which STRUCTURE differentiates more efficiently as distinct genetic clusters compared to GDA's measure of distance between EUR and both AMR and EAS.

3.5.3. Comparisons of 10-Percentile Co-Ancestry Ratio Patterns

To facilitate the evaluation of trends in the detection of co-ancestry using the smallscale BT ancestry panel and the initial assessment of admixture using GDA, the mean co-ancestry ratios per 10percentile group of individuals were plotted. This visualization aimed to smooth the data and provide a final comparison of co-ancestry patterns. The figure labeled S3B displays the co-ancestry proportions derived from the Origins SNPs and BT SNPs, as well as the GDA proportions. When admixture patterns are summarised into percentile groups, it is much easier to see the very close match in estimated co-ancestry ratios between Origins and BT SNP-based STRUCTURE runs. This is particularly evident in the 10th ASW percentile with a three-way co-ancestry pattern, and the 10th PEL percentile with a fourth EAS co-ancestry. However, co-ancestry proportions below 10% regularly fail to be detected by BT (1st ACB percentile, 3rd–5th PEL, 1st–2nd MXL, 9th–10th CLM percentiles). Therefore, it remains prudent to recognise that BT will not consistently detect co-ancestry ratios ≤10%. The presence of EAS co-ancestry at very small proportions in many of the MXL-CLM-PUR BT percentile groups indicates this component should be ignored when it is less than 10% and AMR co-ancestry is present above this ratio at the same time. The percentile group patterns in GDA emphasise that it is not an efficient technique for detecting admixture accurately when co-ancestral ratios are below 20%, so it does not provide an accurate measure of individuals with these proportions and STRUCTURE would be required in all cases, particularly as the bulk of the PEL-MXL-CLM percentile groups show spurious EAS co-ancestry ratios above this threshold value).

3.6. Audit of Additional Variation in BT SNPs from the GnomAD 3.1 Database

The co-amplified flanking SNPs and extra third-substitution alleles amongst both ancestry and appearance binary BT SNPs detected in the gnomAD 3.1 database. Twelve ancestry SNPs and three appearance SNPs had a third substitution allele, which reached the highest allele frequency of only 0.0002 in rs2302013 and rs917115 (both in East Asians). Ancestry SNP rs1063677 and appearance SNP rs12821256 showed all four substitution alleles, with the highest frequency for allele T of 0.0005 in Europeans in the GC SNP rs1063677.

The power of gnomAD to detect low frequency variants across the genome enabled sequence screens that indicated a large number of flanking SNPs within 25 nucleotides of the target site of many BT SNPs. Amongst the 115 ancestry SNPs, 49 had flanking SNPs, while in the 41 appearance (EVC) SNPs, there were 23, notably markers targeted in the SNP-rich MC1R gene. Four ancestry SNPs showed informative combinations of alleles in close proximity which show unlinked allele frequencies between the two loci—in other words, forming population-informative 2-SNP microhaplotypes (i.e., diplotypes). The Chr-3 pair rs1169671-rs76444263 (target SNP in bold), Chr-8 pair rs75064826-rs13280988 and Chr-19 pair rs2337025-rs2337024 all show SAS-informative diplotypes, while the Chr-20 pair rs4809578-

rs310644 has a range of diplotypes, which are most differentiating for AFR and EAS population groups. Microhaplotype rs1169671-rs76444263 combines a tri-allelic and binary SNP, but the latter has low levels of polymorphism so is less informative than the other binary SNP pairs. Diplotype SNP allele combinations can be analysed in Snipper by assigning A, C, G, T allele nomenclature to the alphabetic arrangement of diplotypes, which, for the above binary SNP pairs, would be A=AA, C=AG, G=CA, T=CG combinations; A=AA, C=AG, G=GA, T=GG combinations; and A=AC, C=AT, G=TC, T=TT combinations, respectively. While the phase of each SNP pair's alleles needs to be detected from the sequence data to do this, it indicates the potential extra variant information, which is accessible from MPS analysis of forensic SNPs.

4. AT A GLANCE

The main objective of the VISAGE Consortium is to create a comprehensive forensic intelligence tool using MPS technology. This will involve the development of a complete analytical pipeline.The inclusion of population reference data and predictive algorithms for inferring age, ancestry, and appearance features associated with the genotyped SNPs, along with an optimal sequencing technique suited to the two primary forensic MPS platforms now in use, is necessary.By initially utilizing a prototype tool that incorporates basic age predictors in one multiplex, along with wellestablished predictors for pigmentation phenotype and continental ancestry in another, we were able to lay a solid groundwork for the development of the more advanced VISAGE Enhanced Tool (ET).The ET method involves significant enlargement of all three 'AAA' predictive systems within the identical parallel MPS multiplex setup as BT. This arrangement includes distinct DNA procedures specifically designed for methylation analysis and SNP genotyping.The BT ancestry panel selected the most useful SNPs from many existing forensic ancestry panels, prioritizing the reliability of known MPS sequences and maximizing ancestry informativeness.Due to this, BT has demonstrated exceptional sequencing efficiency in forensic DNA analysis [29,37], and allows for accurate ancestry predictions for populations of continental and South Asian descent with the greatest statistical certainty.

Although we dedicated considerable resources to genotyping BT SNPs in populations addressing several geographic gaps in coverage left by large-scale genomic sequencing projects, many global regions remain to be characterised with new studies. The dynamic system in Snipper, i.e., compiling the largest possible array of population data and allowing the end-user to select which samples extend or modify the standardised reference set, provides flexibility for statistical analyses of BT SNP data. It also allows new population data to be uploaded to the webpages holding reference sets (**http://mathgene.usc.es/snipper/forensic_mps_aims.html**, accessed on 20 August 2021) and the additional populations shown in **File**

S1. Although genetic cluster analyses using STRUCTURE can be challenging for forensic practitioners analysing population data for the first time, in our view, it is the best way to detect and analyse individual co-ancestry in persons with admixed backgrounds. The comparisons of GDA and STRUCTURE made in this study indicate that GDA is not accurate enough to evaluate low level co-ancestry when admixture patterns are complex and an individual has more than two co-ancestries. However, when the BT ancestry SNPs are compared to the much larger panel of Human Origins SNPs, the level of detail obtained using STRUCTURE is well matched and indicates BT SNPs are informative enough to accurately detect co-ancestral components present above 10% proportions.

Furthermore, the meticulousness in choosing the BT ancestry SNPs, considering their documented reliability and sensitivity in previous MPSbased forensic ancestry panels [8,12,18,20,23], has played a crucial role in guaranteeing consistent performance in evaluating both forensic MPS platforms in the future.The VISAGE Consortium has followed SWGDAM guidelines for newly developed forensic DNA techniques, including AmpliSeq chemistry [29], PowerSeq chemistry [37], and ForenSeq chemistry (with a manuscript in submission). This includes ensuring sequencing chemistry, library preparation, and sequence read balance are all in accordance with the guidelines. The consortium has observed these factors in the forensic validations conducted so far.The ET ancestry panel has utilized these identical principles to enhance the multiplex size and expand the spectrum of populations that can be distinguished by ET ancestry SNPs.

5. CONCISE SUMMARY

This article describes the creation of a panel of single nucleotide polymorphisms (SNPs) that can determine a person's ancestry. The panel, called VISAGE Basic Tool (BT), consists of 41 SNPs that predict appearance and 112 SNPs that predict ancestry (with three SNPs shared between the two sets). These SNPs are analyzed using massively parallel sequencing (MPS) technology. In addition, a separate MPS analysis pipeline is used to analyze blood-based age using methylation markers. The SNPs used for the BT ancestry panel were primarily established forensic markers that have demonstrated reliable sequencing performance in MPS. The total magnitude of the SNP multiplex largely aligned with existing forensic MPS assays. SNPs were selected to distinguish individuals belonging to the five primary continental demographic groups: Africa, Europe, East Asia, America, and Oceania. Additionally, the selection was expanded to include differentiation of persons from South Asia. The BT ancestry panel demonstrated zero classification error when analyzed using the Bayes likelihood calculators of the Snipper online analysis portal, based on data from 1000 Genomes and HGDP-CEPH samples from six population groupings. The discriminative ability of the ancestral single nucleotide polymorphisms (SNPs) of BT was carefully equalized to minimize any potential bias in estimating the percentage of shared ancestry in individuals with mixed genetic backgrounds. The balancing process resulted in nearly identical cumulative population-specific divergence values for Africa, Europe, America, and Oceania. East Asia exhibited a somewhat lower value compared to the average, whereas South Asia stood out as an outlier from the other groupings. The African, European, and Native American estimated co-ancestry proportions were compared in the six admixed groups of the 1000 Genomes project. This comparison was done using the BT ancestry panel SNPs and 572,000 Affymetrix Human Origins array SNPs. Co-ancestry proportions that were quite similar were reported, reaching a minimum value of 10%. However, below this threshold, the detection of low-level co-ancestry using BT SNPs was not always reliable. The Snipper analysis portal offers an extensive population dataset for the BT ancestry panel SNPs. This dataset includes a standardized reference dataset of 520 samples, as well as an additional 3445 samples from various genome diversity projects such as 1000 Genomes, HGDP-CEPH, Simons Foundation, and Estonian Biocentre. Additionally, there are 167 samples from in-house genotyping of individuals from Middle East, North, and East African regions, which complement the sampling regimes of the other diversity projects.

Appendix A

Centres and investigators of the VISible Attributes through GEnomics (VISAGE) Consortium, Website: **http://www.visage-h2020.eu/** (accessed on 20 August 2021).

- Erasmus University Medical Center Rotterdam, Rotterdam, The Netherlands: Manfred Kayser, Vivian Kalamara, Arwin Ralf, Athina Vidaki
- Jagiellonian University, Krakow, Poland: Wojciech Branicki, Ewelina Pośpiech, Aleksandra Pisarek
- Universidade de Santiago de Compostela, Santiago de Compostela, Spain: Ángel Carracedo, Maria Victoria Lareu, Christopher Phillips, Ana Freire-Aradas, Ana Mosquera-Miguel, María de la Puente
- Medizinische Universität Innsbruck, Innsbruck, Austria: Walther Parson, Catarina Xavier, Antonia Heidegger, Harald Niederstätter
- Universität zu Köln, Cologne, Germany: Michael Nothnagel, Maria-Alexandra Katsara, Tarek Khellaf
- King's College London, London, UK: Barbara Prainsack, Gabrielle Samuel
- Klinikum der Universität zu Köln, Cologne, Germany: Peter M. Schneider, Theresa E. Gross,
- Jan Fleckhaus, Elaine Cheung.

- Bundeskriminalamt, Wiesbaden, Germany: Ingo Bastisch, Nathalie Schury, Jens Teodoridis,
- Martina Unterländer
- Institut National de Police Scientifique, Lyon, France: François-Xavier Laurent, Caroline
- Bouakaze, Yann Chantrel, Anna Delest, Clémence Hollard, Ayhan Ulus, Julien Vannier
- Netherlands Forensic Institute, The Hague, Netherlands: Titia Sijen, Kris van der Gaag,
- Marina Ventayol-Garcia
- National Forensic Centre, Swedish Police Authority, Linköping, Sweden: Johannes Hedman,
- Klara Junker, Maja Sidstedt
- Metropolitan Police Service, London, United Kingdom: Shazia Khan, Carole E. Ames, Andrew Revoir
- CentralneLaboratoriumKryminalistycznePolicji, Warsaw, Poland: Magdalena Spólnicka, Ewa Kartasinska, Anna Woźniak

REFERENCES

1. Phillips, C. Forensic genetic analysis of bio-geographical ancestry. Forensic Sci. Int. Genet. **2015**, 18, 49–65. **[Google Scholar]** **[CrossRef]**
2. Kayser, M. Forensic DNA Phenotyping: Predicting human appearance from crime scene material for investigative purposes. Forensic Sci. Int. Genet. **2015**, 18, 33–48. **[Google Scholar]** **[CrossRef]** **[PubMed]**
3. Freire-Aradas, A.; Phillips, C.; Lareu, M.V. Forensic individual age estimation with DNA: From initial approaches to methylation tests. Forensic Sci. Rev. **2017**, 29, 121–144. **[Google Scholar]** **[PubMed]**
4. King, T.E.; Fortes, G.G.; Balaresque, P.; Thomas, M.G.; Balding, D.; Delser, P.M.; Neumann, R.; Parson, W.; Knapp, M.; Walsh, S.; et al. Identification of the remains of King Richard III. Nat. Commun. **2014**, 5, 5631. **[Google Scholar]** **[CrossRef]**
5. Walsh, S.; Liu, F.; Ballantyne, K.N.; van Oven, M.; Lao, O.; Kayser, M. IrisPlex: A sensitive DNA tool for accurate prediction of blue and brown eye colour in the absence of ancestry information. Forensic Sci. Int. Genet. **2011**, 5, 170–180. **[Google Scholar]** **[CrossRef]**

6. Walsh, S.; Liu, F.; Wollstein, A.; Kovatsi, L.; Ralf, A.; Kosiniak-Kamysz, A.; Branicki, W.; Kayser, M. The HIrisPlex system for simultaneous prediction of hair and eye colour from DNA. Forensic Sci. Int. Genet. **2013**, 7, 98–115. **[Google Scholar] [CrossRef] [PubMed] [Green Version]**
7. Walsh, S.; Chaitanya, L.; Breslin, K.; Muralidharan, C.; Bronikowska, A.; Pospiech, E.; Koller, J.; Kovatsi, L.; Wollstein, A.; Branicki, W.; et al. Global skin colour prediction from DNA. Hum. Genet. **2017**, 136, 847–863. **[Google Scholar] [CrossRef] [Green Version]**
8. Phillips, C.; Parson, W.; Lundsberg, B.; Santos, C.; Freire-Aradas, A.; Torres, M.; Eduardoff, M.; Børsting, C.; Johansen, P.; Fondevila, M.; et al. Building a forensic ancestry panel from the ground up: The EUROFORGEN Global AIM-SNP set. Forensic Sci. Int. Genet. **2014**, 11, 13–25. **[Google Scholar] [CrossRef] [Green Version]**
9. Phillips, C.; Freire Aradas, A.; Kriegel, A.K.; Fondevila, M.; Bulbul, O.; Santos, C.; Serrulla Rech, F.; Perez Carceles, M.D.; Carracedo, A.; Schneider, P.M.; et al. Eurasiaplex: A forensic SNP assay for differentiating European and South Asian ancestries. Forensic Sci. Int. Genet. **2013**, 7, 359–366. **[Google Scholar] [CrossRef]**
10. Carvalho Gontijo, C.; Porras-Hurtado, L.G.; Freire-Aradas, A.; Fondevila, M.; Santos, C.; Salas, A.; Henao, J.; Isaza, C.; Beltrán, L.; Nogueira Silbiger, V.; et al. PIMA: A population informative multiplex for the Americas. Forensic Sci. Int. Genet. **2020**, 44, 102200. **[Google Scholar] [CrossRef] [Green Version]**
11. Santos, C.; Phillips, C.; Fondevila, M.; Daniel, R.; van Oorschot, R.A.H.; Burchard, E.G.; Schanfield, M.S.; Souto, L.J.; Uacyisrael, J.; Via, M.; et al. Pacifiplex: An ancestry-informative SNP panel centred on Australia and the Pacific region. Forensic Sci. Int. Genet. **2016**, 20, 71–80. **[Google Scholar] [CrossRef] [PubMed]**
12. Phillips, C.; McNevin, D.; Kidd, K.K.; Lagacé, R.; Wootton, S.; de la Puente, M.; Freire-Aradas, A.; Mosquera-Miguel, A.; Eduardoff, M.; Gross, T.; et al. MAPlex-A massively parallel sequencing ancestry analysis multiplex for Asia-Pacific populations. Forensic Sci. Int. Genet. **2019**, 42, 213–226. **[Google Scholar] [CrossRef] [Green Version]**
13. Breslin, K.; Wills, B.; Ralf, A.; Ventayol Garcia, M.; Kukla-Bartoszek, M.; Pospiech, E.; Freire-Aradas, A.; Xavier, C.; Ingold, S.; de La Puente, M.; et al. HIrisPlex-S system for eye, hair, and skin color prediction from DNA: Massively parallel sequencing solutions for two common forensically used platforms. Forensic Sci. Int. Genet. **2019**, 43, 102152. **[Google Scholar] [CrossRef] [PubMed]**

14. Al-Asfi, M.; McNevin, D.; Mehta, B.; Power, D.; Gahan, M.E.; Daniel, R. Assessment of the Precision ID Ancestry Panel. Int. J. Legal. Med. **2018**, 132, 1581–1594. **[Google Scholar] [CrossRef]**

15. The 1000 Genomes Project Consortium; Auton, A.; Brooks, L.D.; Durbin, R.M.; Garrison, E.P.; Kang, H.M.; Korbel, J.O.; Marchini, J.L.; McCarthy, S.; McVean, G.A.; et al. A global reference for human genetic variation. Nature **2015**, 526, 68–74. **[Google Scholar]**

16. Bergström, A.; McCarthy, S.A.; Hui, R.; Almarri, M.A.; Ayub, Q.; Danecek, P.; Chen, Y.; Felkel, S.; Hallast, P.; Kamm, J.; et al. Insights into human genetic variation and population history from 929 diverse genomes. Science **2020**, 367, 1339–1349. **[Google Scholar] [CrossRef]**

17. Byrska-Bishop, M.; Evani, U.S.; Zhao, X.; Basile, A.O.; Abel, H.J.; Regier, A.A.; AndréCorvelo,A.;Clarke,W.E.;Musunuri,R.;Nagulapalli,K.;etal.HighCoverage Whole Genome Sequencing of the Expanded 1000 Genomes Project Cohort Including 602 trios. Available online: **https://www.internationalgenome.org/data-portal/data-collection/30x-grch38; http://ftp.1000genomes.ebi.ac.uk/vol1/ftp/data_collections/1000G_2504_high_coverage/working/20190425_NYGC_GATK/** (accessed on 20 June 2021).

18. Xavier, C.; de la Puente, M.; Phillips, C.; Eduardoff, M.; Heidegger, A.; Mosquera-Miguel, A.; Freire-Aradas, A.; Lagace, R.; Wootton, S.; Power, D.; et al. Forensic evaluation of the Asia Pacific ancestry-informative MAPlex assay. Forensic Sci. Int. Genet. **2020**, 48, 102344. **[Google Scholar] [CrossRef]**

19. Cheung, E.Y.Y.; Phillips, C.; Eduardoff, M.; Lareu, M.V.; McNevin, D. Performance of ancestry-informative SNP and microhaplotype markers. Forensic Sci. Int. Genet. **2019**, 43, 102141. **[Google Scholar] [CrossRef] [PubMed]**

20. Phillips, C.; Amigo, J.; Tillmar, A.O.; Peck, M.A.; de la Puente, M.; Ruiz-Ramírez, J.; Bittner, F.; Idrizbegović, Š.; Wang, Y.; Parsons, T.J.; et al. A compilation of tri-allelic SNPs from 1000 Genomes and use of the most polymorphic loci for a large-scale human identification panel. Forensic Sci. Int. Genet. **2020**, 46, 102232. **[Google Scholar] [CrossRef] [Green Version]**

21. Galanter, J.M.; Fernandez-Lopez, J.C.; Gignoux, C.R.; Barnholtz-Sloan, J.; Fernandez-Rozadilla, C.; Via, M.; Hidalgo-Miranda, A.; Contreras, A.V.; Figueroa, L.U.; Raska, P.; et al. Development of a panel of genome-wide ancestry informative markers to study admixture throughout the Americas. PLoS Genet. **2012**, 8, e1002554. **[Google Scholar] [CrossRef] [PubMed] [Green Version]**

22. Kidd, K.K.; Speed, W.C.; Pakstis, A.J.; Furtado, M.R.; Fang, R.; Madbouly, A.; Maiers, M.; Middha, M.; Friedlaender, F.R.; Kidd, J.R. Progress toward an efficient panel of SNPs for ancestry inference. Forensic Sci. Int. Genet. **2014**, 10, 23–32. **[Google Scholar] [CrossRef] [Green Version]**

23. Pereira, V.; Freire-Aradas, A.; Ballard, D.; Børsting, C.; Diez, V.; Pruszkowska-Przybylska, P.; Ribeiro, J.; Achakzai, N.M.; Aliferi, A.; Bulbul, O.; et al. Development and validation of the EUROFORGEN NAME (North African and Middle Eastern) ancestry panel. Forensic Sci. Int. Genet. **2019**, 42, 260–267. **[Google Scholar] [CrossRef] [PubMed]**

24. Mao, X.; Bigham, A.W.; Mei, R.; Gutierrez, G.; Weiss, K.M.; Brutsaert, T.D.; Leon-Velarde, F.; Moore, L.G.; Vargas, E.; McKeigue, P.M.; et al. A genomewide admixture mapping panel for Hispanic/Latino populations. Am. J. Hum. Genet **2007**, 80, 1171–1178. **[Google Scholar] [CrossRef] [PubMed] [Green Version]**

25. Available online: **http://mathgene.usc.es/Snipper/** (accessed on 20 June 2021).

26. Phillips, C.; Amigo, J.; McNevin, D.; de la Puente, M.; Cheung, E.Y.Y.; Lareu, M.V. Online population data resources for forensic SNP analysis with Massively Parallel Sequencing: An overview of online population data for forensic purposes. In Forensic DNA Analysis: Technological Development and Innovative Applications; Pilli, E., Berti, A., Eds.; CRC Press: Boca Raton, FL, USA, 2021. **[Google Scholar]**

27. Mallick, S.; Li, H.; Lipson, M.; Mathieson, I.; Gymrek, M.; Racimo, F.; Zhao, M.; Chennagiri, N.; Nordenfelt, S.; Tandon, A.; et al. The Simons Genome Diversity Project: 300 genomes from 142 diverse populations. Nature **2016**, 538, 201–206. **[Google Scholar] [CrossRef]**

28. Pagani, L.; Lawson, D.J.; Jagoda, E.; Mörseburg, A.; Eriksson, A.; Mitt, M.; Clemente, F.; Hudjashov, G.; DeGiorgio, M.; Saag, L.; et al. Genomic analyses inform on migration events during the peopling of Eurasia. Nature **2016**, 538, 238–242. **[Google Scholar] [CrossRef] [Green Version]**

29. Xavier, C.; de la Puente, M.; Mosquera-Miguel, A.; Freire-Aradas, A.; Kalamara, V.; Vidaki, A.; Gross, T.; Revoir, A.; Pośpiech, E.; Kartasińska, E.; et al. Development and validation of the VISAGE AmpliSeq Basic Tool to predict appearance and ancestry from DNA. Forensic Sci. Int. Genet. **2020**, 48, 102336. **[Google Scholar] [CrossRef]**

30. Pritchard, J.K.; Stephens, M.; Donnelly, P. Inference of population structure using multilocus genotype data. Genetics **2000**, 155, 945–959. **[Google Scholar] [CrossRef]**

31. Evanno, G.; Regnaut, S.; Goudet, J. Detecting the number of clusters of individuals using the software STRUCTURE: A simulation study. Mol. Ecol. **2005**, 14, 2611–2620. **[Google Scholar] [CrossRef] [Green Version]**

32. Kopelman, N.M.; Mayzel, J.; Jakobsson, M.; Rosenberg, N.A.; Mayrose, I. Clumpak: A program for identifying clustering modes and packaging population structure inferences across K. Mol. Ecol. Resour. **2015**, 15, 1179–1191. **[Google Scholar] [CrossRef] [PubMed] [Green Version]**

33. R: A Language and Environment for Statistical Computing. Available online: **http://www.r-project.org/** (accessed on 20 June 2021).

34. Paradis, E. Pegas: An R package for population genetics with an integrated-modular approach. Bioinformatics **2010**, 26, 419–420. **[Google Scholar] [CrossRef] [Green Version]**

35. Alexander, D.; Novembre, J.; Lange, K. Fast model-based estimation of ancestry in unrelated individuals. Genome Res. **2009**, 19, 1655–1664. **[Google Scholar] [CrossRef] [PubMed] [Green Version]**

36. Cheung, E.Y.Y.; Gahan, M.E.; McNevin, D. Prediction of biogeographical ancestry from genotype: A comparison of classifiers. Int. J. Legal Med. **2017**, 131, 901–912. **[Google Scholar] [CrossRef] [PubMed]**

37. Palencia-Madrid, L.; Xavier, C.; de la Puente, M.; Hohoff, C.; Phillips, C.; Kayser, M.; Parson, W. on behalf of the VISAGE Consortium, Evaluation of the VISAGE Basic Tool for Appearance and Ancestry Prediction Using PowerSeq Chemistry on the MiSeqFGx System. Genes **2020**, 11, 708. **[Google Scholar] [CrossRef] [PubMed]**

10 ON THE IDENTIFICATION OF BODY FLUIDS AND TISSUEs: A CRUCIAL LINK IN THE INVESTIGATION AND SOLUTION OF CRIME

1. INTRODUCTION: AN OVERVIEW

Body fluid and tissue identification can add evidence in criminal investigations by establishing a crucial link between the donor, the cell type and the activities that occurred. In this review, we first provide the forensic context of body fluid and tissue identification which resides in activity-level evaluations, then we discuss methods to locate body fluids at the scene or in the laboratory, which is followed by the major marker methodologies to analyze them. One of these methods is mRNA profiling, and we take a retrospective look at casework details and verdicts for mRNA cases in the Netherlands. This leads us to a criminalistic view on targets that can be accommodated in assays and the interpretation of cell typing results for instance, in mixed stains, which needs a very different approach from the interpretation of DNA results. Lastly, we consider possible other marker types that have been suggested, and practical aspects when introducing cell typing into a forensic laboratory.

1.1. Prosecution and Defense Scenario

Increasingly, cases come to court in which the presence of cellular material of a person is not disputed but the activity that caused the deposition is. The debate then centers around the question 'how did his/her DNA get there'? Forensic scientists approach such questions by performing activity-level evaluations [1,2,3,4,5,6,7,8]. Figure 1 shows activity-level evaluation in the context of forensic human biology analyses. Generalizing, activity-level evaluations weigh the likelihood of the forensic evidence under one scenario (hypothesis 1; H1, also known as prosecution scenario) versus an alternative scenario (hypothesis 2; H2, also known as defense scenario). The two hypotheses need to be formulated well, describe the alleged activities and be mutually exclusive. In the evaluation, the probability of the findings given the propositions is considered (not the probability of the propositions themselves) [1].

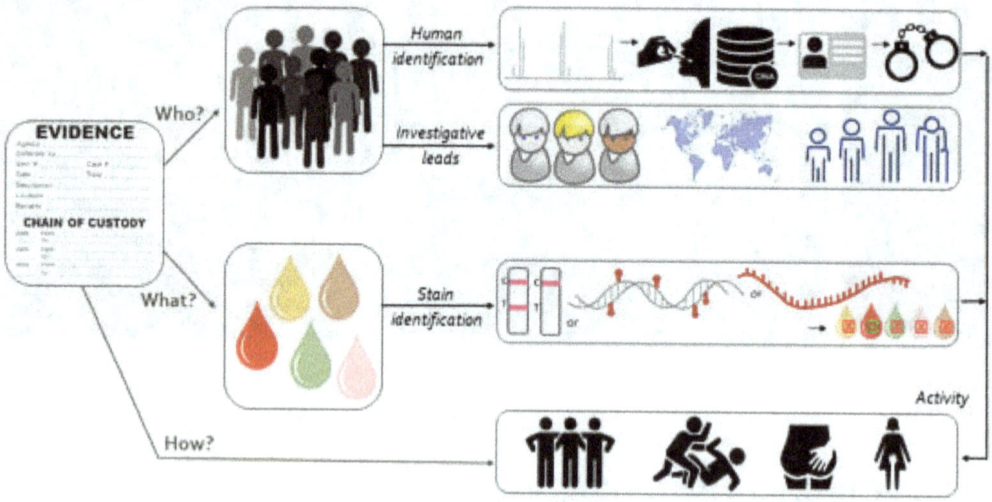

Figure 1. Stain identification in the context of the forensic process showing the link between 'who', 'what' and 'how'.

The 'findings' in the case can relate to cellular material matching victim or suspect which under H1 is indicative of an offensive activity (e.g., blood matching the victim on the blade of a knife indicative of the victim being stabbed; cellular material matching the suspect on the handle of a knife supporting the proposition that the suspect carried out the stabbing). Under H2, this questioned cellular material on the evidentiary item may result from a number of scenarios: (1) the cellular material was deposited not during the offense but at an earlier or later time (the suspect did not stab but picked up the knife after the stabbing); (2) the cellular material was not deposited by direct contact but was the result of secondary (or tertiary or further) transfer (the suspect shook hands with the real perpetrator who then handled the knife in the stabbing); (3) the item on which the cellular material was deposited belongs to the suspect but was used in the offense by another person (the knife (owned by the suspect who uses it to cut food) was handled by the real perpetrator in the stabbing); (4) the cellular material was deposited on the knife in a different way (the victim fell into the knife).

1.2. Addressing Alternative Scenarios

Forensic studies aim to develop approaches to assist in addressing offensive and alternative scenarios. To address deposition during the offense or during an earlier or later encounter, inferring the time since deposition (TSD) may be helpful. For bloodstains, various spectroscopic and chemometric TSD methods have been proposed that rely foremost on changes to hemoglobin [**9,10,11,12,13**]. An approach that would be applicable to more body fluids than blood is based on differences in the degradation over time of distinct RNA molecules outside the human body. Determining relative expression ratios may allow inference of TSD, although robustness is not yet at the level needed for forensic casework [**14,15,16,17,18,19**]. Recently, microbes were explored for TSD purposes of saliva samples with some success, but the high inter-individual variation can surpass the time-dependent variation [**20**].

To address the question of primary deposition or secondary transfer, TPPR (transfer, prevalence, persistence and recovery) issues are studied [**21,22,23,24,25,26,27,28,29,30,31**]. The aspect of transfer appears the most complex among TPPR issues and many studies have gained information on transfer rates, and the various aspects that influence transfer rates such as wet or dried state, application of friction and pressure, smooth or rough surface and size of the stain [**32,33,34,35,36,37,38**]. Generally, probabilistic frameworks are used to guide the evaluation, and Bayesian networks are appreciated for their graphical strength in this evaluative process [**39,40**].

Inferring the body fluid(s) present in stains is, in the context of secondary (or more) transfer, important for two reasons: (1) to assess the cellular content of the primary stain in relation to the DNA recovered from the evidentiary sample as some fluids have very high cellular content (for example nasal secretion), whilst others contain much fewer cells (for instance urine) and (2) to assess whether the body fluid involved is likely to occur in what is suggested) to be the primary location [**41**]. For example, intimate body fluids (vaginal cellular material, menstrual secretion, semen) can be found in underpants of the wearer, but are less expected on hands or touched items [**42,43,44**]. Saliva and nasal secretion, on the other hand, can reside on hands or items, and blood could occur when people have (small) wounds. Organ tissues (for instance, CNS (central nervous system), heart, or adipose tissue), on the other hand, are not expected on hands or on items.

The scenario that another person and not the suspect utilized an item (belonging to the suspect) on which cellular material was deposited in the offense, can relate to objects (e.g., a knife used for stabbing or a bottle that was inserted vaginally) or clothing/ shoes that appear to have been worn during the offense for instance because blood spatter or organ tissue matching the victim found on them. Cell typing of samples from such items may provide the crucial link of the evidentiary item to the alleged crime (the knife carries muscle tissue matching the victim on the blade; the bottle contains vaginal material matching the victim on the bottle neck; the shoe carries CNS tissue matching the head-kicked victim), but the link to the perpetrator needs to be provided by other means. This may be addressed for instance through fingerprint analysis (e.g., on the bottom of the bottle or the handle of the knife), DNA-analysis (e.g., of the shoelaces or the insides of the neck and collar areas of the sweater) or CCTV-footage or witness reports on the suspect acting in the stabbing or wearing the shoes or clothing at the time of the attack.

When a different way for the deposition of the cellular material is proposed (e.g., shooting out of self-defense, intercourse with consent), the evaluation is often at the offense level, which means the domain of the court [**2,45,46**]. With such scenarios, DNA nor cell typing add value in most of the cases.

1.3. Contextualizing Evidentiary Traces

Not only the type of body fluid or organ tissue, but also the location, pattern and amount of cellular material can be relevant for activity-level evaluations or contextualizing the scene. For example, trousers of a suspect may carry multiple bloodstains matching the DNA profile of a deceased person. Bloodstain pattern analysis may reveal a mist-like pattern and diluted bloodstains. RNA analysis of multiple stains could indicate the presence of blood, saliva, and nasal mucosa in various combinations. Together, the location, pattern, amount, and type of detected body fluids indicate expirated blood. Pathology may reveal injuries to the lungs or airways, which could have triggered the victim to expel blood mixed with air from the lungs through the nose or mouth. The combination of identified body fluids, location/ pattern and amounts would support the suspect being in the vicinity of the dying victim expelling blood and would provide less support for a scenario in which the suspect would visit the scene of the crime a day later.

2. LOCATING BIOLOGICAL FORENSIC EVIDENCE

Locating and identifying body fluids and tissues is important for two main reasons: (1) to find traces related to the alleged crime which can then be collected and from which the identity of the perpetrator may be revealed by further testing; (2) to contextualize the traces as explained in Section 1.3 to provide information about what activities may have taken place. This can be done at the scene, where time is limited, using techniques that are mostly presumptive and visual in nature, or in a forensic laboratory (using samples and items collected at the scene) where more detailed analysis is possible.

2.1. At the Scene of the Crime

Here we describe technologies for locating latent biological evidence for use at the scene that can also be used in the laboratory. These include chemiluminescent sprays such as those based on luminol, safer and non-invasive alternative light sources and spectroscopic methods using handheld instruments. Handheld devices, and technologies that are non-destructive to the sample offer the greatest potential as these can be used to rapidly direct investigations and the collection of evidence.

2.1.1. Chemical Sprays for Blood and Semen

Sometimes blood at crime scenes is difficult to see, perhaps there is a very small quantity of diluted blood (cleaning may have taken place), the blood is on a surface that makes it difficult to find (like a dark substrate or upon repainting) or there is a trail of blood-stained shoeprints leading from the scene which are no longer visible. Luminol and the more user-friendly, luminol-derived Bluestar (Bluestar Forensic, Monaco) reagent [**47**], are often used to detect haemoglobin and its derivatives resulting in a blue fluorescence which is captured by photography [**48**]. One disadvantage of such methods includes that the luminescence produced can be faint and short-lived, and in the case of luminol the visualization must be carried out in near darkness [**48**]. Different formulations exist and those that maximise the brightness and longevity of the fluorescence and that have few adverse effects on subsequent tests for blood or on DNA profiling are preferred [**48,49,50,51**]. A more recent development is the proposed use of a click reaction [**52**] between serum albumin and tetraphenylethene maleimide. The reaction is less harsh than that of luminol and BlueStar and produces a stable and sensitive response and shows promise for further development.

To locate semen, alternative light sources (ALS; see **Section 2.1.2**) and acid phosphatase tests are used that suffer from limitations in sensitivity and toxicity, respectively. In 2017, STK Sperm Tracker™ was introduced to the market by AXO Science (Lyon, France) as a human semen-specific test [**53**]. Sperm Tracker is available as a spray for crime scene use and in impregnated sheets for use on larger items. Detection requires a UV light source, that the room or space be darkened, and it must be used before luminol or BlueStar.

2.1.2. Alternative Light Sources

ALS refers to the use of light of different wavelengths, including infrared, to detect forensic evidence in a non-destructive manner, and are often used to assist in the reconstruction of events. The detection of biological evidence is possible because they contain autofluorescent components which allow them to be visualized when illuminated at specific wavelengths.

An early study comparing different laser and ultraviolet light sources for the detection of biological fluids [54] has been followed by the development of many commercially available light sources such as the Polilight® series (Rofin Australia Pty Ltd., Melbourne, VIC, Austraila) and the LED-based Crime-lite® series (Foster and Freeman Ltd., Evesham, UK). A selection of illustrative articles is presented here. In an examination of the utility of the Polilight® [55] stains of blood, semen and saliva, not visible to the eye, were able to be detected and Polilight® performed well when compared to other presumptive screening tests.

As different body fluids and substrates fluoresce at different wavelengths, selecting the best combination of lightsource (wavelength) and filter used for detection is important. By comparing results obtained from five body fluids applied to 29 different materials, the Lumatec Superlight 410 (Lumatec GMBH, Deisenhofen, Germany) was used on fresh stains **[56]** and the same stains after two years **[57]** using different filters. Their findings show that for every combination of substrate, fluid, light source, and filter, except one, there was a specific combination that was best. In general though, stains could still be visualised two years later, using a light source between 415 nm and 460 nm in combination with a yellow or orange filter.

To improve the utility of light sources and photography at crime scenes, a study was conducted **[51]** combining a blue Crime-lite XL light source in combination with a 360° camera to capture semen and saliva stains on a number of different substrates. This study was carried out in a mock crime scene indoor setting using volunteers to examine the images and locate the stains. The colour of the substrate was found to have an effect on the ability to see the stains, however, in general, the combination of light source and camera was effective.

A side by side comparison of the Crime-lite® 82S, Polilight® PL400 and Polilight® PL500 [58] was recently carried out, comparing the sensitivity and performance of each on dilutions of saliva and semen on different fabrics. The LED light source used in the Crime-lite® 82S provided better detection of dilutions of saliva and overall performed better as a screening tool.

Recent developments include combined handheld, UV/Vis/IR multi-wavelength light sources and camera combined, with automatic filter selection all controlled from an integrated touch screen for example the Crime-lite AUTO. This handheld instrument appears to offer a number of advantages for crime scene use, the most obvious of which is the combined handheld unit. See also Section 2.2.3 for an alternative.

2.1.3. Spectroscopic Methods at the Scene

Spectroscopic techniques for locating and identifying body fluids are available, with handheld devices for crime scene use as well as methods requiring laboratory-based equipment **[59]**. Handheld NIR (near infrared) spectrometers have been tested **[60]** with blood and potential applications to other fluids including age estimation **[13]**. NIR spectroscopy is quick and non-destructive with no sample preparation and background fluorescence encountered with **[61]**. In the most recent example **[60]**, the instrument is paired with a mobile phone and software containing the necessary tools to train a variety of statistical models to interpret test data based on machine learning. The best of these models could correctly identify blood in 94% of cases, albeit with a false positive rate of 14% for blood-like substances such as red wine, tomato sauce, and coffee.

Hyperspectral imaging (HSI) is also a non-destructive spectroscopic technique and can be used to "map" large geographical areas as well as smaller items [**62**]. HSI records, as a continuous measurement, electromagnetic spectra over a wide range of wavelengths for every pixel in an image, and from this creates unique spectra. Since 2012 when first proposed as a tool to characterise forensic evidence [**63,64**] HIS has emerged as a potential tool for bloodstain detection.

The identification of blood by HIS is based upon the visualisation of haemoglobin and its components in the 400 to 700 nm range. Changes in the Soret peak observed at 415 nm are used to detect aging of the sample. In a set of fingerprints, aged over a 30 day period, HSI enabled the identification of the blood as well as aging of the prints [**65**].

When comparing a Crime-lite® ML2 ALS instrument (Foster and Freeman Ltd., Evesham, UK) and HIS-NIR imaging using an SWIR3 hyperspectral camera working in the 1000–2500 nm spectral range (Specim Ltd., Oulu, Finland) [66], the resultant images obtained from the HIS-NIR imaging were shown to be superior at revealing the location of body fluid staining in known reference samples, simulated casework samples and on unknown staining on forensic exhibits. Using blood samples and different substrates, spectra were generated [67] that were used to train different classifiers to detect aged bloodstains and most recently a "blood detection dataset" was produced [68] specifically to assist in the challenging task of algorithm development for this new technology.

2.2. At the Forensic Laboratory

In the previous section, we described approaches for locating biological evidence at crime scenes, particularly latent evidence that may not be visible to the naked eye. These methods can also be employed in a forensic laboratory when transportable items are involved. In the remainder of this section, we discuss methods that are primarily laboratory-based for locating biological fluids. These chemical, immunological, and spectroscopic tests are often used to presumptively identify biological fluids before conducting further, more specific testing where necessary.

2.2.1. Chemical and Immunochromatographic Tests

With the exception of microscopic identification of spermatozoa, forensic scientists often rely on sensitive but non-specific chemical tests, based primarily on the activity of enzymes in the target body fluid. Although easy to use, they are not human-specific and are largely presumptive in nature with many examples of false positive reactions reported. For reviews covering this area, see [**69,70,71**]. To supplement these chemical tests, laboratories may use immunochromatographic assays, which include tests for saliva, semen, urine, blood and menstrual blood. Despite advantages of speed, cost and ease of use, these assays are not as suitable for crime scene deployment as they require an extract of a sample to be made and are not an integral part of the DNA profiling process. To date, there is only one report of combining such tests into a format amenable to detecting body fluids in mixtures [72]. The more recent emergence of proteomics in the forensic literature (see Section 7.1.2) and the identification of new candidate markers [73] is likely to drive the development of immunologically-based assays based on multiplexing in a single assay that may be amenable for use at the crime scene.

Immunochromatographic methods can also be used to detect DNA amplicons and direct PCR of *Streptococcus sanguinis* and *Streptococcus salivarius* specific to saliva has been successfully integrated with an immunochromatographic strip detection method [74].

Improvements to the technology for detection have allowed for the development of a protein microarray sensor [**75**] for the detection of semen and vaginal cellular material. Antibodies to semenogelin-2 and anti-17 beta estradiol were immobilised on an array surface. To enhance the signal achieved and increase the sensitivity of the assay, a metal enhanced fluorescence (MEF) approach was taken. The sample containing body fluids was itself labelled with a fluorescent dye and after hybridisation and washing steps the fluorescence signals are detected.

2.2.2. Spectroscopic Techniques

Raman spectroscopy, for which less sensitive handheld devices are available, relies upon the scattering of light by biological compounds. The outputs are complex spectra built up of the multiple components of each fluid. Statistical tools are available and needed to determine the unique spectroscopic profile of the molecular structure of each. Such profiles have been determined for a range of body fluids and tissues of forensic interest, such as blood [**76**], semen, saliva, vaginal fluid and sweat [**77**,**78**].

Early evaluations [**76**] considered factors of forensic interest such as the substrate, within-person variability and time since deposition in blood samples. Blood was able to be detected on luminescent fabrics by first removing the stained area from the substrate. Variability was observed as bloodstains aged and also between and within people. The changes in spectra as a bloodstain ages were further explored [**79**] over a period of 2 years with age predicted with an accuracy of approximately 70%. Statistical models were further improved [**80**] to accommodate environmental factors.

Fourier transform infrared (FT-IR) spectroscopy, routinely used in forensic chemistry, has also been evaluated for biological fluids with an important consideration that any environmental contamination is accounted for. Attenuated total reflectance (ATF) FT-IR spectroscopy [**81**,**82**] has been used to characterise a number of body fluids, accommodating the age of the stain and excluding unexpected non-target components. Similar studies have also been undertaken on semen [**83,84**], with methods developed to identify and avoid interference from a number of environmental factors; on dried urine [**85**] where the gender of the donor was able to be deciphered; and to distinguish between menstrual and peripheral blood [**86**]. The alternative modification, external reflection FT-IR spectroscopy, has also been proposed [**59**] to specifically identify body fluids associated with sexual assault. The effects of different fabric colours and commonly used household substances on identification were also assessed. These instruments are not handheld and, therefore, not compatible with examinations at the crime scene.

2.2.3. A Practical Example

The utility of combining ALS detection with an immunochromatographic test for the presence of prostate-specific antigen (PSA, also known as gamma-seminoprotein, kallikrein-3 or P-30 antigen), on laundered clothing [87] followed by DNA profiling has been demonstrated. In this example, semen stains were located using a Forenscope Mobile Multispectral UV-VIS-IR Imaging System® (Grimed Ltd., Voor, The Netherlands) which, like the Crime Lite AUTO described in Section 2.1.2, combines light source, filters, camera and software in one handheld instrument. Semen stains could be detected and confirmed using both the Forenscope system and the PSA test. High washing temperatures had the biggest impact on the ALS detection, polyester fabric had the biggest detrimental impact on the PSA test. DNA profiling however was successful on all semen samples regardless of washing temperature, detergent or fabric.

3. MAJOR TYPES OF MARKERS AND TECHNOLOGIES EMPLOYED TO DETECT THEM

3.1. RNA Markers

RNA is the link between the genome and protein content of each cell and its expression or its effect on expression of cell type-specific proteins has been widely adopted as a laboratory-based approach for body fluid identification [**69,71,88**] for forensic purposes. Alongside mRNA, small non-coding RNAs have generated significant interest [**89**] to date, which will be described in **Section 7.1.1**. RNA analysis has also been suggested for other forensic applications such as post mortem interval and age of a stain determination [**17,19,90**].

3.1.1. Messenger RNA

There are many examples, over more than twenty years, of messenger RNA (mRNA) being proposed as a confirmatory test for body fluid and tissue identification with an early example being the identification of menstrual blood [**91**]. A selection of the numerous papers published are included here and will assist in directing the reader to further studies.

The stability of RNA in stains of forensic interest was described in 1999 [**92**] with a demonstration of the detection of skin epithelial cells in dried blood cells. This was followed by studies describing stability studies in vaginal swabs, blood, semen and saliva stains [**93**], stains up to 23 years old [**94**] and transcriptome studies showing the persistence of regions of RNA of interest in samples deliberately degraded [**95,96,97**].

To minimise sample loss during testing and optimise the efficiency of the laboratory process, it is important to recover DNA and RNA from the same sample [**98,99,100**]. A recent paper compared a number of different approaches [**101**] and found methods with small modifications to [**98,99**] remained the best. Equally important in minimising sample loss and optimising the laboratory process is the creation of multiplex assays each containing mRNA markers of known specificity [**98,102,103,104,105,106,107**] that can be selected from the literature and online databases [**98,107**] and whole genome expression analysis [**108,109,110**]. Once these factors are considered, then casework and casework applications follow [**111,112,113,114,115**].

Most of the published work depends upon the detection of mRNA markers by reverse transcription PCR (RT PCR) and capillary electrophoresis (CE) [**92,102,103,106,116**]. Real time PCR (qPCR) has also been used [**116,117**] but is somewhat limited by the number of markers that can be multiplexed together (restricted by the availability of fluorescent dyes) and the difficulty in identifying appropriate housekeeping genes, applicable to all included body fluids of interest. More recently, massively parallel sequencing (MPS) has been used to detect multiplexed markers [**118,119,120**] reflecting a shift towards this technology in forensic science [**121**]. The main advantages of MPS is the high multiplexing capacity, that amplicons can have overlapping (small) sizes and that nucleotide variation is detected. These first two features are of importance with forensic traces as they are often of minute amounts and suffer from degradation due to external factors. The forensic importance of analysing sequence variation in RNA amplicons will be discussed in **Section 6.4**. Other techniques for detecting markers are given in **Section 3.1.3**.

3.1.2. Circular RNA

Circular RNAs (circRNAs) are highly expressed [**122,123**] and as they share sequence with the mRNA equivalent to which they are related can also be body fluid/ tissue-specific [**124**]. Because these molecules are closed circular structures, they are very stable and this makes them promising candidates for body fluid identification. In the first report [**125**] of their inclusion for forensic application, microarray expression profiles of circRNAs of venous blood, semen, saliva, vaginal cellular material and menstrual blood samples were produced. Although semen, saliva and venous blood could be distinguished from each other vaginal cellular material and menstrual blood could not.

A further study [**126**] combined mRNA markers with circRNA markers for the same genes (ALAS2 and MMP7), which were markers already used for body fluid identification [**106,127,128**], and demonstrated improvements in the sensitivity and stability of the assay compared to mRNA alone. This was also found in a similar study of circRNA markers in blood, menstrual blood, saliva, semen, urine and vaginal cellular material, using gene targets well known in the mRNA profiling community (for example HTN3 for saliva and CYP2B7P1 for vaginal material) [**129**]. Further investigation resulted in an 18 plex multiplex assay combining circRNAs, mRNAs and housekeeping genes, with good sensitivity and specificity and the potential to identify fluids in degraded samples due to the stability of the circRNA molecules [**129**].

3.1.3. Alternative Techniques to Analyse RNA Markers

Many of the methods and much of the research described above use either RT PCR and CE, qPCR and/or increasingly RNA sequencing to detect the markers under study. These have been described in more detail in a recent review [**88**]. Some examples of newly proposed techniques follow.

Loop mediated isothermal amplification (LAMP) [**130**] can provide higher specificity than PCR because of the use of multiple primers and the higher temperatures at which amplification occurs. In 2015, the first reports of applying LAMP to mRNA body fluid identification [**131**] detected hemoglobin beta as a marker for blood and was followed by similar studies using a direct RT LAMP method to detect the expression of the statherin gene in saliva [**132**] The same markers and the TGM4 gene marker for semen were targeted in the design of an assay for the identification of blood, semen and saliva [**133**]. Extending the format to include vaginal cellular material and azoospermatic semen in a microtitre plate with a metal dye indicator and colorimetric detection, significantly improved the utility of the approach and may make it more suitable to laboratory requiring a higher throughput [**134**].

High resolution melt (HRM) curve analysis measures the melting temperature (Tm) and generates a distinct and characteristic melt curve for each amplicon in a sample. It has been proposed for a number of applications such as a detection method for SNPs [**135**], to detect sequence differences in the hypervariable regions of mtDNA [**136**], to characterise the oral microbiome of different people using

16SrRNA [**137**], as a technique to analyse methylation sensitive sites for body fluid determination [**138**] and as a method to identify mRNA markers in body fluids [**139**] in a multiplex format due to the high resolution of each distinct melt curve for each amplicon.

Since two publications some time ago [**108,140**], the NanoStringR nCounter system (nanoString, Seattle, WA, USA) [**141**] has received little forensic interest. This is somewhat surprising given the strengths of the platform that include a direct assay not involving PCR and measurement of gene expression of up to 800 mRNA candidates in a single multiplex reaction in a semi-automated fashion. These studies successfully tested 18 and 23 markers for body fluids, respectively. [**108,140**]

Similarly, HyBeacon probes [**142**], used for the detection of SNPs and STRs in areas such as clinical diagnostics and food authentication, have received some but not extensive interest. The ParaDNA Body Fluid ID test comprising RT PCR and melt curve detection was successfully evaluated for the detection of mRNA in body fluids of forensic interest [**143**] in combination with the now withdraw/unavailable ParaDNA system (LGC Forensics Teddington, Middlesex, UK) [**144**] for STR detection.

3.2. Epigenetic Markers

Body fluid identification can also be accomplished at the DNA level by examining epigenetic modifications to specific sites on the genome, primarily methylation at the 5′ position of cytosine in a CpG dinucleotide. These sites are known as tissue-based differentially methylated regions (tDMRs) and have been specifically examined for body fluids of forensic interest such as blood, semen, saliva, skin, urine, and vaginal secretions.

Whilst the initial application of epigenetics in forensic science was the identification of body fluids and tissues, methylation analysis has also been proposed for age estimation and differentiation of twins [**145,146,147**]. A range of methods have been applied for identifying appropriate markers, detecting the epigenetic modifications, and assessing the results. A comprehensive review [**146**], describes many of these approaches in more detail.

3.2.1. Marker Selection and Assay Design

With the increasing availability of freely available methylation data, researchers can assess many thousands of CpG sites simultaneously to find candidate markers. For example, the human methylation bead array system (Illumina) was used to screen over 450,000 CpG sites in samples of blood, saliva, and vaginal cellular material [**148,149**]. More recently, overexpressed genes in genome wide expression datasets were combined with heavily methylated gene body CpG islands (CGI) from methylation datasets [**150**]. Further *in silico* analysis of one of these datasets [**149**] was undertaken and four new markers able to discriminate blood (2 markers), vaginal cellular material (1 marker) and buccal cells (1 marker) were found [**151**].

Once identified, primers are designed and ideally markers are multiplexed enabling the simultaneous identification of different fluids/tissues. An example is a PCR multiplex combining CpG sites in the DACT1, USP49, PFN3, and PRMT2 genes to identify spermatozoa and differentiate between menstrual blood and vaginal cellular material from blood and saliva [**148,152**]. This multiplex has been extended to include amplicons for the 16S rRNA gene of bacteria specific oral and vaginal origin, *Veillonellaatypica* and/or *Streptococcus salivarius*, and *Lactobacillus crispatus* and/or *Lactobacillus gasseri* respectively [**153**].

3.2.2. Techniques to Analyse Epigenetic Modifications

Early research focused on the use of methylation-sensitive/ dependent restriction enzymes followed by PCR and CE [**154**]. The advantage of this approach was the ability to co-amplify STRs at a similar level of sensitivity, but drawbacks included incomplete restriction and template degradation, which can distort the methylation ratios that are critical to the interpretation of the results, which was particularly pronounced in low template samples. More recent assays [**155**], therefore, use amplicons with multiple restriction sites.

There are multiple methods to determine the relative methylation levels achieved, and they all start with bisulfite conversion of the DNA and amplification using primers designed to anneal to the converted DNA. Examples are qPCR with HRM [**138,151**] often confirmed with pyrosequencing [**156**], sequencing of cloned products [**150**] and changes in mobility of the PCR amplicons [**157**]. A multiplex methylation SNaPshot approach has been used to identify blood, saliva, semen and vaginal cellular material, and produced successful DNA methylation profiles in aged and mixed samples [**148**]. In a separate study it was successful in the identification of semen, saliva, venous blood and menstrual blood in body fluid mixtures and in crime scene stains [**158**]. Methylation state specificity was achieved using the single-base extension primers of the SNaPshot assay. Amplification refractory mutation system-PCR (ARMS-PCR), otherwise known as allele-based PCR [**159**], in combination with CE was used as an alternative method to test 22 possible markers for venous blood, saliva, semen, menstrual blood, and vaginal cellular material in multiplexes [**160**]. A random forest model was employed and performed well in predicting single source body fluids with high prediction accuracy (99.66%).

The multistep process of bisulfite conversion, PCR and detection by CE or sequencing is vulnerable to variation due to poor sample quality and quantity and especially degradation during the bisulfite conversion step. A new multiplex quantitative RT PCR method to measure the amount of genomic and bisulfite-converted DNA, and the degradation level of the conversion step as well as the conversion efficiency has been described [**161**]. Besides, natural variation in methylation status has been found between individuals, and some tissue-specific differentially methylated regions are susceptible to change due to environmental factors and age. For example, methylation of a CpG site in PRMT2 in blood samples was found to be an age-associated marker, whereas no significant difference based on age was observed for three spermatozoa-specific hypomethylated markers DACT1, USP49, and PRMT2 in men of different ages [**149,152**]. Others have demonstrated that within-person variation in methylation ratios was not observed, but variation was observed between people in an assay designed to identify vaginal cellular material [**157**].

3.3. Microbial Markers

Microbiomes are comprised of the bacterial, archaeal, viral and fungal microbial taxa communities present in/on a location of interest, such as the human body. Microbes have an advantage of high abundance and stability. Microbiomes can be considered as a whole (the human microbiome) or more specifically relating to a more defined location, for example the skin microbiome of humans where different bodily locations (moist armpit, sebaceous facial areas, dry forearm) can be dominated by different species [**162**]. A subset of markers and target organisms can be chosen to represent the fluid/ body site of choice [**153,163**] but it should be noted that different species may perform the same biological function (such as the production of lactic acid in the vagina) and may not function in all individuals [**164,165**]. Even human blood, previously considered to be sterile in a healthy person, may not be so [**166**].

More routine analysis of microbiomes has been made possible by developments in sequencing and related technology. Despite early promise, some challenges remain in adopting this technology for forensic science. In addition to variations between and within people [**164,167,168,169,170**] a key consideration is that microbial communities are strongly influenced by many external factors such as geography, time, season, health, diet, genetic factors, anti-inflammatory drugs and lifestyle [**171,172,173,174,175,176**], and even the presence of pets [**177**]. Consideration of these factors is necessary for any evaluation of microbiomes whether they "match" or not. Many of these factors relating to the human skin microbiome are neatly summarized in [**178,179**] and can be directly applied to all microbiome research and applications. In particular, the potential effects of the presence of contamination in the reagents and consumables used has been highlighted [**180**].

3.3.1. Microbial Markers for Body Fluid Identification

Many possible applications of the analysis of microbiomes are described in a recent review [**181**]. These include the identification of people [**182,183,184**]; establishing links with personal possessions such as phones and shoes [**185,186,187**]; forensic botany (including environmental DNA), in which analysis of the phyllosphere and soil can provide links between people and crime scene locations [**171,188,189,190**]; and the identification of microflora specific to different body locations such as saliva [**191**].

Many studies have focused on specific body sites/ fluids for example the microbiomes of saliva [**192,193**], faeces [**194**], the vagina [**164,195**] with recent publications focusing on distinguishing between different sources of blood (menstrual, venous, fingerpick and nasal) [**196,197**] and semen [**198**]. *Lactobacillus* species have been incorporated into mRNA multiplexes and collaborative exercises [**163,199**] and in multiplexed methylation -sensitive restriction enzyme PCR assays [**153**]. Interpretation of the presence of such markers should proceed with care as microorganisms can be detected on non-target body locations, probably either from their high abundance and/or carry-over [**104**]. Unsurprisingly, vaginal samples and menstrual blood are unable to be distinguished and share metagenomic profiles [**196,200**], and in one study, samples taken from the penis the vaginal markers responded while no female DNA was detected [**168**].

In an extension from simply identifying bacteria representative of the oral cavity, it was [**201**] recognized that identifying them could be used to distinguish between expirated bloodstains (such as those forced by airflow out of the nose or mouth) and impact spatter, providing what could be an additional crucial piece of information for an investigation (see **Section 1.3**).

3.3.2. Technologies to Analyze Microbial Markers

For the identification of microbial profiles specific to body locations, sequencing of the 16S rRNA gene is typically carried out, with the profiles found to be diagnostic of the area sampled. Saliva, skin, peripheral blood, menstrual blood, faeces and semen have all been tested in this way [**169,200,202**]. Whole genome shotgun sequencing has been suggested to outperform 16S rRNA analysis because of higher accuracy [**203**], but this comes with higher costs.

Not all assays are based on the 16S rRNA gene or on sequencing. For example microarrays targeting multiple genes across a range of known microorganisms have been described [**164,168**] and a qPCR assay [**193**] has been developed to detect three bacteria (*Streptococcus salivarius, Streptococcus sanguinis*, and *Neisseria subflava*) known to be present in the oral cavity. A similar microarray-based method has been described [**194**] for targeting the 16S rRNA, GroEL and 18S rRNA genes of a number of microorganisms present in faeces and other forensically relevant fluids.

4. RETROSPECTIVE ANALYSIS OF RNA TYPING IN FORENSIC CASEWORK

4.1. Requests and Results for RNA Typing in Casework

Forensic casework comes in great diversity, and questions can be put forward that cannot be addressed with existing methodologies. This feeds the development of new methods, like RNA typing assays which were especially triggered by the limitations for the tests for vaginal cellular material and menstrual secretion [**72,204,205,206,207**] and the difficulties to apply immunohistochemical staining for organ tissues to samplings from bullets where the tissue tends to reside in the grooves [**208**]. It is interesting to reflect, in a retrospective manner, on which forensic questions RNA typing assays are applied in actual forensic casework, and whether this corresponds to the questions that initially triggered the development of the assays.

RNA typing has been applied regularly at the Netherlands Forensic Institute since 2012. RNA was extracted in 452 cases and in 238 of these cases, RNA typing was performed (in the other 214 cases, RNA was extracted but RNA typing was not (yet) requested by police or prosecution). In 178 cases (75%) body fluid typing was performed and in 60 cases (25%) organ typing. On average, RNA is extracted for four samples per case. To study the context and details of cases in which RNA typing was performed, the details of 27 body fluid cases analyzed in 2020 were examined. All 27 cases were sexual assaults, of which 25 questioned the presence of vaginal cellular material (note that at the NFI presumptive tests are used to assess the presence of blood, saliva, and seminal fluid). The 26th case aimed to discern menstrual or peripheral blood in a vaginal sampling of an assaulted female and the 27th case questioned the presence of semen or seminal fluid on the genitals of an adolescent female (generally the presence of semen is not assessed through RNA typing but microscopic analysis and differential extraction is used). Thus, in the Netherlands, RNA body fluid typing is mostly applied in sexual assault cases to assess the presence of vaginal cellular material.

In the 25 cases that assessed vaginal cellular material, 56 samples were analyzed of which 19 resulted in vaginal cellular material detected (13 cases). In nine samples (four cases), saliva was detected (one of these samples, a penile swab, was also positive for vaginal cellular material; the other saliva-positive samples were all finger/nail dirt samplings). The corresponding DNA profiles of 53 of these 56 samples were mixed male/female profiles, while three showed no male (amelogenin Y) DNA and a full female profile (samplings from paper tissue, condom, or finger). The male/female ratio at the amelogenin locus in these mixed samples varied from 0.8 to 178, but this bore no relation to whether vaginal cellular material was seen or not. This is not unexpected as these are casework specimens, not ground truth data, and the female component may derive from other cells, for example skin cells, which are no longer included in the NFI body fluid RNA assay used in 2020.

4.2. RNA Typing Results in Verdicts

The ultimate value of RNA typing is best assessed by regarding verdicts after trial procedures (the proof is in the pudding). In the Dutch registry of verdicts **[209]**, 21 cases can be found in which RNA typing was actively considered in the verdict by the judge (note that not all verdicts are taken up in the registry and that the judge decided on the use of the RNA results in the context of all evidence presented, in most cases without data on prevalence of such RNA results in alternative scenarios).

Ten cases were sexual assaults and 11 cases were not. For the sexual assaults, in nine cases the presence of vaginal cellular material was of importance; in one case menstrual secretion. These body fluids were found four times on a penis, three times on a finger/nail dirt, once in underpants of a male, once on the outside of a condom and once on an inserted item (in this case a piece of ginger; a cultural punishment by a father). In eight of these ten cases, the defense presented alternative scenarios: once the timing of deposition was questioned ("the forensic report does not state when the menstrual secretion was deposited on the penis"). In six cases, secondary transfer was suggested: Three times vaginal material was supposedly picked up from either an item carrying vaginal material, or from being nearby the victim's vagina or from an unspecified source and then transferred to the penis. Vaginal cells on fingers of the suspect were suggested to originate from the victim touching her vagina and then shaking hands with the suspect, or from an unspecified activity. Vaginal cells in male underpants were suggested to originate from assisting the victim during vomiting after which her cellular material was transferred to his penis and underpants after a toilet visit (RNA typing was performed much later so the alternative scenario focused on explaining the female DNA). For a case with the presence of vaginal cells on the outside of a condom, the alternative scenario was that the father masturbated using a condom and that the results of vaginal cells and DNA-match with the adolescent daughter should be ignored as the mother was not included in the comparison (note that the DNA-profile fully matched the daughter).

These alternative scenarios follow three of the four general scenarios proposed in **Section 1.1**. These were: (1) 'time of deposition', (2) 'secondary transfer' and (3) 'innocent explanation'; 'another person performed the crime' was not proposed. This makes sense as most of the evidentiary items involved body parts such as finger/nail dirt or penis.

In the remaining 11 verdicts considering RNA typing results, the evidentiary items included two bullets, two knives, a baseball bat, five pieces of clothing and a bed sheet. The cellular material found on these items matched the victim(s) in all 11 cases. Of the 11 cases, nine cases were analyzed for organ tissues and two for body fluids. Both multiplexes contain markers for blood, and in all 11 cases, blood was present in the stains analyzed. In four cases, CNS tissue was found as well (not necessarily in all evidentiary stains analyzed within a case; all four cases involved samplings taken from clothing). In five cases, skeletal muscle was detected (both cases that involved a knife, one of the cases involving a bullet and two cases involving clothing: for these latter two cases, CNS was observed in stains analyzed within the case as well). In one of the two cases analyzed for body fluids, besides blood, saliva was found in a mist-like pattern indicating expirated blood (this case was analyzed using a body fluid assay not yet carrying nasal mucosa markers).

The alternative scenarios put forward by the defense fall into three categories: once the time of deposition was questioned (this was for the case in which expirated blood was implied; the suspect was suggested to have visited the scene a day later when the victims had already died). Five times it was suggested that another person was involved (twice handling the knife, three times wearing the clothing that contained CNS material matching the victim). Five times another explanation was given (the suspect shot at a car not at the victim; the victim started shooting first so it was self-defense; the victim fell of the stairs (for the case in which blood was found on a baseball bat); the injuries were self-inflicted and the large puddles of blood on the bed sheets were staged by using animal or menstrual blood (this was the second case analyzed by body fluid typing); the CNS and blood on the clothing of the suspect are not shown to be the result of violence (no suggestion was given how CNS did end up on trousers and a shirt). For these cases, the alternative scenarios follow three of the four general scenarios proposed in **Section 1.1**. These were: (1) 'time of deposition', (2) 'another person performed the crime' and (3) 'innocent explanation'; 'secondary transfer' was not proposed. This makes sense, as in these cases, generous amounts of cellular material matching the victim(s) were found for which it is more difficult to invoke secondary transfer.

5. A CRIMINALISTIC VIEW ON TARGETS TO BE INCLUDED IN A CELL TYPING ASSAY

Basically, there are two main reasons to include markers for a body fluid or an organ tissue in a cell typing assay: (1) the cell type can be questioned in forensic cases and (2) the cell type can be informative to an alternative, innocent explanation.

5.1. Cell Types Questioned in Forensic Cases

From the case descriptions in **Section 4.1**, it is evident that in sexual assault allegations, most often the presence of vaginal cellular material and menstrual secretions is questioned.

Semen (spermatozoa and/or seminal fluid) can be involved as well, generally in three circumstances: (1) as questioned body fluid in a sample in which semen is expected to be the predominant body fluid such as in a ejaculation stain on the body or clothing of the victim or inside a condom; (2) as a questioned body fluid in a sample containing a surplus amount of other cellular material such as in a vaginal, oral or rectal sample taken from the victim; or (3) as a background body fluid in a penile swab or finger/nail dirt sample that is examined for the presence of, for example, vaginal cellular material.

Under circumstance (1), semen will be the predominant cell type, and, in most cases, microscopic analysis will suffice to show presence of spermatozoa and generate a DNA profile for the semen donor. In circumstance (2), when a surplus amount of cellular material of the victim is present, differential extraction (DE), (in which a mild lysis to extract nucleic acids from non-spermatozoa cells, followed by a strong lysis to extract nucleic acids of the spermatozoa) is likely performed. Since the presence of semen is questioned, most often this DE method will suffice and produce a sperm fraction from which a DNA profile informative for the semen donor is derived. When confirmation of the presence of spermatozoa in the sperm fraction is needed, various methods can be applied such as microscopic analysis or MSRE analysis **[154,155,210,211]** on DNA extracted from the sperm fraction **[212]**

This is different in circumstance (3), where semen may be present in such amounts that it masks the presence of other body fluids. Here, it would be useful to apply a DE method that not only extracts DNA but also RNA and analyze the non-sperm RNA fraction for cell types other than spermatozoa (note that seminal fluid RNA will end up in this non-sperm RNA fraction as well). However, DE is hard to combine with RNA extraction as RNases are active during the mild lysis step unless an ample amount of strong RNase inhibitors is used **[104]**.

Other body fluids of which the presence may be questioned, are saliva and peripheral blood. For blood, molecular analyses are mostly applied for discerning peripheral blood and menstrual secretion. Saliva may be assessed in allegations of licking, which means that often body locations are sampled (breasts, genitals, mouth), and mixed DNA profiles are expected. To assess allegations of anal penetration, the identification of a rectal mucosa marker was described recently **[213]**. A rectal mucosa marker is to be preferred over markers for fecal matter as rectal mucosa provides a more direct link to invasive activities. Finding a marker specific for rectal mucosa is challenging since many body cavities and tubular organs in the human body are lined by mucous membranes (for instance, along the respiratory, digestive, and urogenital tract), an epithelial tissue that secretes mucus. Thus, specificity of mucous membrane genes may be an issue, they may prove general mucosa markers or cross-react with some other body fluid derived from a mucous membrane **[98,214]**.

5.2. Cell Types Informing on an Alternative Scenario

The second reason to include markers for a specific body fluid in a cell typing assay is to inform an alternative, innocent explanation for the findings. Nasal secretion has a high cellular content and may therefore leave detectable amounts after secondary transfer, which may be proposed as an alternative scenario (H1: vaginal penetration by penis; H2: victim sneezes in hand, shakes hand of the suspect, suspect touches his penis during toilet visit). Thus, nasal secretion markers have been identified and included in body fluid typing assays [**104,215**]. In addition, the presence of nasal secretion and blood in a sample may indicate nosebleed blood, that can be a spontaneous occurrence not connected to a crime. Occasionally, nasal secretion may be among the questioned body fluid such as in case of expiration of blood (here saliva markers will also be informative) or when a nosebleed is caused in a fight.

Other body fluids for which markers have been identified are urine and sweat [**128,216,217,218**]. These two body fluids have a relatively low cellular amount and are likely of limited importance. Urine may contribute some cellular material in underpants; sweat can be deposited together with skin. Skin was one of the earlier cell types for which mRNA markers were identified [**98,219,220,221,222**], probably because contact traces are frequently submitted for forensic analyses. However, forensic practice in the Netherlands has shown that there is hardly any value in showing the presence of skin, as skin residues reside in almost all submitted samples. The presence of skin and DNA of a person of interest may be regarded mistakenly as an indication of direct contact, and due to the abundance of epithelial material in public and private items [**42**], secondary transfer is within the bound of possibility.

For the assessment of cases of violence, various tissue types can be included. CNS tissue (brain and spinal cord) is highly important to include in the assays because of the often-lethal consequences. Other organs such as liver, heart, kidney, lung, trachea, intestine, stomach, spleen can be included for chest and abdominal injuries, but blood, muscular tissue and/or adipose are informative for injuries anywhere on a body [**223,224,225**].

5.3. Fluids and Tissues Carry Multiple Cell Types

In a human body, there are ~210 cell types [**226**], and body fluids and organs contain several types of cells (semen may be an exception as semen carries besides spermatozoa only few other cell types).

As evidentiary stains may be minute, not all cell types may be represented in a sample, so it can be opportune to include markers for various cell types from one tissue or fluid in an assay. For example, CNS tissue comprises two major tissues: grey matter and white matter. Grey matter (~10% of the tissue in the brain volume) consists mainly of neuronal cell bodies (and unmyelinated axons and glial cells), while white matter (the deeper layer) mainly contains myelinated axons (and astrocytes and oligodendrocytes that produce myelin) [**227**]. Whether an evidentiary stain carries predominantly grey or white matter, will affect which markers can respond.

With body fluids, samplings may have a more even distribution of cell types, due to the liquid constitution. These have different biological functions that affect their localization. For example, red blood cells function within the blood (amongst others for carriage of oxygen) while white blood cells act mostly outside of the bloodstream (immune system). As a consequence, white blood cells crawl into the lymphatic system by a process denoted extravasation [**228**]). The lymphatic system is an extensive drainage network and several other forensically relevant body fluids may thereby carry white blood cells (e.g., nasal secretion [**228**]).

It is crucial to understand the biological function and performance on other body fluids or tissues for markers included in a cell typing assay.

6. INTERPRETATION OF CELL TYPING RESULTS

Generally, an evidentiary stain that is subjected for cell type analysis is also submitted for DNA profiling as one wishes to infer what cell type is donated by which person. This invokes a three-way interpretation: (1) the DNA profile; (2) the cell typing data and 3) the combination aiming to associate donor and cell type. The interpretation of DNA profiles has progressed tremendously through the application of probabilistic software [**229,230,231,232,233**] that use information on the number of contributors, allele frequencies, peak height, drop-in, dropout, degradation and more to provide a weight of evidence in the form of a likelihood ratio (LR). The LR includes a person of interest under H1 (H2 generally calculates the likelihood for an unknown, unrelated person). With the interpretation of cell typing data, several issues are to be considered: (1) limitations in sensitivity; (2) constraints for specificity; (3) degradation in evidentiary stains; (4) complications in case of a mixture of cell types and (5) providing an evidential value. These issues are discussed below, followed by developments on the association of donor and cell type.

6.1. Sensitivity, Specificity and Degradation Issues Affecting Interpretation

Ideally, a cell typing method has similar sensitivity for all cell types assessed in an assay, and a similar sensitivity as DNA profiling so that for all donors that give DNA information cell type information is derived as well. Over time, DNA profiling has become more and more sensitive and a full DNA profile can be generated from DNA amounts that equate to a few cells. The sensitivity of cell typing depends greatly on the type of marker that is used. DNA-based markers (those assessing methylation status) will at best be as sensitive as DNA profiling as both analyze features of the two genomic DNA copies. MSRE analysis [**154,155,210,211**] indeed approaches the sensitivity of DNA profiling, but methods that rely on a bisulfite conversion are much less sensitive as a large portion of DNA is lost during the conversion [**146,147**].

RNA and protein/ enzyme markers are expressed and translated from DNA and may be several folds more abundant than DNA although expression levels can vary highly for different genes, and abundance is further influenced by stability/ turnover rates. Environmental and physiological factors may cause variation between people and over time (an infection will increase the number of white blood cells and the mRNAs these cells contain). Thus, it appears inevitable that the sensitivity of markers targeting either the same or different body fluids will vary [**121**] despite careful marker selection and assay optimization. An extreme example is semen from an azoospermic male, which will provide RNA and proteins for seminal fluid but little DNA (or spermatozoa mRNAs/ proteins). Thorough validation by which understanding of marker performance is obtained is of pivotal importance.

Specificity issues can relate to human-specificity or tissue-specificity [**234**]. Methods that analyze nucleic acids, can most often be designed to be human (or at least primate)-specific, which is less feasible for tests based on enzyme activity or antibodies. Processes such as readthrough or spurious transcription giving rise to non-specific background expression of mRNAs may result in signals above the detection threshold for the assay, especially when samples are over-amplified (by using too much input or too many amplification cycles). Technological imperfections can also cause non-specific signals like remnants of DNA in RNA assays (this is only an issue when it is not possible to design cDNA-specific amplicons with for instance one primer spanning an exon-exon boundary) or incomplete bisulfite conversion in methylation-based assays. The most difficult form of non-specificity is when markers cross-react with cell types other than the intended cell type. This occurs more with body fluids than with organs. For instance, saliva, nasal secretion and vaginal material are produced in body cavities (oral, nasal, vaginal) that are all lined with mucous membranes. These can, as previously mentioned, give rise to expression of the same mucous markers in these body fluids (denoted general mucosa markers [**98**]). These non-specific responses can show inter-individual variation: mRNA vaginal markers were detected in nasal secretions in many donors, with no relation to gender or having a cold [**104**]. As with sensitivity, thorough validation with different donors is highly important to understand marker performance.

Outside the human body, factors such as high humidity, UV radiation and/or high temperature can invoke degradation of nucleic acids, especially when stains have not fully dried. DNA is more resistant to hydrolysis than RNA, as the 2'-OH group can attack the 3'-phosphate, leading to hydrolytic cleavage of the phosphodiester bond, which may lead to samples providing a DNA but no or hardly an RNA profile [**97**]. Amplicons in RNA assays are therefore generally shorter (preferably under ~150 base pairs) than in DNA typing (up to ~450 base pairs). Intramolecular base pairing within RNA molecules (not only G:C and A:U but also G:U) may result in secondary and tertiary structures that provide more stability to certain regions, and amplicons targeting such stable RNA regions (StaRs) [**95,235**] may enhance RNA profiling. DNA methylation assays have the advantage of using the same nucleic acid as used for DNA profiling, so there is no difference in stability (the methylation marks remain stable also in body fluids deposited outside a human body [**236**]).

6.2. Interpretation of Mixed Samples

RNA casework has shown that most evidentiary samples contain multiple fluids/tissues, particularly with body fluid typing and less so with organ typing. One cause is that many samplings are taken from body locations (penis, fingers) or fabrics (clothing, bedding) that are likely to carry skin and other body fluid depositions. Moreover, the contributions may be highly unbalanced. To work on mixtures, markers should best respond in on-off modus meaning that a signal is obtained when the body fluid is present and not when a body fluid is absent. This can be achieved with RNA-based assays when markers are selected that show a large difference in expression between target and non-target tissues. Over-amplification needs to be avoided and detection thresholds need to be set.

For methylation-based assays, application to mixtures depends on the technology that is chosen. With MSRE, CpG targets are selected that are only methylated in the target tissue (this does not need to be a 100% methylation). PCR product can only be generated when the restriction enzyme is unable to cut the DNA due to methylation of the restriction site [**237**].

When methylation levels are assessed quantitively, for instance by sequencing bisulfite-converted DNA, it is highly complex to set interpretation guidelines for mixed samples. For example, when a chosen marker shows on average a 50% methylation rate in vaginal mucosa and 10% in other cell types, a 20% methylation level for the marker in an evidentiary sample can occur in different ways: (1) no vaginal mucosa is present and the methylation level of the other cell types (skin and/or semen) turns out higher than the average of 10%; (2) vaginal mucosa is present and no other cell types and the 20% methylation rate is an outlier for vaginal mucosa; (3) vaginal mucosa is mixed with other cell types for which a ratio of 1:3 would nicely explain the methylation rate of 20%. In this example, the DNA profile may be informative as a female donor will correspond to vaginal mucosa and the male donor to semen (if detected), but assumptions may need to made, for example, that no saliva from either one of the donors is present. When choosing a methodology for casework application, its suitability for mixed samples needs to be considered to enable appropriate interpretation.

6.3. Reporting Cell Typing Results

In expert reports, cell typing results are generally given as 'indication for the presence of' when genetic markers or tests for a body fluid or organ tissue are observed. With RNA typing, interpretation thresholds are applied as both drop-in and dropout may occur, due to limitations in sensitivity and specificity described above. These interpretation thresholds can include a numerical scoring [**238**], or a strategy of using replicates and a 50% rule in which at least half of the markers over all replicates need to be detected [**111**]. All have the drawback that they represent a 'fall-of-the-cliff' method, which means that the detection of one marker more or less may change the interpretation of the results.

Nowadays, the general trend in forensic reporting is to provide an evidential value, for example by presenting a likelihood ratio; the probability of the evidence given two competing hypotheses, H1 and H2. Formulating H1 can be straightforward ('the sample contains vaginal cellular material'); formulating H2 is more complex as it could be 'the sample does not contain vaginal cellular material' or 'the sample contains another body fluid'. These hypotheses follow the simplifying assumption of one body fluid per sample. More realistic hypotheses consider mixtures and could be formulated as H1: 'the sample contains vaginal cellular material, and possibly other body fluids' and H2: 'the sample does not contain vaginal cellular material, but other body fluids' (note that one could also specify these other body fluids). Conditioning on cellular material assumed to be present (for instance, because the sample is a penile swab) would generate hypotheses like H1: 'the sample contains vaginal cellular material, and penile skin and possibly other body fluids' and H2: 'the sample does not contain vaginal cellular material, but penile skin and possibly other body fluids'.

Some statistical approaches have been proposed for body fluid typing; for organ typing, a multivariate statistical model was trained [**120,239,240,241,242**]. The basis of such models is an experimental dataset consisting of ground truth data, that should be casework representative. This is challenging as casework includes a wide range of samples for which the true composition is not known. It is not trivial to prepare such a dataset, and the LR should be calibrated to suit the size of the dataset (note that for DNA datasets the allele frequencies are used, while with RNA datasets an RNA profile is considered in its entirety). Reporting the LR in a verbal scale rather than a numerical value, seems more appropriate. Clearly, further development is needed, although the developments are promising.

6.4. Associating Donor and Body Fluid

A challenge for any forensic RNA typing method is the association of donor and body fluid. Complications are that one body fluid can be given by multiple donors and/or one donor can give multiple body fluids. Even with simple mixtures of two donors each giving one body fluid, it was shown that peak heights in DNA and RNA profiles cannot be used straightforwardly [**97**]. Only with gender-specific body fluids (vaginal cellular material and semen) and the involvement (or assumption) of one donor of that gender, is association of donor and body fluid possible. This introduces the risk of an association fallacy [**2,243**]. Thus, alternative procedures are being developed like SNPs (single nucleotide polymorphisms) in transcribed regions (RNA-SNPs) [**242,244,245,246**]. The concept is that the RNA indicates which cell type is present and that, as the RNA is transcribed from DNA, the genetic variation within this transcribed region provides information on the identity of the donor. First, which cell types are present is assessed, then the genotype for the RNA-SNPs of the donors that are assumed to be present are derived by genotyping their reference DNA (since this is DNA, there is no need to provide the body fluid questioned) and lastly the RNA of the stain is sequenced to see what SNPs are present in the transcribed mRNA to see if/ who of the donors matches this sequence.

This is a developing area with multiple challenges at hand: (1) SNPs can affect the stability or transcription level of RNAs, so the genotypes at the DNA and RNA level may not align (for instance one appears heterozygous at the DNA level but since the presence of a SNP affects RNA stability or expression level, one appears homozygous at the RNA level; (2) linked SNPs should be regarded according to their genetic phase (equivalent to a microhaplotype), which may be complicated when different SNPs reside in different amplicons; (3) the approach is only to be explored for samples in which all donors can be assumed as there is no clear strategy/consensus yet on how to deal with unknown donors. It is probably best to limit the approach initially to two-person mixtures.

CpG-SNPs (SNPs nearby CpGs indicative of cell types) have also been described [**247,248**]. Methods not depending on bisulfite conversion (such as MSRE) may be most practical to use to detect these as the bisulfite conversion will affect all non-methylated cytosines complicating SNP detection and primer design. A MS-HRM assay targeting DACT1 that is hypomethylated in semen was used [**249**] to determine if it was possible to associate semen with a DNA profile in a mixture. Some progress was made, and it was possible to determine whether the semen compromised the majority, almost half, or was in the minority of the components in a mixed fluid.

7. FURTHER CONSIDERATIONS

7.1. Other Marker Types and Technologies That Have Been Explored

7.1.1. Non-Coding RNAs

Various non-coding RNAs have been explored as markers for body fluid and tissue identification.

miRNAs are a class of small RNA molecules, 18–25 nucleotides in length, which are involved in the regulation (repression) of mRNA translation and stability [**69,71**]. with various forensic applications including body fluid identification [**250**].

Adult-specific roles for miRNAs (adult physiology, cancer development or suppression) have been described in various stem cell populations [**251**] and show continuous/ steady expression. This means these markers may be less specific for body fluid and tissue identification than might be suggested by the highly specific expression patterns seen in embryos [**252**]. Additionally, since human miRNAs generally interact through limited base pairing of only a few bases in the 5' part of the miRNA, a miRNA can bind to many targets. Conversely, an mRNA may be targeted by several (different) miRNAs. For these reasons, a key limitation of miRNAs is their specificity. Nonetheless, many studies have proposed miRNAs for body fluids such as blood, saliva, menstrual blood and semen [**253,254,255,256,257**] and body tissues including brain, liver, skeletal muscle and skin [**258**]. miRNAs are stable [**259**] and have been shown to be detectable in forensic-like samples when treated to a range of environmental conditions [**218,260**] after laundering [**261**].

Methods to analyze miRNAs primarily include miRNA expression profiles to identify candidate markers, followed by qPCR to test specificity [**253,255,256,258,262**]. Some approaches include the extraction and analysis of miRNA and DNA together [**263**] and multiplexed miRNA panels [**264**] able to discriminate between venous blood, menstrual blood, semen, and saliva. High throughput sequencing of miRNAs from body fluid samples has also been used to identify new candidates [**265**]. Statistical methods and reference (endogenous) miRNA markers [**262**] are needed to measure miRNA expression with qPCR. Recently classification algorithms have been applied to the interpretation of miRNA profiles as detection is not a simple yes–no answer [**259**].

The longest known class of small non-coding RNA are the piwi-interacting RNA (piRNA), 26–31 nucleotides in length. Their role is in the transcriptional and post-transcriptional silencing of transposable elements which may be differentially expressed in different body fluids making them suitable candidates for identifying body fluids (although transposon silencing is foremost important in the germline where piRNAs were initially found [**266**]). Two papers [**267,268**] describe the characterization by RNA sequencing of piRNA expression profiles and the selection of three piRNA markers (piR-hsa-27622, piR-hsa-1207 and piR-hsa-27493) that distinguish between venous blood and menstrual blood and a further two (piR-hsa-27493 and piR-hsa-26591) to distinguish between saliva and vaginal material, implemented as TaqMan RT-qPCR assays.

Short interfering RNA (siRNA) are another class of small non-coding RNA with a role in gene expression [**269**]. To date there are no reports of their use as markers in forensic science, perhaps because their role is to interfere with the expression of specific genes, by degrading RNA after transcription, rather than to promote the expression or modification of specific transcripts.

Long non-coding RNAs (lncRNAs) are RNA transcripts not translated into proteins that appear to be involved in the regulation of gene expression. Approximately 78% of them are tissue-based compared to approximately 18% of mRNA transcripts. One of the best studied is the X-inactive-based transcript (XIST) involved in X-chromosome inactivation [**270**,**271**]. To date, XIST has been incorporated into an assay [**272**] to positively identify male and female cell material in forensic samples with a second study [**273**] further testing the assay on forensic type samples.

7.1.2. Proteome

All body fluids and tissues contain unique proteomes, derived from the expression of mRNAs (see **Section 3.1.1**) in turn derived from the genome. In the past, unique proteins of each body fluid or tissue type have been detected and presumptively identified by determination of the enzyme activity (acid phosphatase for example) or immunological properties (RSID tests (Independent Forensics, Lombard, IL, USA) for example). More recently technological developments in proteomics, as for genomics, have highlighted potential benefits for forensic identification purposes and useful reviews of the forensic potential have been published [**274**,**275**,**276**].

Mass spectrometry (MS) is the analytical method of choice with advantages including high sensitivity and specificity [**277**]. Generally, candidate markers are found by *de novo* analysis or from reference proteomes, then validated by testing on known samples. By detecting multiple peptides in a single assay from more than one protein per fluid, the assay can be considered not only confirmatory but also human-based and suitable for mixtures. Sensitive and specific assays have been developed including blood, semen, seminal fluid, saliva, vaginal/ menstrual fluid and urine [**277**,**278**,**279**,**280**] using methods such as matrix-assisted laser desorption/ionization (MALDI) MS [**277**], quadrupole time-of-flight MS [**278**,**279**] MALDI MS Profiling and Imaging [**281**] and MALDI time-of-flight MS [**282**] from samples as diverse as blood-stained finger marks [**281**] and blood and vaginal cellular material under fingernails [**282**], although difficulties in identifying urine recovered from substrates and semen samples that had been mixed with lubricants were found [**280**]. A challenge to be addressed is that the protein content of each fluid/ tissue varies considerably, and whilst it is possible to detect very small amounts of blood in saliva, the opposite was not true [**277,278,279**].

MS methods tend to be destructive to the sample, however in a recent report [**283**] a new approach, sheath-flow probe electrospray ionisation MS was used, which allows stains to be sampled with no preparation or sample destruction bar the initial small amount taken. In the research which examined blood, saliva and urine, alterations were observed in the spectra over time suggesting that this approach could also be used to age a stain.

The relationship between the proteome and the genome offers the possibility for proteomic “genotyping” [**284,285**] in a similar manner to the suggested RNA SNP and CpG SNP approaches described in **Section 6.4**. This has clear advantages when DNA in a sample is compromised in quality and quantity such as in a hair shaft, as proteins are more stable and resistant to damage and decay than DNA. Genetic variations in human DNA can be linked to mutations found in hair proteins (genetically variant peptides (GVPs) referred to as single amino acid polymorphisms, SAPs, which in turn can be associated with their DNA counterparts (missense SNPs). GVPs containing SAPs can be identified by mapping these peptide sequences using MS and results have been obtained from short lengths of human hair [**275,286**]. Not only could this approach be used to “identify” and link individuals, but it can also be used to infer ancestry as SNP profiles varied between ancestral groups.

7.1.3. Aptamers

Aptamers are single-stranded oligonucleotides or peptides that are selected using SELEX (systematic evolution of ligands by exponential enrichment) in a sequential process to bind their target molecules in a highly specific and sensitive manner. Initial studies used RNA aptamers [**287,288**], with the first description of a DNA aptamer in 1992 [**289**] and the first XNA aptamer capable of binding to a small molecule (ochratoxin A) in 2018 [**290**]. Aptamers have a number of advantages over assays such as the immunochromatogenic-based methods described in **Section 2.2.1**. Consistent aptamer synthesis methods, more straightforward functionalization, equivalent binding affinities and cheaper long term and stable production are all factors.

Aptamers are now widely used as biosensors in a large number of fields [**291,292**] with significant and recent examples seen for the rapid detection of SARS-CoV-2 [**293,294**] and have potential for the use in forensic science [**295**]. Aptamers have been developed to detect PSA [**296**], hemoglobin [**297**] and more recently, aptamers to detect spermatozoa have been described using a combination of Cell-

SELEX and massively parallel sequencing technologies [**295**]. Once suitably specific and sensitive aptamers are obtained, they can be built into a range of sensors for detection many of them suitable for field deployment.

8. AT A GLANCE

Body fluid and body tissue identification are important in forensic science as they can provide key evidence in a criminal investigation and may assist the court in reaching conclusions. Establishing a link between identifying the fluid or tissue and the DNA profile adds further weight to this evidence. Many forensic laboratories retain techniques for the identification of biological fluids that have been widely used for some time. More recently, many different biomarkers and technologies have been proposed for identification of body fluids and tissues of forensic relevance some of which are now used in forensic casework. Here, we summarize the role of body fluid/ tissue identification in the evaluation of forensic evidence, describe how such evidence is detected at the crime scene and in the laboratory, elaborate different technologies available to do this, and reflect real life experiences.

9. CONCISE SUMMARY

Preferably, body fluid typing and DNA profiling (to answer the what and the who question) are analyzed on the exact same sample. This can be achieved when the DNA extract is used for cell type inference (as with methylation analysis) or when RNA is extracted from a fraction normally discarded during DNA extraction (like a flow through fraction when binding DNA to a silica column). Case reports have been published for both methylation [**298**] and RNA-based assays [**299**]. The advantage of using DNA for body fluid typing is that no additional extraction procedure is needed; the disadvantage is that less DNA remains for further analyses such as Y-STR profiling, mtDNA analysis or the prediction of age, ancestry, appearance. Microbiome analysis can use either DNA or RNA. The global COVID-19 pandemic has stimulated the development of assays that may find their use in forensic analysis such as multiplexed and extraction-free amplification assays [**300**], which may provide RNA-based tests prior to DNA extraction and analysis that may present the opportunity of triage. Such extraction-free methods [**301**] present pioneering opportunities beyond advancements such as one-step RT-PCR methods that simplify current methodology [**302**].

Introducing cell typing methodologies in a forensic laboratory requires extensive validation, implementation of interpretation and reporting, and explaining results for judiciary. This comes with additional costs (also because the technique itself may ask quite some hands-on laboratory work) and it has been suggested that it is best performed or outsourced to specialized laboratories.

REFERENCES

1. Taylor, D.; Kokshoorn, B.; Biedermann, A. Evaluation of Forensic Genetics Findings given Activity Level Propositions: A Review. *Forensic Sci. Int. Genet.* **2018**, *36*, 34–49. **[Google Scholar] [CrossRef] [Green Version]**
2. Meakin, G.E.; Kokshoorn, B.; Oorschot, R.A.H.; Szkuta, B. Evaluating Forensic DNA Evidence: Connecting the Dots. *WIREs Forensic Sci.* **2021**, *3*, e1404. **[Google Scholar] [CrossRef]**
3. Gill, P.; Hicks, T.; Butler, J.M.; Connolly, E.; Gusmão, L.; Kokshoorn, B.; Morling, N.; van Oorschot, R.A.H.; Parson, W.; Prinz, M.; et al. DNA Commission of the International Society for Forensic Genetics: Assessing the Value of Forensic Biological Evidence—Guidelines Highlighting the Importance of Propositions: Part I: Evaluation of DNA Profiling Comparisons given (Sub-) Source Propositions. *Forensic Sci. Int. Genet.* **2018**, *36*, 189–202. **[Google Scholar] [CrossRef] [Green Version]**
4. Gill, P.; Hicks, T.; Butler, J.M.; Connolly, E.; Gusmão, L.; Kokshoorn, B.; Morling, N.; van Oorschot, R.A.H.; Parson, W.; Prinz, M.; et al. DNA Commission of the International Society for Forensic Genetics: Assessing the Value of Forensic Biological Evidence—Guidelines Highlighting the Importance of Propositions. Part II: Evaluation of Biological Traces Considering Activity Level Propositions. *Forensic Sci. Int. Genet.* **2020**, *44*, 102186. **[Google Scholar] [CrossRef] [Green Version]**
5. Jackson, G.; Biedermann, A. "Source" or "Activity" What Is the Level of Issue in a Criminal Trial? *Significance* **2019**, *16*, 36–39. **[Google Scholar] [CrossRef]**
6. Pope, S.; Biedermann, A. Editorial: The Dialogue Between Forensic Scientists, Statisticians and Lawyers About Complex Scientific Issues for Court. *Front. Genet.* **2020**, *11*, 704. **[Google Scholar] [CrossRef]**
7. Puch-Solis, R.; Pope, S. Interpretation of DNA Data within the Context of UK Forensic Science—Evaluation. *Emerg. Top. Life Sci.* **2021**, *5*, 405–413. **[Google Scholar] [CrossRef]**
8. Pope, S.; Puch-Solis, R. Interpretation of DNA Data within the Context of UK Forensic Science—Investigation. *Emerg. Top. Life Sci.* **2021**, *5*, 395–404. **[Google Scholar] [CrossRef] [PubMed]**
9. Lin, H.; Zhang, Y.; Wang, Q.; Li, B.; Huang, P.; Wang, Z. Estimation of the Age of Human Bloodstains under the Simulated Indoor and Outdoor Crime Scene Conditions by ATR-FTIR Spectroscopy. *Sci. Rep.* **2017**, *7*, 13254. **[Google Scholar] [CrossRef]**

10. Stotesbury, T.; Cossette, M.-L.; Newell-Bell, T.; Shafer, A.B.A. An Exploratory Time Since Deposition Analysis of Whole Blood Using Metrics of DNA Degradation and Visible Absorbance Spectroscopy. *Pure Appl. Geophys.* **2021**, *178*, 735–743. **[Google Scholar] [CrossRef]**

11. Weber, A.R.; Lednev, I.K. Crime Clock—Analytical Studies for Approximating Time since Deposition of Bloodstains. *Forensic Chem.* **2020**, *19*, 100248. **[Google Scholar] [CrossRef]**

12. Bremmer, R.H.; Nadort, A.; van Leeuwen, T.G.; van Gemert, M.J.C.; Aalders, M.C.G. Age Estimation of Blood Stains by Hemoglobin Derivative Determination Using Reflectance Spectroscopy. *Forensic Sci. Int.* **2011**, *206*, 166–171. **[Google Scholar] [CrossRef] [PubMed]**

13. Edelman, G.; van Leeuwen, T.G.; Aalders, M.C.G. Hyperspectral Imaging for the Age Estimation of Blood Stains at the Crime Scene. *Forensic Sci. Int.* **2012**, *223*, 72–77. **[Google Scholar] [CrossRef] [PubMed]**

14. Alshehhi, S.; Haddrill, P.R. Estimating Time since Deposition Using Quantification of RNA Degradation in Body Fluid-Specific Markers. *Forensic Sci. Int.* **2019**, *298*, 58–63. **[Google Scholar] [CrossRef] [Green Version]**

15. Alshehhi, S.; Haddrill, P.R. Evaluating the Effect of Body Fluid Mixture on the Relative Expression Ratio of Blood-Specific RNA Markers. *Forensic Sci. Int.* **2020**, *307*, 110116. **[Google Scholar] [CrossRef]**

16. Fu, J.; Allen, R.W. A Method to Estimate the Age of Bloodstains Using Quantitative PCR. *Forensic Sci. Int. Genet.* **2019**, *39*, 103–108. **[Google Scholar] [CrossRef]**

17. Heneghan, N.; Fu, J.; Pritchard, J.; Payton, M.; Allen, R.W. The Effect of Environmental Conditions on the Rate of RNA Degradation in Dried Blood Stains. *Forensic Sci. Int. Genet.* **2021**, *51*, 102456. **[Google Scholar] [CrossRef]**

18. Weinbrecht, K.D.; Fu, J.; Payton, M.E.; Allen, R.W. Time-Dependent Loss of mRNA Transcripts from Forensic Stains. *Res. Rep. Forensic Med. Sci.* **2017**, *7*, 1–12. **[Google Scholar] [CrossRef] [Green Version]**

19. Salzmann, A.P.; Russo, G.; Kreutzer, S.; Haas, C. Degradation of Human mRNA Transcripts over Time as an Indicator of the Time since Deposition (TsD) in Biological Crime Scene Traces. *Forensic Sci. Int. Genet.* **2021**, *53*, 102524. **[Google Scholar] [CrossRef]**

20. Díez López, C.; Kayser, M.; Vidaki, A. Estimating the Time Since Deposition of Saliva Stains With a Targeted Bacterial DNA Approach: A Proof-of-Principle Study. *Front. Microbiol.* **2021**, *12*, 1102. **[Google Scholar] [CrossRef]**

21. Gill, P.; Bleka, Ø.; Roseth, A.; Fonneløp, A.E. An LR Framework Incorporating Sensitivity Analysis to Model Multiple Direct and Secondary Transfer Events on Skin Surface. *Forensic Sci. Int. Genet.* **2021**, *53*, 102509. **[Google Scholar]** **[CrossRef]** **[PubMed]**

22. Puliatti, L.; Handt, O.; Taylor, D. The Level of DNA an Individual Transfers to Untouched Items in Their Immediate Surroundings. *Forensic Sci. Int. Genet.* **2021**, *54*, 102561. **[Google Scholar]** **[CrossRef]**

23. Saric, N.; Fabien, L.; Fischer, J.; Hermelin, A.; Massonnet, G.; Burnier, C. A Preliminary Investigation of Transfer of Condom Lubricants in the Vaginal Matrix. *Forensic Sci. Int.* **2021**, *325*, 110847. **[Google Scholar]** **[CrossRef]**

24. Kelly, P.; Connolly, E. The Prevalence and Persistence of Saliva in Vehicles. *Forensic Sci. Int. Genet.* **2021**, *53*, 102530. **[Google Scholar]** **[CrossRef]**

25. Reither, J.B.; Gray, E.; Durdle, A.; Conlan, X.A.; van Oorschot, R.A.H.; Szkuta, B. Investigation into the Prevalence of Background DNA on Flooring within Houses and Its Transfer to a Contacting Surface. *Forensic Sci. Int.* **2021**, *318*, 110563. **[Google Scholar]** **[CrossRef]**

26. Thornbury, D.; Goray, M.; van Oorschot, R.A.H. Indirect DNA Transfer without Contact from Dried Biological Materials on Various Surfaces. *Forensic Sci. Int. Genet.* **2021**, *51*, 102457. **[Google Scholar]** **[CrossRef]**

27. Tanzhaus, K.; Reiß, M.-T.; Zaspel, T. "I've Never Been at the Crime Scene!"—Gloves as Carriers for Secondary DNA Transfer. *Int. J. Legal Med.* **2021**, *135*, 1385–1393. **[Google Scholar]** **[CrossRef]**

28. Burrill, J.; Kombara, A.; Daniel, B.; Frascione, N. Exploration of Cell-Free DNA (CfDNA) Recovery for Touch Deposits. *Forensic Sci. Int. Genet.* **2021**, *51*, 102431. **[Google Scholar]** **[CrossRef]** **[PubMed]**

29. Schyma, C.; Madea, B.; Müller, R.; Zieger, M.; Utz, S.; Grabmüller, M. DNA-Free Does Not Mean RNA-Free—The Unwanted Persistence of RNA. *Forensic Sci. Int.* **2021**, *318*, 110632. **[Google Scholar]** **[CrossRef]**

30. Ménard, H.; Cole, C.; Gray, A.; Mudie, R.; Klu, J.K.; Nic Daéid, N. Creation of a Universal Experimental Protocol for the Investigation of Transfer and Persistence of Trace Evidence: Part 1—From Design to Implementation for Particulate Evidence. *Forensic Sci. Int. Synerg.* **2021**, *3*, 100165. **[Google Scholar]** **[CrossRef]** **[PubMed]**

31. Samie, L.; Taroni, F.; Champod, C. Estimating the Quantity of Transferred DNA in Primary and Secondary Transfers. *Sci. Justice J. Forensic Sci. Soc.* **2020**, *60*, 128–135. **[Google Scholar]** **[CrossRef]** **[PubMed]** **[Green Version]**

32. van Oorschot, R.A.H.; Szkuta, B.; Meakin, G.E.; Kokshoorn, B.; Goray, M. DNA Transfer in Forensic Science: A Review. *Forensic Sci. Int. Genet.* **2019**, *38*, 140–166. **[Google Scholar] [CrossRef] [PubMed]**

33. Goray, M.; Eken, E.; Mitchell, R.J.; van Oorschot, R.A.H. Secondary DNA Transfer of Biological Substances under Varying Test Conditions. *Forensic Sci. Int. Genet.* **2010**, *4*, 62–67. **[Google Scholar] [CrossRef] [PubMed]**

34. Goray, M.; van Oorschot, R.A.H.; Mitchell, J.R. DNA Transfer within Forensic Exhibit Packaging: Potential for DNA Loss and Relocation. *Forensic Sci. Int. Genet.* **2012**, *6*, 158–166. **[Google Scholar] [CrossRef]**

35. Verdon, T.J.; Mitchell, R.J.; van Oorschot, R.A.H. The Influence of Substrate on DNA Transfer and Extraction Efficiency. *Forensic Sci. Int. Genet.* **2013**, *7*, 167–175. **[Google Scholar] [CrossRef]**

36. Szkuta, B.; Harvey, M.L.; Ballantyne, K.N.; van Oorschot, R.A.H. DNA Transfer by Examination Tools—A Risk for Forensic Casework? *Forensic Sci. Int. Genet.* **2015**, *16*, 246–254. **[Google Scholar] [CrossRef]**

37. McColl, D.L.; Harvey, M.L.; van Oorschot, R.A.H. DNA Transfer by Different Parts of a Hand. *Forensic Sci. Int. Genet. Suppl. Ser.* **2017**, *6*, e29–e31. **[Google Scholar] [CrossRef] [Green Version]**

38. Lehmann, V.J.; Mitchell, R.J.; Ballantyne, K.N.; van Oorschot, R.A.H. Following the Transfer of DNA: How Far Can It Go? *Forensic Sci. Int. Genet. Suppl. Ser.* **2013**, *4*, e53–e54. **[Google Scholar] [CrossRef]**

39. Taylor, D.; Biedermann, A.; Samie, L.; Pun, K.-M.; Hicks, T.; Champod, C. Helping to Distinguish Primary from Secondary Transfer Events for Trace DNA. *Forensic Sci. Int. Genet.* **2017**, *28*, 155–177. **[Google Scholar] [CrossRef] [Green Version]**

40. Taylor, D.; Samie, L.; Champod, C. Using Bayesian Networks to Track DNA Movement through Complex Transfer Scenarios. *Forensic Sci. Int. Genet.* **2019**, *42*, 69–80. **[Google Scholar] [CrossRef]**

41. Bouzga, M.M.; Dørum, G.; Gundersen, K.; Kohler, P.; Hoff-Olsen, P.; Fonneløp, A.E. Is It Possible to Predict the Origin of Epithelial Cells?—A Comparison of Secondary Transfer of Skin Epithelial Cells versus Vaginal Mucous Membrane Cells by Direct Contact. *Sci. Justice* **2020**, *60*, 234–242. **[Google Scholar] [CrossRef]**

42. van den Berge, M.; Ozcanhan, G.; Zijlstra, S.; Lindenbergh, A.; Sijen, T. Prevalence of Human Cell Material: DNA and RNA Profiling of Public and Private Objects and after Activity Scenarios. *Forensic Sci. Int. Genet.* **2016**, *21*, 81–89. **[Google Scholar] [CrossRef] [PubMed]**

43. Van den Berge, M.; van de Merwe, L.; Sijen, T. DNA Transfer and Cell Type Inference to Assist Activity Level Reporting: Post-Activity Background Samples as a Control in Dragging Scenario. *Forensic Sci. Int. Genet. Suppl. Ser.* **2017**, *6*, e591–e592. **[Google Scholar] [CrossRef] [Green Version]**

44. Burrill, J.; Daniel, B.; Frascione, N. Illuminating Touch Deposits through Cellular Characterization of Hand Rinses and Body Fluids with Nucleic Acid Fluorescence. *Forensic Sci. Int. Genet.* **2020**, *46*, 102269. **[Google Scholar] [CrossRef]**

45. Cook, R.; Evett, I.W.; Jackson, G.; Jones, P.J.; Lambert, J.A. A Model for Case Assessment and Interpretation. *Sci. Justice* **1998**, *38*, 151–156. **[Google Scholar] [CrossRef]**

46. Evett, I.W.; Jackson, G.; Lambert, J.A. More on the Hierarchy of Propositions: Exploring the Distinction between Explanations and Propositions. *Sci. Justice* **2000**, *40*, 3–10. **[Google Scholar] [CrossRef]**

47. Blum, L.J.; EsperanÇA, P.; Rocquefelte, S. A New High-Performance Reagent and Procedure for Latent Bloodstain Detection Based on Luminol Chemiluminescence. *Can. Soc. Forensic Sci. J.* **2006**, *39*, 81–99. **[Google Scholar] [CrossRef]**

48. Quinones, I.; Sheppard, D.; Harbison, S.; Elliot, D. Comparative Analysis of Luminol Formulations. *Can. Soc. Forensic Sci. J.* **2007**, *40*, 53–63. **[Google Scholar] [CrossRef]**

49. Finnis, J.; Lewis, J.; Davidson, A. Comparison of Methods for Visualizing Blood on Dark Surfaces. *Sci. Justice* **2013**, *53*, 178–186. **[Google Scholar] [CrossRef]**

50. Patel, G.; Hopwood, A. An Evaluation of Luminol Formulations and Their Effect on DNA Profiling. *Int. J. Leg. Med.* **2013**, *127*, 723–729. **[Google Scholar] [CrossRef] [PubMed]**

51. Sheppard, K.; Cassella, J.P.; Fieldhouse, S.; King, R. The Adaptation of a 360° Camera Utilising an Alternate Light Source (ALS) for the Detection of Biological Fluids at Crime Scenes. *Sci. Justice J. Forensic Sci. Soc.* **2017**, *57*, 239–249. **[Google Scholar] [CrossRef] [PubMed]**

52. Wang, Z.; Zhang, P.; Liu, H.; Zhao, Z.; Xiong, L.; He, W.; Kwok, R.T.K.; Lam, J.W.Y.; Ye, R.; Tang, B.Z. Robust Serum Albumin-Responsive AIEgen Enables Latent Bloodstain Visualization in High Resolution and Reliability for Crime Scene Investigation. *ACS Appl. Mater. Interfaces* **2019**, *11*, 17306–17312. **[Google Scholar] [CrossRef]**

53. Borges, E.; Degiuli, A.; Desrentes, S.; Popielarz, C.; Blum, L.J.; Marquette, C.A. Evaluation of the SPERM TRACKER™ for Semen Stains Localization on Fabrics. *J. Forensic Res.* **2017**, *8*. **[Google Scholar] [CrossRef]**

54. Auvdel, M.J. Comparison of Laser and Ultraviolet Techniques Used in the Detection of Body Secretions. *J. Forensic Sci.* **1987**, *32*, 326–345. **[Google Scholar] [CrossRef] [PubMed] [Green Version]**

55. Vandenberg, N.; van Oorschot, R.A.H. The Use of Polilight® in the Detection of Seminal Fluid, Saliva, and Bloodstains and Comparison with Conventional Chemical-Based Screening Tests. *J. Forensic Sci.* **2006**, *51*, 361–370. **[Google Scholar] [CrossRef] [PubMed]**

56. Sterzik, V.; Panzer, S.; Apfelbacher, M.; Bohnert, M. Searching for Biological Traces on Different Materials Using a Forensic Light Source and Infrared Photography. *Int. J. Leg. Med.* **2016**, *130*, 599–605. **[Google Scholar] [CrossRef]**

57. Sterzik, V.; Hinderberger, P.; Panzer, S.; Bohnert, M. Visualizing Old Biological Traces on Different Materials without Using Chemicals. *Int. J. Leg. Med.* **2018**, *132*, 35–41. **[Google Scholar] [CrossRef]**

58. Tay, J.; Joudo, J.; Tran, T.; Ta, H.; Botting, J.; Liew, Y.; Cooper, P.; Rye, M. Comparison of Crime-Lite® 82S, Polilight® PL400 and Polilight® PL500 for the Detection of Semen and Saliva Stains. *Aust. J. Forensic Sci.* **2020**, *53*, 483–493. **[Google Scholar] [CrossRef]**

59. Zapata, F.; de la Ossa, M.Á.F.; García-Ruiz, C. Differentiation of Body Fluid Stains on Fabrics Using External Reflection Fourier Transform Infrared Spectroscopy (FT-IR) and Chemometrics. *Appl. Spectrosc.* **2016**, *70*, 654–665. **[Google Scholar] [CrossRef]**

60. Morillas, A.V.; Gooch, J.; Frascione, N. Feasibility of a Handheld near Infrared Device for the Qualitative Analysis of Bloodstains. *Talanta* **2018**, *184*, 1–6. **[Google Scholar] [CrossRef] [PubMed] [Green Version]**

61. Pereira, J.F.Q.; Silva, C.S.; Vieira, M.J.L.; Pimentel, M.F.; Braz, A.; Honorato, R.S. Evaluation and Identification of Blood Stains with Handheld NIR Spectrometer. *Microchem. J.* **2017**, *133*, 561–566. **[Google Scholar] [CrossRef]**

62. Edelman, G.J.; van Leeuwen, T.G.; Aalders, M.C.G. Hyperspectral Imaging of the Crime Scene for Detection and Identification of Blood Stains. In Proceedings of the Algorithms and Technologies for Multispectral, Hyperspectral, and Ultraspectral Imagery XIX, Baltimore, MD, USA, 18 May 2013; Volume 8743, pp. 47–53. **[Google Scholar]**

63. Edelman, G.; Manti, V.; Ruth, S.; van Leeuwen, T.; Aalders, M.C.G. Identification and Age Estimation of Blood Stains on Colored Backgrounds by near Infrared Spectroscopy. *Forensic Sci. Int.* **2012**, *220*, 239–244. **[Google Scholar] [CrossRef]**

64. Edelman, G.; Gaston, E.; van Leeuwen, T.; Cullen, P.J.; Aalders, M.C.G. Hyperspectral Imaging for Non-Contact Analysis of Forensic Traces. *Forensic Sci. Int.* **2012**, *223*, 28–39. **[Google Scholar] [CrossRef] [PubMed] [Green Version]**
65. Cadd, S.; Li, B.; Beveridge, P.; O'Hare, W.T.; Islam, M. Age Determination of Blood-Stained Fingerprints Using Visible Wavelength Reflectance Hyperspectral Imaging. *J. Imaging* **2018**, *4*, 141. **[Google Scholar] [CrossRef] [Green Version]**
66. Malegori, C.; Alladio, E.; Oliveri, P.; Manis, C.; Vincenti, M.; Garofano, P.; Barni, F.; Berti, A. Identification of Invisible Biological Traces in Forensic Evidences by Hyperspectral NIR Imaging Combined with Chemometrics. *Talanta* **2020**, *215*, 120911. **[Google Scholar] [CrossRef]**
67. Zulfiqar, M.; Ahmad, M.; Sohaib, A.; Mazzara, M.; Distefano, S. Hyperspectral Imaging for Bloodstain Identification. *Sensors* **2021**, *21*, 3045. **[Google Scholar] [CrossRef] [PubMed]**
68. Romaszewski, M.; Głomb, P.; Sochan, A.; Cholewa, M. A Dataset for Evaluating Blood Detection in Hyperspectral Images. *Forensic Sci. Int.* **2021**, *320*, 110701. **[Google Scholar] [CrossRef]**
69. Sijen, T. Molecular Approaches for Forensic Cell Type Identification: On mRNA, MiRNA, DNA Methylation and Microbial Markers. *Forensic Sci. Int. Genet.* **2015**, *18*, 21–32. **[Google Scholar] [CrossRef]**
70. Sakurada, K.; Watanabe, K.; Akutsu, T. Current Methods for Body Fluid Identification Related to Sexual Crime: Focusing on Saliva, Semen, and Vaginal Fluid. *Diagnostics* **2020**, *10*, 693. **[Google Scholar] [CrossRef]**
71. Harbison, S.A.; Fleming, R.I. Forensic Body Fluid Identification: State of the Art. *Res. Rep. Forensic Med. Sci.* **2016**, *6*, 11–23. **[Google Scholar] [CrossRef] [Green Version]**
72. Holtkötter, H.; Schwender, K.; Wiegand, P.; Peiffer, H.; Vennemann, M. Improving Body Fluid Identification in Forensic Trace Evidence—Construction of an Immunochromatographic Test Array to Rapidly Detect up to Five Body Fluids Simultaneously. *Int. J. Leg. Med.* **2018**, *132*, 83–90. **[Google Scholar] [CrossRef] [PubMed]**
73. de Beijer, R.P.; de Graaf, C.; van Weert, A.; van Leeuwen, T.G.; Aalders, M.C.G.; van Dam, A. Identification and Detection of Protein Markers to Differentiate between Forensically Relevant Body Fluids. *Forensic Sci. Int.* **2018**, *290*, 196–206. **[Google Scholar] [CrossRef]**

74. Lee, J.W.; Jung, J.Y.; Lim, S.-K. Simple and Rapid Identification of Saliva by Detection of Oral Streptococci Using Direct Polymerase Chain Reaction Combined with an Immunochromatographic Strip. *Forensic Sci. Int. Genet.* **2018**, *33*, 155–160. **[Google Scholar] [CrossRef]**

75. Abbas, N.; Lu, X.; Badshah, M.A.; In, J.B.; Heo, W.I.; Park, K.Y.; Lee, M.-K.; Kim, C.H.; Kang, P.; Chang, W.-J.; et al. Development of a Protein Microarray Chip with Enhanced Fluorescence for Identification of Semen and Vaginal Fluid. *Sensors* **2018**, *18*, 3874. **[Google Scholar] [CrossRef] [Green Version]**

76. Boyd, S.; Bertino, M.F.; Seashols, S.J. Raman Spectroscopy of Blood Samples for Forensic Applications. *Forensic Sci. Int.* **2011**, *208*, 124–128. **[Google Scholar] [CrossRef] [PubMed]**

77. Virkler, K.; Lednev, I.K. Raman Spectroscopic Signature of Semen and Its Potential Application to Forensic Body Fluid Identification. *Forensic Sci. Int.* **2009**, *193*, 56–62. **[Google Scholar] [CrossRef]**

78. Casey, T.; Mistek, E.; Halámková, L.; Lednev, I.K. Raman Spectroscopy for Forensic Semen Identification: Method Validation vs. Environmental Interferences. *Vib. Spectrosc.* **2020**, *109*, 103065. **[Google Scholar] [CrossRef]**

79. Doty, K.C.; Muro, C.K.; Lednev, I.K. Predicting the Time of the Crime: Bloodstain Aging Estimation for up to Two Years. *Forensic Chem.* **2017**, *5*, 1–7. **[Google Scholar] [CrossRef]**

80. Rosenblatt, R.; Halámková, L.; Doty, K.C.; de Oliveira, E.A.C.; Lednev, I.K. Raman Spectroscopy for Forensic Bloodstain Identification: Method Validation vs. Environmental Interferences. *Forensic Chem.* **2019**, *16*, 100175. **[Google Scholar] [CrossRef]**

81. Takamura, A.; Watanabe, K.; Akutsu, T.; Ozawa, T. Soft and Robust Identification of Body Fluid Using Fourier Transform Infrared Spectroscopy and Chemometric Strategies for Forensic Analysis. *Sci. Rep.* **2018**, *8*, 8459. **[Google Scholar] [CrossRef] [PubMed]**

82. Orphanou, C.-M. The Detection and Discrimination of Human Body Fluids Using ATR FT-IR Spectroscopy. *Forensic Sci. Int.* **2015**, *252*, e10–e16. **[Google Scholar] [CrossRef]**

83. Sharma, S.; Chophi, R.; Singh, R. Forensic Discrimination of Menstrual Blood and Peripheral Blood Using Attenuated Total Reflectance (ATR)-Fourier Transform Infrared (FT-IR) Spectroscopy and Chemometrics. *Int. J. Leg. Med.* **2020**, *134*, 63–77. **[Google Scholar] [CrossRef]**

84. Zha, S.; Wei, X.; Fang, R.; Wang, Q.; Lin, H.; Zhang, K.; Zhang, H.; Liu, R.; Li, Z.; Huang, P.; et al. Estimation of the Age of Human Semen Stains by Attenuated Total Reflection Fourier Transform Infrared Spectroscopy: A Preliminary Study. *Forensic Sci. Res.* **2020**, *5*, 119–125. **[Google Scholar] [CrossRef]**

85. Takamura, A.; Halamkova, L.; Ozawa, T.; Lednev, I.K. Phenotype Profiling for Forensic Purposes: Determining Donor Sex Based on Fourier Transform Infrared Spectroscopy of Urine Traces. *Anal. Chem.* **2019**, *91*, 6288–6295. **[Google Scholar] [CrossRef]**

86. Mistek-Morabito, E.; Lednev, I.K. Discrimination of Menstrual and Peripheral Blood Traces Using Attenuated Total Reflection Fourier Transform-Infrared (ATR FT-IR) Spectroscopy and Chemometrics for Forensic Purposes. *Anal. Bioanal. Chem.* **2021**, *413*, 2513–2522. **[Google Scholar] [CrossRef]**

87. Karadayi, S.; Moshfeghi, E.; Arasoglu, T.; Karadayi, B. Evaluating the Persistence of Laundered Semen Stains on Fabric Using a Forensic Light Source System, Prostate-Specific Antigen Semiquant Test and DNA Recovery-Profiling. *Med. Sci. Law* **2020**, *60*, 122–130. **[Google Scholar] [CrossRef] [PubMed]**

88. Lynch, C.; Fleming, R. RNA-Based Approaches for Body Fluid Identification in Forensic Science. *WIREs Forensic Sci.* **2021**, *3*, e1407. **[Google Scholar] [CrossRef]**

89. El-Mogy, M.; Lam, B.; Haj-Ahmad, T.A.; McGowan, S.; Yu, D.; Nosal, L.; Rghei, N.; Roberts, P.; Haj-Ahmad, Y. Diversity and Signature of Small RNA in Different Bodily Fluids Using next Generation Sequencing. *BMC Genom.* **2018**, *19*, 408. **[Google Scholar] [CrossRef] [PubMed]**

90. Na, J.-Y. Estimation of the Post-Mortem Interval Using MicroRNA in the Bones. *J. Forensic Leg. Med.* **2020**, *75*, 102049. **[Google Scholar] [CrossRef] [PubMed]**

91. Bauer, M.; Patzelt, D. Evaluation of Mrna Markers for the Identification of Menstrual Blood. *J. Forensic Sci.* **2002**, *47*, 1278–1282. **[Google Scholar] [CrossRef]**

92. Bauer, M.; Kraus, A.; Patzelt, D. Detection of Epithelial Cells in Dried Blood Stains by Reverse Transcriptase-Polymerase Chain Reaction. *J. Forensic Sci.* **1999**, *44*, 1232–1236. **[Google Scholar] [CrossRef]**

93. Setzer, M.; Juusola, J.; Ballantyne, J. Recovery and Stability of RNA in Vaginal Swabs and Blood, Semen, and Saliva Stains. *J. Forensic Sci.* **2008**, *53*, 296–305. **[Google Scholar] [CrossRef]**

94. Kohlmeier, F.; Schneider, P.M. Successful mRNA Profiling of 23 Years Old Blood Stains. *Forensic Sci. Int. Genet.* **2012**, *6*, 274–276. **[Google Scholar] [CrossRef]**

95. Lin, M.-H.; Jones, D.F.; Fleming, R. Transcriptomic Analysis of Degraded Forensic Body Fluids. *Forensic Sci. Int. Genet.* **2015**, *17*, 35–42. **[Google Scholar] [CrossRef] [PubMed]**

96. Salzmann, A.P.; Russo, G.; Aluri, S.; Haas, C. Transcription and Microbial Profiling of Body Fluids Using a Massively Parallel Sequencing Approach. *Forensic Sci. Int. Genet.* **2019**, *43*, 102149. **[Google Scholar] [CrossRef] [PubMed]**

97. Harteveld, J.; Lindenbergh, A.; Sijen, T. RNA Cell Typing and DNA Profiling of Mixed Samples: Can Cell Types and Donors Be Associated? *Sci. Justice* **2013**, *53*, 261–269. **[Google Scholar] [CrossRef]**

98. Lindenbergh, A.; de Pagter, M.; Ramdayal, G.; Visser, M.; Zubakov, D.; Kayser, M.; Sijen, T. A Multiplex (m)RNA-Profiling System for the Forensic Identification of Body Fluids and Contact Traces. *Forensic Sci. Int. Genet.* **2012**, *6*, 565–577. **[Google Scholar] [CrossRef] [PubMed]**

99. Bowden, A.; Fleming, R.; Harbison, S. A Method for DNA and RNA Co-Extraction for Use on Forensic Samples Using the Promega DNA IQ™ System. *Forensic Sci. Int. Genet.* **2011**, *5*, 64–68. **[Google Scholar] [CrossRef]**

100. Alvarez, M.; Juusola, J.; Ballantyne, J. An mRNA and DNA Co-Isolation Method for Forensic Casework Samples. *Anal. Biochem.* **2004**, *335*, 289–298. **[Google Scholar] [CrossRef]**

101. Wang, S.; Shanthan, G.; Bouzga, M.M.; Dinh, H.M.T.; Haas, C.; Fonneløp, A.E. Evaluating the Performance of Five Up-to-Date DNA/RNA Co-Extraction Methods for Forensic Application. *Forensic Sci. Int.* **2021**, *328*, 110996. **[Google Scholar] [CrossRef] [PubMed]**

102. Juusola, J.; Ballantyne, J. Multiplex mRNA Profiling for the Identification of Body Fluids. *Forensic Sci. Int.* **2005**, *152*, 1–12. **[Google Scholar] [CrossRef]**

103. Akutsu, T.; Watanabe, K.; Takamura, A.; Sakurada, K. Evaluation of Skin- or Sweat-Characteristic mRNAs for Inferring the Human Origin of Touched Contact Traces. *Leg. Med.* **2018**, *33*, 36–41. **[Google Scholar] [CrossRef]**

104. van den Berge, M.; Bhoelai, B.; Harteveld, J.; Matai, A.; Sijen, T. Advancing Forensic RNA Typing: On Non-Target Secretions, a Nasal Mucosa Marker, a Differential Co-Extraction Protocol and the Sensitivity of DNA and RNA Profiling. *Forensic Sci. Int. Genet.* **2016**, *20*, 119–129. **[Google Scholar] [CrossRef] [PubMed]**

105. Cossu, C.; Germann, U.; Kratzer, A.; Bär, W.; Haas, C. How Specific Are the Vaginal Secretion mRNA-Markers HBD1 and MUC4? *Forensic Sci. Int. Genet. Suppl. Ser.* **2009**, *2*, 536–537. **[Google Scholar] [CrossRef]**

106. Richard, M.L.L.; Harper, K.A.; Craig, R.L.; Onorato, A.J.; Robertson, J.M.; Donfack, J. Evaluation of mRNA Marker Specificity for the Identification of Five Human Body Fluids by Capillary Electrophoresis. *Forensic Sci. Int. Genet.* **2012**, *6*, 452–460. **[Google Scholar] [CrossRef]**

107. Fleming, R.I.; Harbison, S. The Development of a mRNA Multiplex RT-PCR Assay for the Definitive Identification of Body Fluids. *Forensic Sci. Int. Genet.* **2010**, *4*, 244–256. **[Google Scholar] [CrossRef]**

108. Park, J.-L.; Park, S.-M.; Kim, J.-H.; Lee, H.-C.; Lee, S.-H.; Woo, K.-M.; Kim, S.-Y. Forensic Body Fluid Identification by Analysis of Multiple RNA Markers Using NanoString Technology. *Genom. Inform.* **2013**, *11*, 277–281. **[Google Scholar] [CrossRef] [Green Version]**

109. Hanson, E.; Ingold, S.; Haas, C.; Ballantyne, J. Targeted Multiplexed next Generation RNA Sequencing Assay for Tissue Source Determination of Forensic Samples. *Forensic Sci. Int. Genet. Suppl. Ser.* **2015**, *5*, e441–e443. **[Google Scholar] [CrossRef]**

110. Zubakov, D.; Hanekamp, E.; Kokshoorn, M.; van IJcken, W.; Kayser, M. Stable RNA Markers for Identification of Blood and Saliva Stains Revealed from Whole Genome Expression Analysis of Time-Wise Degraded Samples. *Int. J. Leg. Med.* **2008**, *122*, 135–142. **[Google Scholar] [CrossRef] [Green Version]**

111. Lindenbergh, A.; Maaskant, P.; Sijen, T. Implementation of RNA Profiling in Forensic Casework. *Forensic Sci. Int. Genet.* **2013**, *7*, 159–166. **[Google Scholar] [CrossRef]**

112. Tozzo, P.; Nespeca, P.; Spigarolo, G.; Caenazzo, L. The Importance of Distinguishing Menstrual and Peripheral Blood in Forensic Casework: A Case Report. *Am. J. Forensic Med. Pathol.* **2018**, *39*, 337–340. **[Google Scholar] [CrossRef]**

113. Fabbri, M.; Venturi, M.; Talarico, A.; Inglese, R.; Gaudio, R.M.; Neri, M. mRNA Profiling: Application to an Old Casework. *Forensic Sci. Int. Genet. Suppl. Ser.* **2017**, *6*, e380–e382. **[Google Scholar] [CrossRef] [Green Version]**

114. Fox, A.; Gittos, M.; Harbison, S.A.; Fleming, R.; Wivell, R. Exploring the Recovery and Detection of Messenger RNA and DNA from Enhanced Fingermarks in Blood. *Sci. Justice* **2014**, *54*, 192–198. **[Google Scholar] [CrossRef]**

115. Lux, C.; Schyma, C.; Madea, B.; Courts, C. Identification of Gunshots to the Head by Detection of RNA in Backspatter Primarily Expressed in Brain Tissue. *Forensic Sci. Int.* **2014**, *237*, 62–69. **[Google Scholar] [CrossRef] [PubMed]**

116. Haas, C.; Klesser, B.; Maake, C.; Bär, W.; Kratzer, A. mRNA Profiling for Body Fluid Identification by Reverse Transcription Endpoint PCR and Realtime PCR. *Forensic Sci. Int. Genet.* **2009**, *3*, 80–88. **[Google Scholar] [CrossRef] [PubMed]**

117. Nussbaumer, C.; Gharehbaghi-Schnell, E.; Korschineck, I. Messenger RNA Profiling: A Novel Method for Body Fluid Identification by Real-Time PCR. *Forensic Sci. Int.* **2006**, *157*, 181–186. **[Google Scholar] [CrossRef]**

118. Ingold, S.; Dørum, G.; Hanson, E.; Berti, A.; Branicki, W.; Brito, P.; Elsmore, P.; Gettings, K.B.; Giangasparo, F.; Gross, T.E.; et al. Body Fluid Identification Using a Targeted mRNA Massively Parallel Sequencing Approach—Results of a EUROFORGEN/EDNAP Collaborative Exercise. *Forensic Sci. Int. Genet.* **2018**, *34*, 105–115. **[Google Scholar] [CrossRef] [Green Version]**

119. Hanson, E.; Ingold, S.; Haas, C.; Ballantyne, J. Messenger RNA Biomarker Signatures for Forensic Body Fluid Identification Revealed by Targeted RNA Sequencing. *Forensic Sci. Int. Genet.* **2018**, *34*, 206–221. **[Google Scholar] [CrossRef]**

120. Dørum, G.; Ingold, S.; Hanson, E.; Ballantyne, J.; Snipen, L.; Haas, C. Predicting the Origin of Stains from next Generation Sequencing mRNA Data. *Forensic Sci. Int. Genet.* **2018**, *34*, 37–48. **[Google Scholar] [CrossRef] [PubMed]**

121. Haas, C.; Neubauer, J.; Salzmann, A.P.; Hanson, E.; Ballantyne, J. Forensic Transcriptome Analysis Using Massively Parallel Sequencing. *Forensic Sci. Int. Genet.* **2021**, *52*, 102486. **[Google Scholar] [CrossRef] [PubMed]**

122. Salzman, J.; Gawad, C.; Wang, P.L.; Lacayo, N.; Brown, P.O. Circular RNAs Are the Predominant Transcript Isoform from Hundreds of Human Genes in Diverse Cell Types. *PLoS ONE* **2012**, *7*, e30733. **[Google Scholar] [CrossRef] [Green Version]**

123. Guo, J.U.; Agarwal, V.; Guo, H.; Bartel, D.P. Expanded Identification and Characterization of Mammalian Circular RNAs. *Genome Biol.* **2014**, *15*, 409. **[Google Scholar] [CrossRef]**

124. Salzman, J.; Chen, R.E.; Olsen, M.N.; Wang, P.L.; Brown, P.O. Cell-Type Specific Features of Circular RNA Expression. *PLOS Genet.* **2013**, *9*, e1003777. **[Google Scholar] [CrossRef]**

125. Song, F.; Luo, H.; Xie, M.; Zhu, H.; Hou, Y. Microarray Expression Profile of Circular RNAs in Human Body Fluids. *Forensic Sci. Int. Genet. Suppl. Ser.* **2017**, *6*, e55–e56. **[Google Scholar] [CrossRef] [Green Version]**

126. Zhang, Y.; Liu, B.; Shao, C.; Xu, H.; Xue, A.; Zhao, Z.; Shen, Y.; Tang, Q.; Xie, J. Evaluation of the Inclusion of Circular RNAs in mRNA Profiling in Forensic Body Fluid Identification. *Int. J. Leg. Med.* **2018**, *132*, 43–52. **[Google Scholar] [CrossRef]**

127. Juusola, J.; Ballantyne, J. mRNA Profiling for Body Fluid Identification by Multiplex Quantitative RT-PCR *. *J. Forensic Sci.* **2007**, *52*, 1252–1262. **[Google Scholar] [CrossRef] [PubMed]**

128. Liu, B.; Yang, Q.; Meng, H.; Shao, C.; Jiang, J.; Xu, H.; Sun, K.; Zhou, Y.; Yao, Y.; Zhou, Z.; et al. Development of a Multiplex System for the Identification of Forensically Relevant Body Fluids. *Forensic Sci. Int. Genet.* **2020**, *47*, 102312. **[Google Scholar] [CrossRef]**

129. Baonian, L.; Song, F.; Yang, Q.; Zhou, Y.; Chengchen, S.; Shen, Y.; Zhao, Z.; Tang, Q.; Hou, Y.; Xie, J. Characterization of Tissue-Specific Biomarkers with the Expression of CircRNAs in Forensically Relevant Body Fluids. *Int. J. Leg. Med.* **2019**, *133*, 1321–1331. **[Google Scholar] [CrossRef]**

130. Notomi, T.; Okayama, H.; Masubuchi, H.; Yonekawa, T.; Watanabe, K.; Amino, N.; Hase, T. Loop-Mediated Isothermal Amplification of DNA. *Nucleic Acids Res.* **2000**, *28*, e63. **[Google Scholar] [CrossRef] [PubMed] [Green Version]**

131. Su, C.-W.; Li, C.-Y.; Lee, J.C.-I.; Ji, D.-D.; Li, S.-Y.; Daniel, B.; Syndercombe-Court, D.; Linacre, A.; Hsieh, H.-M. A Novel Application of Real-Time RT-LAMP for Body Fluid Identification: Using HBB Detection as the Model. *Forensic Sci. Med. Pathol.* **2015**, *11*, 208–215. **[Google Scholar] [CrossRef]**

132. Tsai, L.-C.; Su, C.-W.; Lee, J.C.-I.; Lu, Y.-S.; Chen, H.-C.; Lin, Y.-C.; Linacre, A.; Hsieh, H.-M. The Detection and Identification of Saliva in Forensic Samples by RT-LAMP. *Forensic Sci. Med. Pathol.* **2018**, *14*, 469–477. **[Google Scholar] [CrossRef]**

133. Satoh, T.; Kouroki, S.; Ogawa, K.; Tanaka, Y.; Matsumura, K.; Iwase, S. Development of MRNA-Based Body Fluid Identification Using Reverse Transcription Loop-Mediated Isothermal Amplification. *Anal. Bioanal. Chem.* **2018**, *410*, 4371–4378. **[Google Scholar] [CrossRef]**

134. Jackson, K.R.; Layne, T.; Dent, D.A.; Tsuei, A.; Li, J.; Haverstick, D.M.; Landers, J.P. A Novel Loop-Mediated Isothermal Amplification Method for Identification of Four Body Fluids with Smartphone Detection. *Forensic Sci. Int. Genet.* **2020**, *45*, 102195. **[Google Scholar] [CrossRef]**

135. Mehta, B.; Daniel, R.; McNevin, D. HRM and SNaPshot as Alternative Forensic SNP Genotyping Methods. *Forensic Sci. Med. Pathol.* **2017**, *13*, 293–301. **[Google Scholar] [CrossRef] [PubMed]**

136. Rocha, A.D.S.; De Amorim, I.S.S.; Simão, T.D.A.; Fonseca, A.D.S.; Garrido, R.G.; Mencalha, A.L. High-Resolution Melting (HRM) of Hypervariable Mitochondrial DNA Regions for Forensic Science. *J. Forensic Sci.* **2018**, *63*, 536–540. **[Google Scholar] [CrossRef]**

137. Wang, S.; Song, F.; Wang, Y.; Huang, Y.; Xie, B.; Luo, H. High Resolution Melting Analysis (HRM) Based on 16SrRNA as a Tool for Personal Identification with the Human Oral Microbiome. *Forensic Sci. Int. Genet. Suppl. Ser.* **2019**, *7*, 161–163. **[Google Scholar] [CrossRef]**

138. Alghanim, H.; Balamurugan, K.; McCord, B. Development of DNA Methylation Markers for Sperm, Saliva and Blood Identification Using Pyrosequencing and QPCR/HRM. *Anal. Biochem.* **2020**, *611*, 113933. **[Google Scholar] [CrossRef]**

139. Hanson, E.K.; Ballantyne, J. Rapid and Inexpensive Body Fluid Identification by RNA Profiling-Based Multiplex High Resolution Melt (HRM) Analysis. *F1000Research* **2014**, *2*, 281. **[Google Scholar] [CrossRef]**

140. Danaher, P.; White, R.L.; Hanson, E.K.; Ballantyne, J. Facile Semi-Automated Forensic Body Fluid Identification by Multiplex Solution Hybridization of NanoString® Barcode Probes to Specific MRNA Targets. *Forensic Sci. Int. Genet.* **2015**, *14*, 18–30. **[Google Scholar] [CrossRef]**

141. Malkov, V.A.; Serikawa, K.A.; Balantac, N.; Watters, J.; Geiss, G.; Mashadi-Hossein, A.; Fare, T. Multiplexed Measurements of Gene Signatures in Different Analytes Using the NanostringNcounter™ Assay System. *BMC Res. Notes* **2009**, *2*, 80. **[Google Scholar] [CrossRef] [PubMed] [Green Version]**

142. French, D.J.; Archard, C.L.; Brown, T.; McDowell, D.G. HyBeaconTM Probes: A New Tool for DNA Sequence Detection and Allele Discrimination. *Mol. Cell. Probes* **2001**, *15*, 363–374. **[Google Scholar] [CrossRef] [PubMed]**

143. Blackman, S.; Stafford-Allen, B.; Hanson, E.K.; Panasiuk, M.; Brooker, A.-L.; Rendell, P.; Ballantyne, J.; Wells, S. Developmental Validation of the ParaDNA® Body Fluid ID System—A Rapid Multiplex MRNA-Profiling System for the Forensic Identification of Body Fluids. *Forensic Sci. Int. Genet.* **2018**, *37*, 151–161. **[Google Scholar] [CrossRef] [PubMed]**

144. Blackman, S.; Dawnay, N.; Ball, G.; Stafford-Allen, B.; Tribble, N.; Rendell, P.; Neary, K.; Hanson, E.K.; Ballantyne, J.; Kallifatidis, B.; et al. Developmental Validation of the ParaDNA® Intelligence System—A Novel Approach to DNA Profiling. *Forensic Sci. Int. Genet.* **2015**, *17*, 137–148. **[Google Scholar] [CrossRef] [Green Version]**

145. Hong, S.R.; Jung, S.-E.; Lee, E.H.; Shin, K.-J.; Yang, W.I.; Lee, H.Y. DNA Methylation-Based Age Prediction from Saliva: High Age Predictability by Combination of 7 CpG Markers. *Forensic Sci. Int. Genet.* **2017**, *29*, 118–125. **[Google Scholar] [CrossRef] [PubMed]**

146. Vidaki, A.; Kayser, M. Recent Progress, Methods and Perspectives in Forensic Epigenetics. *Forensic Sci. Int. Genet.* **2018**, *37*, 180–195. **[Google Scholar] [CrossRef]**

147. Kader, F.; Ghai, M.; Olaniran, A.O. Characterization of DNA Methylation-Based Markers for Human Body Fluid Identification in Forensics: A Critical Review. *Int. J. Leg. Med.* **2020**, *134*, 1–20. **[Google Scholar] [CrossRef]**

148. Lee, H.Y.; An, J.H.; Jung, S.-E.; Oh, Y.N.; Lee, E.Y.; Choi, A.; Yang, W.I.; Shin, K.-J. Genome-Wide Methylation Profiling and a Multiplex Construction for the Identification of Body Fluids Using Epigenetic Markers. *Forensic Sci. Int. Genet.* **2015**, *17*, 17–24. **[Google Scholar] [CrossRef] [PubMed]**

149. Park, J.-L.; Kwon, O.-H.; Kim, J.H.; Yoo, H.-S.; Lee, H.-C.; Woo, K.-M.; Kim, S.-Y.; Lee, S.-H.; Kim, Y.S. Identification of Body Fluid-Specific DNA Methylation Markers for Use in Forensic Science. *Forensic Sci. Int. Genet.* **2014**, *13*, 147–153. **[Google Scholar] [CrossRef]**

150. Ghai, M.; Naidoo, N.; Evans, D.L.; Kader, F. Identification of Novel Semen and Saliva Specific Methylation Markers and Its Potential Application in Forensic Analysis. *Forensic Sci. Int. Genet.* **2020**, *49*, 102392. **[Google Scholar] [CrossRef]**

151. Antunes, J.; Gauthier, Q.; Aguiar-Pulido, V.; Duncan, G.; McCord, B. A Data-Driven, High-Throughput Methodology to Determine Tissue-Specific Differentially Methylated Regions Able to Discriminate Body Fluids. *Electrophoresis* **2021**, *42*, 1168–1176. **[Google Scholar] [CrossRef]**

152. An, J.H.; Choi, A.; Shin, K.-J.; Yang, W.I.; Lee, H.Y. DNA Methylation-Specific Multiplex Assays for Body Fluid Identification. *Int. J. Leg. Med.* **2013**, *127*, 35–43. **[Google Scholar] [CrossRef]**

153. Choi, A.; Shin, K.-J.; Yang, W.I.; Lee, H.Y. Body Fluid Identification by Integrated Analysis of DNA Methylation and Body Fluid-Specific Microbial DNA. *Int. J. Leg. Med.* **2014**, *128*, 33–41. **[Google Scholar] [CrossRef] [PubMed]**

154. Frumkin, D.; Wasserstrom, A.; Budowle, B.; Davidson, A. DNA Methylation-Based Forensic Tissue Identification. *Forensic Sci. Int. Genet.* **2011**, *5*, 517–524. **[Google Scholar] [CrossRef] [PubMed]**

155. Liu, K.-L.; Tsai, L.-C.; Lin, Y.-C.; Huang, N.-E.; Yang, L.-J.; Su, C.-W.; Lee, J.C.-I.; Linacre, A.; Hsieh, H.-M. Identification of Spermatozoa Using a Novel 3-Plex MSRE-PCR Assay for Forensic Examination of Sexual Assaults. *Int. J. Leg. Med.* **2020**, *134*, 1991–2004. **[Google Scholar] [CrossRef]**

156. Vidaki, A.; Giangasparo, F.; Court, D.S. Discovery of Potential DNA Methylation Markers for Forensic Tissue Identification Using Bisulphite Pyrosequencing. *Electrophoresis* **2016**, *37*, 2767–2779. **[Google Scholar] [CrossRef] [Green Version]**

157. Doi, M.; Nishimukai, H.; Asano, M. Application of Fragment Analysis Based on Methylation Status Mobility Difference to Identify Vaginal Secretions. *Sci. Justice* **2021**, *61*, 384–390. **[Google Scholar] [CrossRef]**

158. Holtkötter, H.; Beyer, V.; Schwender, K.; Glaub, A.; Johann, K.S.; Schürenkamp, M.; Sibbing, U.; Banken, S.; Wiegand, P.; Pfeiffer, H.; et al. Independent Validation of Body Fluid-Specific CpG Markers and Construction of a Robust Multiplex Assay. *Forensic Sci. Int. Genet.* **2017**, *29*, 261–268. **[Google Scholar] [CrossRef] [Green Version]**

159. Newton, C.R.; Graham, A.; Heptinstall, L.E.; Powell, S.J.; Summers, C.; Kalsheker, N.; Smith, J.C.; Markham, A.F. Analysis of Any Point Mutation in DNA. The Amplification Refractory Mutation System (ARMS). *Nucleic Acids Res.* **1989**, *17*, 2503–2516. **[Google Scholar] [CrossRef]**

160. Tian, H.; Bai, P.; Tan, Y.; Li, Z.; Peng, D.; Xiao, X.; Zhao, H.; Zhou, Y.; Liang, W.; Zhang, L. A New Method to Detect Methylation Profiles for Forensic Body Fluid Identification Combining ARMS-PCR Technique and Random Forest Model. *Forensic Sci. Int. Genet.* **2020**, *49*, 102371. **[Google Scholar] [CrossRef] [PubMed]**

161. Hong, S.R.; Shin, K.-J. Bisulfite-Converted DNA Quantity Evaluation: A Multiplex Quantitative Real-Time PCR System for Evaluation of Bisulfite Conversion. *Front. Genet.* **2021**, *12*, 173. **[Google Scholar] [CrossRef]**

162. Schommer, N.N.; Gallo, R.L. Structure and Function of the Human Skin Microbiome. *Trends Microbiol.* **2013**, *21*, 660–668. **[Google Scholar] [CrossRef] [Green Version]**

163. Fleming, R.I.; Harbison, S. The Use of Bacteria for the Identification of Vaginal Secretions. *Forensic Sci. Int. Genet.* **2010**, *4*, 311–315. **[Google Scholar] [CrossRef]**

164. Benschop, C.C.G.; Quaak, F.C.A.; Boon, M.E.; Sijen, T.; Kuiper, I. Vaginal Microbial Flora Analysis by next Generation Sequencing and Microarrays; Can Microbes Indicate Vaginal Origin in a Forensic Context? *Int. J. Leg. Med.* **2012**, *126*, 303–310. **[Google Scholar] [CrossRef]**

165. Ravel, J.; Gajer, P.; Abdo, Z.; Schneider, G.M.; Koenig, S.S.K.; McCulle, S.L.; Karlebach, S.; Gorle, R.; Russell, J.; Tacket, C.O.; et al. Vaginal Microbiome of Reproductive-Age Women. *Proc. Natl. Acad. Sci. USA* **2011**, *108*, 4680–4687. **[Google Scholar] [CrossRef] [Green Version]**

166. Castillo, D.J.; Rifkin, R.F.; Cowan, D.A.; Potgieter, M. The Healthy Human Blood Microbiome: Fact or Fiction? *Front. Cell. Infect. Microbiol.* **2019**, *9*, 148. **[Google Scholar] [CrossRef] [Green Version]**

167. Huse, S.M.; Ye, Y.; Zhou, Y.; Fodor, A.A. A Core Human Microbiome as Viewed through 16S RRNA Sequence Clusters. *PLoS ONE* **2012**, *7*, e34242. **[Google Scholar] [CrossRef] [PubMed] [Green Version]**

168. Quaak, F.C.A.; van Duijn, T.; Hoogenboom, J.; Kloosterman, A.D.; Kuiper, I. Human-Associated Microbial Populations as Evidence in Forensic Casework. *Forensic Sci. Int. Genet.* **2018**, *36*, 176–185. **[Google Scholar] [CrossRef] [PubMed]**

169. Hanssen, E.N.; Avershina, E.; Rudi, K.; Gill, P.; Snipen, L. Body Fluid Prediction from Microbial Patterns for Forensic Application. *Forensic Sci. Int. Genet.* **2017**, *30*, 10–17. **[Google Scholar] [CrossRef]**

170. Human Microbiome Project Consortium. Structure, Function and Diversity of the Healthy Human Microbiome. *Nature* **2012**, *486*, 207–214. **[Google Scholar] [CrossRef] [Green Version]**

171. Ishak, S.; Dormontt, E.; Young, J.M. Microbiomes in Forensic Botany: A Review. *Forensic Sci. Med. Pathol.* **2021**, *17*, 297–307. **[Google Scholar] [CrossRef] [PubMed]**

172. Damaso, N.; Mendel, J.; Mendoza, M.; von Wettberg, E.J.; Narasimhan, G.; Mills, D. Bioinformatics Approach to Assess the Biogeographical Patterns of Soil Communities: The Utility for Soil Provenance. *J. Forensic Sci.* **2018**, *63*, 1033–1042. **[Google Scholar] [CrossRef] [PubMed]**

173. Cho, H.-W.; Eom, Y.-B. Forensic Analysis of Human Microbiome in Skin and Body Fluids Based on Geographic Location. *Front. Cell. Infect. Microbiol.* **2021**, *11*, 695191. **[Google Scholar] [CrossRef] [PubMed]**

174. Badgley, A.J.; Jesmok, E.M.; Foran, D.R. Time Radically Alters Ex Situ Evidentiary Soil 16S Bacterial Profiles Produced Via Next-Generation Sequencing. *J. Forensic Sci.* **2018**, *63*, 1356–1365. **[Google Scholar] [CrossRef] [PubMed]**

175. Signoretto, C.; Bianchi, F.; Burlacchini, G.; Sivieri, F.; Spratt, D.; Canepari, P. Drinking Habits Are Associated with Changes in the Dental Plaque Microbial Community. *J. Clin. Microbiol.* **2010**, *48*, 347–356. **[Google Scholar] [CrossRef] [PubMed] [Green Version]**

176. Rogers, M.A.M.; Aronoff, D.M. The Influence of Non-Steroidal Anti-Inflammatory Drugs on the Gut Microbiome. *Clin. Microbiol. Infect.* **2016**, *22*, 178.e1. **[Google Scholar] [CrossRef] [Green Version]**

177. Kates, A.E.; Jarrett, O.; Skarlupka, J.H.; Sethi, A.; Duster, M.; Watson, L.; Suen, G.; Poulsen, K.; Safdar, N. Household Pet Ownership and the Microbial Diversity of the Human Gut Microbiota. *Front. Cell. Infect. Microbiol.* **2020**, *10*, 73. **[Google Scholar] [CrossRef] [PubMed] [Green Version]**

178. Neckovic, A.; van Oorschot, R.A.H.; Szkuta, B.; Durdle, A. Challenges in Human Skin Microbial Profiling for Forensic Science: A Review. *Genes* **2020**, *11*, 1015. **[Google Scholar] [CrossRef]**

179. Kim, D.; Hofstaedter, C.E.; Zhao, C.; Mattei, L.; Tanes, C.; Clarke, E.; Lauder, A.; Sherrill-Mix, S.; Chehoud, C.; Kelsen, J.; et al. Optimizing Methods and Dodging Pitfalls in Microbiome Research. *Microbiome* **2017**, *5*, 52. **[Google Scholar] [CrossRef]**

180. Salter, S.J.; Cox, M.J.; Turek, E.M.; Calus, S.T.; Cookson, W.O.; Moffatt, M.F.; Turner, P.; Parkhill, J.; Loman, N.J.; Walker, A.W. Reagent and Laboratory Contamination Can Critically Impact Sequence-Based Microbiome Analyses. *BMC Biol.* **2014**, *12*, 87. **[Google Scholar] [CrossRef] [Green Version]**

181. Robinson, J.M.; Pasternak, Z.; Mason, C.E.; Elhaik, E. Forensic Applications of Microbiomics: A Review. *Front. Microbiol.* **2021**, *11*, 3455. **[Google Scholar] [CrossRef]**

182. Schmedes, S.E.; Woerner, A.E.; Novroski, N.M.M.; Wendt, F.R.; King, J.L.; Stephens, K.M.; Budowle, B. Targeted Sequencing of Clade-Specific Markers from Skin Microbiomes for Forensic Human Identification. *Forensic Sci. Int. Genet.* **2018**, *32*, 50–61. **[Google Scholar] [CrossRef]**

183. Woerner, A.E.; Novroski, N.M.M.; Wendt, F.R.; Ambers, A.; Wiley, R.; Schmedes, S.E.; Budowle, B. Forensic Human Identification with Targeted Microbiome Markers Using Nearest Neighbor Classification. *Forensic Sci. Int. Genet.* **2019**, *38*, 130–139. **[Google Scholar] [CrossRef] [PubMed]**

184. Fierer, N.; Lauber, C.L.; Zhou, N.; McDonald, D.; Costello, E.K.; Knight, R. Forensic Identification Using Skin Bacterial Communities. *Proc. Natl. Acad. Sci. USA* **2010**, *107*, 6477–6481. **[Google Scholar] [CrossRef] [Green Version]**

185. Meadow, J.F.; Altrichter, A.E.; Green, J.L. Mobile Phones Carry the Personal Microbiome of Their Owners. *PeerJ* **2014**, *2*, e447. **[Google Scholar] [CrossRef] [PubMed] [Green Version]**

186. Goga, H. Comparison of Bacterial DNA Profiles of Footwear Insoles and Soles of Feet for the Forensic Discrimination of Footwear Owners. *Int. J. Leg. Med.* **2012**, *126*, 815–823. **[Google Scholar] [CrossRef]**

187. Lax, S.; Hampton-Marcell, J.T.; Gibbons, S.M.; Colares, G.B.; Smith, D.; Eisen, J.A.; Gilbert, J.A. Forensic Analysis of the Microbiome of Phones and Shoes. *Microbiome* **2015**, *3*, 21. **[Google Scholar] [CrossRef] [Green Version]**

188. Young, J.M.; Linacre, A. Massively Parallel Sequencing Is Unlocking the Potential of Environmental Trace Evidence. *Forensic Sci. Int. Genet.* **2021**, *50*, 102393. **[Google Scholar] [CrossRef]**

189. Allwood, J.S.; Fierer, N.; Dunn, R.R. The Future of Environmental DNA in Forensic Science. *Appl. Environ. Microbiol.* **2020**, *86*, e01504-19. **[Google Scholar] [CrossRef] [PubMed]**

190. Giampaoli, S.; Berti, A.; Di Maggio, R.M.; Pilli, E.; Valentini, A.; Valeriani, F.; Gianfranceschi, G.; Barni, F.; Ripani, L.; Spica, V.R. The Environmental Biological Signature: NGS Profiling for Forensic Comparison of Soils. *Forensic Sci. Int.* **2014**, *240*, 41–47. **[Google Scholar] [CrossRef]**

191. Costello, E.K.; Lauber, C.L.; Hamady, M.; Fierer, N.; Gordon, J.I.; Knight, R. Bacterial Community Variation in Human Body Habitats across Space and Time. *Science* **2009**, *326*, 1694–1697. **[Google Scholar] [CrossRef] [Green Version]**

192. Leake, S.L.; Pagni, M.; Falquet, L.; Taroni, F.; Greub, G. The Salivary Microbiome for Differentiating Individuals: Proof of Principle. *Microbes Infect.* **2016**, *18*, 399–405. **[Google Scholar] [CrossRef] [Green Version]**

193. Jung, J.Y.; Yoon, H.K.; An, S.; Lee, J.W.; Ahn, E.-R.; Kim, Y.-J.; Park, H.-C.; Lee, K.; Hwang, J.H.; Lim, S.-K. Rapid Oral Bacteria Detection Based on Real-Time PCR for the Forensic Identification of Saliva. *Sci. Rep.* **2018**, *8*, 10852. **[Google Scholar] [CrossRef]**

194. Quaak, F.C.A.; de Graaf, M.-L.M.; Weterings, R.; Kuiper, I. Microbial Population Analysis Improves the Evidential Value of Faecal Traces in Forensic Investigations. *Int. J. Leg. Med.* **2017**, *131*, 45–51. **[Google Scholar] [CrossRef]**

195. Akutsu, T.; Motani, H.; Watanabe, K.; Iwase, H.; Sakurada, K. Detection of Bacterial 16S Ribosomal RNA Genes for Forensic Identification of Vaginal Fluid. *Leg. Med.* **2012**, *14*, 160–162. **[Google Scholar] [CrossRef] [PubMed]**

196. Díez López, C.; Montiel González, D.; Haas, C.; Vidaki, A.; Kayser, M. Microbiome-Based Body Site of Origin Classification of Forensically Relevant Blood Traces. *Forensic Sci. Int. Genet.* **2020**, *47*, 102280. **[Google Scholar] [CrossRef]**

197. López, C.D.; Vidaki, A.; Ralf, A.; González, D.M.; Radjabzadeh, D.; Kraaij, R.; Uitterlinden, A.G.; Haas, C.; Lao, O.; Kayser, M. Novel Taxonomy-Independent Deep Learning Microbiome Approach Allows for Accurate Classification of Different Forensically Relevant Human Epithelial Materials. *Forensic Sci. Int. Genet.* **2019**, *41*, 72–82. **[Google Scholar] [CrossRef] [PubMed]**

198. Yao, T.; Han, X.; Guan, T.; Wang, Z.; Zhang, S.; Liu, C.; Liu, C.; Chen, L. Effect of Indoor Environmental Exposure on Seminal Microbiota and Its Application in Body Fluid Identification. *Forensic Sci. Int.* **2020**, *314*, 110417. **[Google Scholar] [CrossRef]**

199. Haas, C.; Hanson, E.; Anjos, M.J.; Ballantyne, K.N.; Banemann, R.; Bhoelai, B.; Borges, E.; Carvalho, M.; Courts, C.; De Cock, G.; et al. RNA/DNA Co-Analysis from Human Menstrual Blood and Vaginal Secretion Stains: Results of a Fourth and Fifth Collaborative EDNAP Exercise. *Forensic Sci. Int. Genet.* **2014**, *8*, 203–212. **[Google Scholar] [CrossRef] [Green Version]**

200. Dobay, A.; Haas, C.; Fucile, G.; Downey, N.; Morrison, H.G.; Kratzer, A.; Arora, N. Microbiome-Based Body Fluid Identification of Samples Exposed to Indoor Conditions. *Forensic Sci. Int. Genet.* **2019**, *40*, 105–113. **[Google Scholar] [CrossRef] [PubMed]**

201. Donaldson, A.E.; Taylor, M.C.; Cordiner, S.J.; Lamont, I.L. Using Oral Microbial DNA Analysis to Identify ExpiratedBloodspatter. *Int. J. Leg. Med.* **2010**, *124*, 569–576. **[Google Scholar] [CrossRef]**

202. Giampaoli, S.; Berti, A.; Valeriani, F.; Gianfranceschi, G.; Piccolella, A.; Buggiotti, L.; Rapone, C.; Valentini, A.; Ripani, L.; Spica, V.R. Molecular Identification of Vaginal Fluid by Microbial Signature. *Forensic Sci. Int. Genet.* **2012**, *6*, 559–564. **[Google Scholar] [CrossRef]**

203. Ranjan, R.; Rani, A.; Metwally, A.; McGee, H.S.; Perkins, D.L. Analysis of the Microbiome: Advantages of Whole Genome Shotgun versus 16S Amplicon Sequencing. *Biochem. Biophys. Res. Commun.* **2016**, *469*, 967–977. **[Google Scholar] [CrossRef] [PubMed] [Green Version]**

204. Holtkötter, H.; Dierig, L.; Schürenkamp, M.; Sibbing, U.; Pfeiffer, H.; Vennemann, M. Validation of an Immunochromatographic D-Dimer Test to Presumptively Identify Menstrual Fluid in Forensic Exhibits. *Int. J. Leg. Med.* **2015**, *129*, 37–41. **[Google Scholar] [CrossRef]**

205. Holtkötter, H.; Filho, C.R.D.; Schwender, K.; Stadler, C.; Vennemann, M.; Pacheco, A.C.; Roca, G. Forensic Differentiation between Peripheral and Menstrual Blood in Cases of Alleged Sexual Assault—Validating an Immunochromatographic Multiplex Assay for Simultaneous Detection of Human Hemoglobin and D-Dimer. *Int. J. Leg. Med.* **2018**, *132*, 683–690. **[Google Scholar] [CrossRef] [PubMed]**

206. Giampaoli, S.; Alessandrini, F.; Berti, A.; Ripani, L.; Choi, A.; Crab, R.; De Vittori, E.; Egyed, B.; Haas, C.; Lee, H.Y.; et al. Forensic Interlaboratory Evaluation of the ForFLUID Kit for Vaginal Fluids Identification. *J. Forensic Leg. Med.* **2014**, *21*, 60–63. **[Google Scholar] [CrossRef] [PubMed]**

207. Hausmann, R.; Pregler, C.; Schellmann, B. The Value of the Lugol's Iodine Staining Technique for the Identification of Vaginal Epithelial Cells. *Int. J. Leg. Med.* **1994**, *106*, 298–301. **[Google Scholar] [CrossRef]**

208. Nichols, C.A.; Sens, M.A. Recovery and Evaluation by Cytologic Techniques of Trace Material Retained on Bullets. *Am. J. Forensic Med. Pathol.* **1990**, *11*, 17–34. **[Google Scholar] [CrossRef] [PubMed]**

209. Uitspraken. Available online: **https://www.rechtspraak.nl/Uitspraken/Paginas/default.aspx** (accessed on 12 September 2021).

210. Lin, Y.-C.; Tsai, L.-C.; Lee, J.C.-I.; Liu, K.-L.; Tzen, J.T.-C.; Linacre, A.; Hsieh, H.-M. Novel Identification of Biofluids Using a Multiplex Methylation-Specific PCR Combined with Single-Base Extension System. *Forensic Sci. Med. Pathol.* **2016**, *12*, 128–138. **[Google Scholar] [CrossRef]**

211. Wasserstrom, A.; Frumkin, D.; Davidson, A.; Shpitzen, M.; Herman, Y.; Gafny, R. Demonstration of DSI-Semen—A Novel DNA Methylation-Based Forensic Semen Identification Assay. *Forensic Sci. Int. Genet.* **2013**, *7*, 136–142. **[Google Scholar] [CrossRef]**

212. Iwasaki, M.; Kubo, S.-I.; Ogata, M.; Nakasono, I. A Demonstration of Spermatozoa on Vaginal Swabs after Complete Destruction of the Vaginal Cell Deposits. *J. Forensic Sci.* **1989**, *34*, 659–664. **[Google Scholar] [CrossRef]**

213. Bamberg, M.; Dierig, L.; Kulstein, G.; Kunz, S.N.; Schmidt, M.; Hadrys, T.; Wiegand, P. Development and Validation of an MRNA-Based Multiplex Body Fluid Identification Workflow and a Rectal Mucosa Marker Pilot Study. *Forensic Sci. Int. Genet.* **2021**, *54*, 102542. **[Google Scholar] [CrossRef] [PubMed]**

214. Zubakov, D.; Kokshoorn, M.; Kloosterman, A.; Kayser, M. New Markers for Old Stains: Stable MRNA Markers for Blood and Saliva Identification from up to 16-Year-Old Stains. *Int. J. Leg. Med.* **2009**, *123*, 71–74. **[Google Scholar] [CrossRef] [PubMed] [Green Version]**

215. Chirnside, O.; Lemalu, A.; Fleming, R. Identification of Nasal Mucosa Markers for Forensic MRNA Body Fluid Determination. *Forensic Sci. Int. Genet.* **2020**, *48*, 102317. **[Google Scholar] [CrossRef]**

216. Xu, Y.; Xie, J.; Cao, Y.; Zhou, H.; Ping, Y.; Chen, L.; Gu, L.; Hu, W.; Bi, G.; Ge, J.; et al. Development of Highly Sensitive and Specific MRNA Multiplex System (XCYR1) for Forensic Human Body Fluids and Tissues Identification. *PLoS ONE* **2014**, *9*, e100123. **[Google Scholar] [CrossRef] [PubMed]**

217. Sakurada, K.; Akutsu, T.; Fukushima, H.; Watanabe, K.; Yoshino, M. Detection of Dermcidin for Sweat Identification by Real-Time RT-PCR and ELISA. *Forensic Sci. Int.* **2010**, *194*, 80–84. **[Google Scholar] [CrossRef]**

218. Layne, T.R.; Green, R.A.; Lewis, C.A.; Nogales, F.; Cruz, T.C.D.; Zehner, Z.E.; Seashols-Williams, S.J. MicroRNA Detection in Blood, Urine, Semen, and Saliva Stains After Compromising Treatments. *J. Forensic Sci.* **2019**, *64*, 1831–1837. **[Google Scholar] [CrossRef]**

219. Visser, M.; Zubakov, D.; Ballantyne, K.N.; Kayser, M. MRNA-Based Skin Identification for Forensic Applications. *Int. J. Leg. Med.* **2011**, *125*, 253–263. **[Google Scholar] [CrossRef] [Green Version]**

220. Hanson, E.; Haas, C.; Jucker, R.; Ballantyne, J. Identification of Skin in Touch/Contact Forensic Samples by Messenger RNA Profiling. *Forensic Sci. Int. Genet. Suppl. Ser.* **2011**, *3*, e305–e306. **[Google Scholar] [CrossRef]**

221. Haas, C.; Hanson, E.; Banemann, R.; Bento, A.M.; Berti, A.; Carracedo, Á.; Courts, C.; Cock, G.D.; Drobnic, K.; Fleming, R.; et al. RNA/DNA Co-Analysis from Human Skin and Contact Traces—Results of a Sixth Collaborative EDNAP Exercise. *Forensic Sci. Int. Genet.* **2015**, *16*, 139–147. **[Google Scholar] [CrossRef]**

222. van den Berge, M.; Carracedo, A.; Gomes, I.; Graham, E.A.M.; Haas, C.; Hjort, B.; Hoff-Olsen, P.; Maroñas, O.; Mevåg, B.; Morling, N.; et al. A Collaborative European Exercise on MRNA-Based Body Fluid/Skin Typing and Interpretation of DNA and RNA Results. *Forensic Sci. Int. Genet.* **2014**, *10*, 40–48. **[Google Scholar] [CrossRef] [Green Version]**

223. Lindenbergh, A.; van den Berge, M.; Oostra, R.-J.; Cleypool, C.; Bruggink, A.; Kloosterman, A.; Sijen, T. Development of a MRNA Profiling Multiplex for the Inference of Organ Tissues. *Int. J. Leg. Med.* **2013**, *127*, 891–900. **[Google Scholar] [CrossRef]**

224. Hanson, E.; Ballantyne, J. Human Organ Tissue Identification by Targeted RNA Deep Sequencing to Aid the Investigation of Traumatic Injury. *Genes* **2017**, *8*, 319. **[Google Scholar] [CrossRef] [Green Version]**

225. Euteneuer, J.; Courts, C. Ten Years of Molecular Ballistics—a Review and a Field Guide. *Int. J. Leg. Med.* **2021**, *135*, 1121–1136. **[Google Scholar] [CrossRef]**

226. Alberts, B.; Johnson, A.; Lewis, J.; Raff, M.; Roberts, K.; Walter, P. *Molecular Biology of the Cell*, 4th ed.; Garland Science: New York, NY, USA, 2002; ISBN 978-0-8153-3218-3. **[Google Scholar]**

227. Mathiesen, C.; Thomsen, K.; Lauritzen, M. Integrated Measurements of Electrical Activity, Oxygen Tension, Blood Flow, and Ca2+-Signaling in Rodents In Vivo. In *Brain Energy Metabolism. Neuromethods*; Hirrlinger, J., Waagepetersen, H., Eds.; Humana Press: New York, NY, USA, 2014; Volume 90. **[Google Scholar] [CrossRef]**

228. Jackson, D.G. Leucocyte Trafficking via the Lymphatic Vasculature—Mechanisms and Consequences. *Front. Immunol.* **2019**, *10*, 471. **[Google Scholar] [CrossRef]**

229. Slagter, M.; Kruise, D.; van Ommen, L.; Hoogenboom, J.; Steensma, K.; de Jong, J.; Hovers, P.; Parag, R.; van der Linden, J.; Kneppers, A.L.J.; et al. The DNAxs Software Suite: A Three-Year Retrospective Study on the Development, Architecture, Testing and Implementation in Forensic Casework. *Forensic Sci. Int. Rep.* **2021**, *3*, 100212. **[Google Scholar] [CrossRef]**

230. McNevin, D.; Wright, K.; Barash, M.; Gomes, S.; Jamieson, A.; Chaseling, J. Proposed Framework for Comparison of Continuous Probabilistic Genotyping Systems amongst Different Laboratories. *Forensic Sci.* **2021**, *1*, 33–45. **[Google Scholar] [CrossRef]**

231. Bleka, Ø.; Storvik, G.; Gill, P. EuroForMix: An Open Source Software Based on a Continuous Model to Evaluate STR DNA Profiles from a Mixture of Contributors with Artefacts. *Forensic Sci. Int. Genet.* **2016**, *21*, 35–44. **[Google Scholar] [CrossRef] [Green Version]**

232. Bright, J.-A.; Cheng, K.; Kerr, Z.; McGovern, C.; Kelly, H.; Moretti, T.R.; Smith, M.A.; Bieber, F.R.; Budowle, B.; Coble, M.D.; et al. STRmix™ Collaborative Exercise on DNA Mixture Interpretation. *Forensic Sci. Int. Genet.* **2019**, *40*, 1–8. **[Google Scholar] [CrossRef] [PubMed]**

233. Coble, M.D.; Bright, J.-A. Probabilistic Genotyping Software: An Overview. *Forensic Sci. Int. Genet.* **2019**, *38*, 219–224. **[Google Scholar] [CrossRef]**

234. van den Berge, M.; Sijen, T. Extended Specificity Studies of MRNA Assays Used to Infer Human Organ Tissues and Body Fluids. *Electrophoresis* **2017**, *38*, 3155–3160. **[Google Scholar] [CrossRef] [PubMed]**

235. Lin, M.-H.; Albani, P.P.; Fleming, R. Degraded RNA Transcript Stable Regions (StaRs) as Targets for Enhanced Forensic RNA Body Fluid Identification. *Forensic Sci. Int. Genet.* **2016**, *20*, 61–70. **[Google Scholar] [CrossRef] [PubMed]**

236. Sasaki, A.; Kim, B.; Murphy, K.E.; Matthews, S.G. Impact of Ex Vivo Sample Handling on DNA Methylation Profiles in Human Cord Blood and Neonatal Dried Blood Spots. *Front. Genet.* **2020**, *11*, 224. **[Google Scholar] [CrossRef]**

237. Lin, Y.-C.; Tsai, L.-C.; Lee, J.C.-I.; Su, C.-W.; Tzen, J.T.-C.; Linacre, A.; Hsieh, H.-M. Novel Identification of Biofluids Using a Multiplex Methylation Sensitive Restriction Enzyme-PCR System. *Forensic Sci. Int. Genet.* **2016**, *25*, 157–165. **[Google Scholar] [CrossRef] [PubMed]**

238. Roeder, A.D.; Haas, C. MRNA Profiling Using a Minimum of Five MRNA Markers per Body Fluid and a Novel Scoring Method for Body Fluid Identification. *Int. J. Leg. Med.* **2013**, *127*, 707–721. **[Google Scholar] [CrossRef] [PubMed]**

239. Iacob, D.; Fürst, A.; Hadrys, T. A Machine Learning Model to Predict the Origin of Forensically Relevant Body Fluids. *Forensic Sci. Int. Genet. Suppl. Ser.* **2019**, *7*, 392–394. **[Google Scholar] [CrossRef]**

240. de Zoete, J.; Curran, J.; Sjerps, M. A Probabilistic Approach for the Interpretation of RNA Profiles as Cell Type Evidence. *Forensic Sci. Int. Genet.* **2016**, *20*, 30–44. **[Google Scholar] [CrossRef] [PubMed]**

241. Ypma, R.J.F.; Wijk, P.A.M.; Gill, R.; Sjerps, M.; van den Berge, M. Calculating LRs for Presence of Body Fluids from MRNA Assay Data in Mixtures. *Forensic Sci. Int. Genet.* **2021**, *52*, 102455. **[Google Scholar] [CrossRef]**

242. Hanson, E.; Ingold, S.; Dorum, G.; Haas, C.; Lagace, R.; Ballantyne, J. Assigning Forensic Body Fluids to DNA Donors in Mixed Samples by Targeted RNA/DNA Deep Seqeuncing of Coding Region SNPs Using Ion Torrent Technology. *Forensic Sci. Int. Genet. Suppl. Ser.* **2019**, *7*, 23–24. **[Google Scholar] [CrossRef]**

243. Gill, P. Misleading DNA Evidence: Reasons for Miscarriages of Justice. *Int. Comment. Evid.* **2012**, *10*, 55–71. **[Google Scholar] [CrossRef]**

244. Wang, S.; Wang, Z.; Tao, R.; Song, F.; Hou, Y. Validating the Consistency of CSNPs Analysis Results between DNA and RNA Using SNaPshot Method. *Forensic Sci. Int. Genet. Suppl. Ser.* **2019**, *7*, 76–78. **[Google Scholar] [CrossRef]**

245. Ingold, S.; Dørum, G.; Hanson, E.; Ballantyne, J.; Haas, C. Assigning Forensic Body Fluids to Donors in Mixed Body Fluids by Targeted RNA/DNA Deep Sequencing of Coding Region SNPs. *Int. J. Leg. Med.* **2020**, *134*, 473–485. **[Google Scholar] [CrossRef] [PubMed]**

246. Ingold, S.; Haas, C.; Dørum, G.; Hanson, E.; Ballantyne, J. Association of a Body Fluid with a DNA Profile by Targeted RNA/DNA Deep Sequencing. *Forensic Sci. Int. Genet. Suppl. Ser.* **2017**, *6*, e112–e113. **[Google Scholar] [CrossRef] [Green Version]**

247. Li, Z.; Li, J.; Li, Y.; Liu, N.; Liu, F.; Ren, J.; Yun, K.; Yan, J.; Zhang, G. Development of a Multiplex Methylation-Sensitive Restriction Enzyme-Based SNP Typing System for Deconvolution of Semen-Containing Mixtures. *Int. J. Leg. Med.* **2021**, *135*, 1281–1294. **[Google Scholar] [CrossRef] [PubMed]**

248. Watanabe, K.; Taniguchi, K.; Akutsu, T. Development of a DNA Methylation-Based Semen-Specific SNP Typing Method: A New Approach for Genotyping from a Mixture of Body Fluids. *Forensic Sci. Int. Genet.* **2018**, *37*, 227–234. **[Google Scholar] [CrossRef]**

249. Fujimoto, S.; Hamano, Y.; Ichioka, K.; Manabe, S.; Hirai, E.; Ogawa, O.; Tamaki, K. Rapid Semen Identification from Mixed Body Fluids Using Methylation-Sensitive High-Resolution Melting Analysis of the DACT1 Gene. *Leg. Med.* **2021**, *48*, 101806. **[Google Scholar] [CrossRef]**

250. Rocchi, A.; Chiti, E.; Maiese, A.; Turillazzi, E.; Spinetti, I. MicroRNAs: An Update of Applications in Forensic Science. *Diagnostics* **2021**, *11*, 32. **[Google Scholar] [CrossRef]**

251. Sun, K.; Lai, E.C. Adult-Specific Functions of Animal MicroRNAs. *Nat. Rev. Genet.* **2013**, *14*, 535–548. **[Google Scholar] [CrossRef]**

252. Wienholds, E.; Kloosterman, W.P.; Miska, E.; Alvarez-Saavedra, E.; Berezikov, E.; de Bruijn, E.; Horvitz, H.R.; Kauppinen, S.; Plasterk, R.H.A. MicroRNA Expression in Zebrafish Embryonic Development. *Science* **2005**, *309*, 310–311. **[Google Scholar] [CrossRef] [Green Version]**

253. Omelia, E.J.; Uchimoto, M.L.; Williams, G. Quantitative PCR Analysis of Blood- and Saliva-Specific MicroRNA Markers Following Solid-Phase DNA Extraction. *Anal. Biochem.* **2013**, *435*, 120–122. **[Google Scholar] [CrossRef] [Green Version]**

254. Hanson, E.K.; Lubenow, H.; Ballantyne, J. Identification of Forensically Relevant Body Fluids Using a Panel of Differentially Expressed MicroRNAs. *Anal. Biochem.* **2009**, *387*, 303–314. **[Google Scholar] [CrossRef]**

255. Zubakov, D.; Boersma, A.W.M.; Choi, Y.; van Kuijk, P.F.; Wiemer, E.A.C.; Kayser, M. MicroRNA Markers for Forensic Body Fluid Identification Obtained from Microarray Screening and Quantitative RT-PCR Confirmation. *Int. J. Leg. Med.* **2010**, *124*, 217–226. **[Google Scholar] [CrossRef] [PubMed] [Green Version]**

256. Park, J.-L.; Park, S.-M.; Kwon, O.-H.; Lee, H.; Kim, J.; Seok, H.H.; Lee, W.S.; Lee, S.-H.; Kim, Y.S.; Woo, K.-M.; et al. Microarray Screening and QRT-PCR Evaluation of MicroRNA Markers for Forensic Body Fluid Identification. *Electrophoresis* **2014**, *35*, 3062–3068. **[Google Scholar] [CrossRef]**

257. Li, Z.; Bai, P.; Peng, D.; Wang, H.; Guo, Y.; Jiang, Y.; He, W.; Tian, H.; Yang, Y.; Huang, Y.; et al. Screening and Confirmation of MicroRNA Markers for Distinguishing between Menstrual and Peripheral Blood. *Forensic Sci. Int. Genet.* **2017**, *30*, 24–33. **[Google Scholar] [CrossRef]**

258. Sauer, E.; Extra, A.; Cachée, P.; Courts, C. Identification of Organ Tissue Types and Skin from Forensic Samples by MicroRNA Expression Analysis. *Forensic Sci. Int. Genet.* **2017**, *28*, 99–110. **[Google Scholar] [CrossRef] [PubMed]**

259. Liu, Y.; He, H.; Xiao, Z.-X.; Ji, A.; Ye, J.; Sun, Q.; Cao, Y. A Systematic Analysis of miRNA Markers and Classification Algorithms for Forensic Body Fluid Identification. *Brief. Bioinform.* **2021**, *22*. **[Google Scholar] [CrossRef]**

260. Zhao, C.; Zhao, M.; Zhu, Y.; Zhang, L.; Zheng, Z.; Wang, Q.; Li, Y.; Zhang, P.; Zhu, S.; Ding, S.; et al. The Persistence and Stability of miRNA in Bloodstained Samples under Different Environmental Conditions. *Forensic Sci. Int.* **2021**, *318*, 110594. **[Google Scholar] [CrossRef] [PubMed]**

261. Mayes, C.; Houston, R.; Seashols-Williams, S.; LaRue, B.; Hughes-Stamm, S. The Stability and Persistence of Blood and Semen MRNA and miRNA Targets for Body Fluid Identification in Environmentally Challenged and Laundered Samples. *Leg. Med.* **2019**, *38*, 45–50. **[Google Scholar] [CrossRef] [Green Version]**

262. Sirker, M.; Fimmers, R.; Schneider, P.M.; Gomes, I. Evaluating the Forensic Application of 19 Target MicroRNAs as Biomarkers in Body Fluid and Tissue Identification. *Forensic Sci. Int. Genet.* **2017**, *27*, 41–49. **[Google Scholar] [CrossRef]**

263. Van der Meer, D.; Uchimoto, M.L.; Williams, G. Simultaneous Analysis of Micro-RNA and DNA for Determining the Body Fluid Origin of DNA Profiles. *J. Forensic Sci.* **2013**, *58*, 967–971. **[Google Scholar] [CrossRef] [PubMed]**

264. Mayes, C.; Seashols-Williams, S.; Hughes-Stamm, S. A Capillary Electrophoresis Method for Identifying Forensically Relevant Body Fluids Using miRNAs. *Leg. Med.* **2018**, *30*, 1–4. **[Google Scholar] [CrossRef] [PubMed]**

265. Seashols-Williams, S.; Lewis, C.; Calloway, C.; Peace, N.; Harrison, A.; Hayes-Nash, C.; Fleming, S.; Wu, Q.; Zehner, Z.E. High-Throughput miRNA Sequencing and Identification of Biomarkers for Forensically Relevant Biological Fluids. *Electrophoresis* **2016**, *37*, 2780–2788. **[Google Scholar] [CrossRef]**

266. Parhad, S.S.; Theurkauf, W.E. Rapid Evolution and Conserved Function of the PiRNA Pathway. *Open Biol.* **2019**, *9*, 180181. **[Google Scholar] [CrossRef] [PubMed] [Green Version]**

267. Wang, S.; Wang, Z.; Tao, R.; He, G.; Liu, J.; Li, C.; Hou, Y. The Potential Use of Piwi-Interacting RNA Biomarkers in Forensic Body Fluid Identification: A Proof-of-Principle Study. *Forensic Sci. Int. Genet.* **2019**, *39*, 129–135. **[Google Scholar] [CrossRef]**

268. Wang, S.; Wang, Z.; Tao, R.; Wang, M.; Liu, J.; He, G.; Yang, Y.; Xie, M.; Zou, X.; Hou, Y. Expression Profile Analysis of Piwi-Interacting RNA in Forensically Relevant Biological Fluids. *Forensic Sci. Int. Genet.* **2019**, *42*, 171–180. **[Google Scholar] [CrossRef]**

269. Dana, H.; Chalbatani, G.M.; Mahmoodzadeh, H.; Karimloo, R.; Rezaiean, O.; Moradzadeh, A.; Mehmandoost, N.; Moazzen, F.; Mazraeh, A.; Marmari, V.; et al. Molecular Mechanisms and Biological Functions of SiRNA. *Int. J. Biomed. Sci. IJBS* **2017**, *13*, 48–57. **[Google Scholar]**

270. Staedtler, F.; Hartmann, N.; Letzkus, M.; Bongiovanni, S.; Scherer, A.; Marc, P.; Johnson, K.J.; Schumacher, M.M. Robust and Tissue-Independent Gender-Specific Transcript Biomarkers. *Biomarkers* **2013**, *18*, 436–445. **[Google Scholar] [CrossRef] [PubMed]**

271. Ng, K.; Pullirsch, D.; Leeb, M.; Wutz, A. *Xist* and the Order of Silencing. *EMBO Rep.* **2007**, *8*, 34–39. **[Google Scholar] [CrossRef] [PubMed] [Green Version]**

272. Van den Berge, M.; Sijen, T. A Male and Female RNA Marker to Infer Sex in Forensic Analysis. *Forensic Sci. Int. Genet.* **2017**, *26*, 70–76. **[Google Scholar] [CrossRef]**

273. Hassan, F.M.; Razik, H.A.A.; Wadie, M.S.; Abdelfattah, D.S. XIST and RPS4Y1 Long Non-Coding RNA Transcriptome as Sex Biomarkers in Different Body Fluids. *Egypt. J. Forensic Sci.* **2019**, *9*, 16. **[Google Scholar] [CrossRef]**

274. Merkley, E.D.; Wunschel, D.S.; Wahl, K.L.; Jarman, K.H. Applications and Challenges of Forensic Proteomics. *Forensic Sci. Int.* **2019**, *297*, 350–363. **[Google Scholar] [CrossRef]**

275. Merkley, E.D. *Applications in Forensic Proteomics: Protein Identification and Profiling*; ACS Symposium Series; American Chemical Society: Washington, DC, USA, 2020. **[Google Scholar]**

276. Parker, G.J.; McKiernan, H.E.; Legg, K.M.; Goecker, Z.C. Forensic Proteomics. *Forensic Sci. Int. Genet.* **2021**, *54*, 102529. **[Google Scholar] [CrossRef]**

277. Yang, H.; Zhou, B.; Deng, H.; Prinz, M.; Siegel, D. Body Fluid Identification by Mass Spectrometry. *Int. J. Leg. Med.* **2013**, *127*, 1065–1077. **[Google Scholar] [CrossRef] [PubMed]**

278. Legg, K.M.; Powell, R.; Reisdorph, N.; Reisdorph, R.; Danielson, P.B. Discovery of Highly Specific Protein Markers for the Identification of Biological Stains. *Electrophoresis* **2014**, *35*, 3069–3078. **[Google Scholar] [CrossRef] [PubMed]**

279. Legg, K.M.; Powell, R.; Reisdorph, N.; Reisdorph, R.; Danielson, P.B. Verification of Protein Biomarker Specificity for the Identification of Biological Stains by Quadrupole Time-of-Flight Mass Spectrometry. *Electrophoresis* **2017**, *38*, 833–845. **[Google Scholar] [CrossRef]**

280. McKiernan, H.E.; Danielson, P.B.; Brown, C.O.; Signaevsky, M.; Westring, C.G.; Legg, K.M. Developmental Validation of a Multiplex Proteomic Assay for the Identification of Forensically Relevant Biological Fluids. *Forensic Sci. Int.* **2021**, *326*, 110908. **[Google Scholar] [CrossRef]**

281. Bradshaw, R.; Bleay, S.; Clench, M.R.; Francese, S. Direct Detection of Blood in Fingermarks by MALDI MS Profiling and Imaging. *Sci. Justice* **2014**, *54*, 110–117. **[Google Scholar] [CrossRef]**

282. Kamanna, S.; Henry, J.; Voelcker, N.H.; Linacre, A.; Kirkbride, K.P. Direct Identification of Forensic Body Fluids Using Matrix-Assisted Laser Desorption/Ionization Time-of-Flight Mass Spectrometry. *Int. J. Mass Spectrom.* **2016**, *397–398*, 18–26. **[Google Scholar] [CrossRef]**

283. Rankin-Turner, S.; Ninomiya, S.; Reynolds, J.C.; Hiraoka, K. Sheath-Flow Probe Electrospray Ionization (SfPESI) Mass Spectrometry for the Rapid Forensic Analysis of Human Body Fluids. *Anal. Methods* **2019**, *11*, 3633–3640. **[Google Scholar] [CrossRef] [Green Version]**

284. Parker, G.J.; Leppert, T.; Anex, D.S.; Hilmer, J.K.; Matsunami, N.; Baird, L.; Stevens, J.; Parsawar, K.; Durbin-Johnson, B.P.; Rocke, D.M.; et al. Demonstration of Protein-Based Human Identification Using the Hair Shaft Proteome. *PLoS ONE* **2016**, *11*, e0160653. **[Google Scholar] [CrossRef]**

285. Goecker, Z.C.; Salemi, M.R.; Karim, N.; Phinney, B.S.; Rice, R.H.; Parker, G.J. Optimal Processing for Proteomic Genotyping of Single Human Hairs. *Forensic Sci. Int. Genet.* **2020**, *47*, 102314. **[Google Scholar] [CrossRef] [PubMed]**

286. Chu, F.; Mason, K.E.; Anex, D.S.; Jones, A.D.; Hart, B.R. Hair Proteome Variation at Different Body Locations on Genetically Variant Peptide Detection for Protein-Based Human Identification. *Sci. Rep.* **2019**, *9*, 7641. **[Google Scholar] [CrossRef]**

287. Tuerk, C.; Gold, L. Systematic Evolution of Ligands by Exponential Enrichment: RNA Ligands to Bacteriophage T4 DNA Polymerase. *Science* **1990**, *249*, 505–510. **[Google Scholar] [CrossRef] [PubMed]**

288. Ellington, A.D.; Szostak, J.W. In Vitro Selection of RNA Molecules That Bind Specific Ligands. *Nature* **1990**, *346*, 818–822. **[Google Scholar] [CrossRef]**

289. Bock, L.C.; Griffin, L.C.; Latham, J.A.; Vermaas, E.H.; Toole, J.J. Selection of Single-Stranded DNA Molecules That Bind and Inhibit Human Thrombin. *Nature* **1992**, *355*, 564–566. **[Google Scholar] [CrossRef] [PubMed]**

290. Rangel, A.E.; Chen, Z.; Ayele, T.M.; Heemstra, J.M. In Vitro Selection of an XNA Aptamer Capable of Small-Molecule Recognition. *Nucleic Acids Res.* **2018**, *46*, 8057–8068. **[Google Scholar] [CrossRef] [PubMed]**

291. Bunka, D.H.J.; Stockley, P.G. Aptamers Come of Age—At Last. *Nat. Rev. Microbiol.* **2006**, *4*, 588–596. **[Google Scholar] [CrossRef]**

292. Song, S.; Wang, L.; Li, J.; Fan, C.; Zhao, J. Aptamer-Based Biosensors. *TrAC Trends Anal. Chem.* **2008**, *27*, 108–117. **[Google Scholar] [CrossRef]**

293. Chen, Z.; Wu, Q.; Chen, J.; Ni, X.; Dai, J. A DNA Aptamer Based Method for Detection of SARS-CoV-2 Nucleocapsid Protein. *Virol. Sin.* **2020**, *35*, 351–354. **[Google Scholar] [CrossRef]**

294. Abrego-Martinez, J.C.; Jafari, M.; Chergui, S.; Pavel, C.; Che, D.; Siaj, M. Aptamer-Based Electrochemical Biosensor for Rapid Detection of SARS-CoV-2: Nanoscale Electrode-Aptamer-SARS-CoV-2 Imaging by Photo-Induced Force Microscopy. *Biosens. Bioelectron.* **2022**, *195*, 113595. **[Google Scholar] [CrossRef]**

295. Gooch, J.; Tungsirisurp, S.; Costanzo, H.; Napier, R.; Frascione, N. Generating Aptamers towards Human Sperm Cells Using Massively Parallel Sequencing. *Anal. Bioanal. Chem.* **2021**, *413*, 5821–5834. **[Google Scholar] [CrossRef] [PubMed]**

296. Satoh, T.; Kouroki, S.; Kitamura, Y.; Ihara, T.; Matsumura, K.; Iwase, S. Detection of Prostate-Specific Antigen in Semen Using DNA Aptamers: An Application of Nucleic Acid Aptamers in Forensic Body Fluid Identification. *Anal. Methods* **2020**, *12*, 2703–2709. **[Google Scholar] [CrossRef] [PubMed]**

297. Lin, H.-I.; Wu, C.-C.; Yang, C.-H.; Chang, K.-W.; Lee, G.-B.; Shiesh, S.-C. Selection of Aptamers Specific for Glycated Hemoglobin and Total Hemoglobin Using On-Chip SELEX. *Lab. Chip* **2015**, *15*, 486–494. **[Google Scholar] [CrossRef] [PubMed]**

298. Choung, C.M.; Lee, J.W.; Park, J.H.; Kim, C.H.; Park, H.-C.; Lim, S.-K. A Forensic Case Study for Body Fluid Identification Using DNA Methylation Analysis. *Leg. Med.* **2021**, *51*, 101872. **[Google Scholar] [CrossRef]**

299. Cortellini, V.; Brescia, G.; Cerri, N.; Verzeletti, A. Simultaneous DNA and RNA Profiling in a Case of Sexual Assault in a 3-Year-Old Child: Forensic Genetics Solves the Crime. *Leg. Med.* **2020**, *47*, 101727. **[Google Scholar] [CrossRef]**

300. Byrnes, S.A.; Gallagher, R.; Steadman, A.; Bennett, C.; Rivera, R.; Ortega, C.; Motley, S.T.; Jain, P.; Weigl, B.H.; Connelly, J.T. Multiplexed and Extraction-Free Amplification for Simplified SARS-CoV-2 RT-PCR Tests. *Anal. Chem.* **2021**, *93*, 4160–4165. **[Google Scholar] [CrossRef] [PubMed]**

301. Verheij, S.; Harteveld, J.; Sijen, T. A Protocol for Direct and Rapid Multiplex PCR Amplification on Forensically Relevant Samples. *Forensic Sci. Int. Genet.* **2012**, *6*, 167–175. **[Google Scholar] [CrossRef] [PubMed]**

302. Yang, Q.; Liu, B.; Zhou, Y.; Yao, Y.; Zhou, Z.; Li, H.; Shao, C.; Sun, K.; Xu, H.; Tang, Q.; et al. Evaluation of One-Step RT-PCR Multiplex Assay for Body Fluid Identification. *Int. J. Leg. Med.* **2021**, *135*, 1727–1735. **[Google Scholar] [CrossRef] [PubMed]**

www.ingramcontent.com/pod-product-compliance
Lightning Source LLC
LaVergne TN
LVHW062215200926
848484LV00006B/1402